S0-BXB-723

ALCOHOLISM:
A REVIEW OF ITS CHARACTERISTICS, ETIOLOGY, TREATMENTS, AND CONTROVERSIES

ALCOHOLISM:
A REVIEW OF ITS CHARACTERISTICS, ETIOLOGY, TREATMENTS, AND CONTROVERSIES

by

Irving M. Maltzman
UCLA, U.S.A.

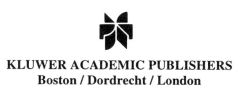

KLUWER ACADEMIC PUBLISHERS
Boston / Dordrecht / London

Distributors for North, Central and South America:
Kluwer Academic Publishers
101 Philip Drive
Assinippi Park
Norwell, Massachusetts 02061 USA
Telephone (781) 871-6600
Fax (781) 871-6528
E-Mail <kluwer@wkap.com>

Distributors for all other countries:
Kluwer Academic Publishers Group
Distribution Centre
Post Office Box 322
3300 AH Dordrecht, THE NETHERLANDS
Telephone 31 78 6392 392
Fax 31 78 6546 474
E-Mail <services@wkap.nl>

 Electronic Services <http://www.wkap.nl>

Library of Congress Cataloging-in-Publication Data

Maltzman, Irving.
   Alcoholism: a review of its characteristics, etiology, treatments, and controversies/by
Irving M. Maltzman.
     p.; cm.
  Includes bibliographical references and index.
  ISBN 0-7923-8656-6 (alk. paper)
  1. Alcoholism. I. Title.
  [DNLM: 1. Alcoholism. WM 274 M261a 1999]
  RC565 . M24 1999
  616.86'1--dc21

                             99-046028

Copyright © 2000 by Kluwer Academic Publishers

All rights reserved. No part of this publication may be reproduced, stored in a retrieval system or transmitted in any form or by any means, mechanical, photo-copying, recording, or otherwise, without the prior written permission of the publisher, Kluwer Academic Publishers, 101 Philip Drive, Assinippi Park, Norwell, Massachusetts 02061

Printed on acid-free paper.

Printed in the United States of America

Contents

AUGUSTANA UNIVERSITY COLLEGE
LIBRARY

PREFACE

Definitions

At the outset I wish to make my usage of the term "alcoholic" and "alcoholism" clear. "Alcoholic" is not synonymous with "heavy drinker". The latter is a mischievous, ambiguous term. I do not use it. The term "alcoholic" in this book has a specific meaning, originally clarified by Jellinek with the qualifier of *gamma* alcoholic. I use the term here as either referring to a gamma alcoholic, in the context of a discussion of Jellinek, or as synonymous with the usage specified by current Diagnostic and Statistical Manuals such as DSM-IV. The term "alcoholism" is not used in DSM-IV. It has been replaced by "dependence" and applies to the negative consequences of excessive use of a variety of different drugs including alcohol. Usage of the term "alcoholism" or "alcohol dependence" has been broadened to include negative social as well bio-behavioral consequences. Loss of control is the sine qua non for alcoholism or alcohol dependence as expressed by a number of negative social consequences reflected in DSM-IV.

I use the term "problem drinker" as synonymous with "alcohol abuse" in DSM-IV or alpha and beta alcoholism in Jellinek's formulation (1960). I find "problem drinker" simpler and less awkward than "alpha" and "beta", or "alcohol abuse". As I use the term "problem drinker" it is *not* synonymous with "alcoholic" or "alcohol dependence". It refers to a qualitatively different condition, one which does not show loss of control although there are negative social consequences. The distinction should become clearer as you progress through the book.

Table P-1. DSM-IV Criteria For Substance (Alcohol) Dependence And Abuse.

Dependence

A maladaptive pattern of substance use leading to clinically significant impairment or distress as manifested by three (or more) of the following occurring at any time in the same 12-month period:

1. tolerance as defined by either of the following:
   a. need for markedly increased amounts of the substance to achieve intoxication or desired effect
   b. markedly diminished effect with continued use of the same amount of the substance
2. withdrawal, as manifested by either of the following:
   a. the characteristic withdrawal syndrome for the substance...
   b. the same (or a closely related) substance is taken to relieve or avoid withdrawal symptoms
3. the substance is often taken in larger amounts or over a longer period than was intended

4. there is a persistent desire or unsuccessful efforts to cut down or control substance use
5. a great deal of time is spent in activities necessary to obtain the substance... or recover from its effects
6. important social, occupational, or recreational activities are given up or reduced because of substance use
7. the substance use is continued despite knowledge of having a persistent or recurrent physical or psychological problem that is likely to have been caused or exacerbated by the substance (e.g., ... continued drinking despite recognition that an ulcer was made worse by alcohol consumption)

Specify if:
With Physiological Dependence:
>   evidence of tolerance or withdrawal (i.e., either Item 1 or 2 is present)

Without Physiological Dependence:
>   no evidence of tolerance or withdrawal (i.e., neither Item 1 nor 2 is present)

Abuse

A. A maladaptive pattern of substance use leading to clinically significant impairment or distress, as manifested by one (or more) of the following, occurring within a 12-month period:
1. recurrent substance use resulting in a failure to fulfill major role obligations at work, school, or home (e.g., repeated absences or poor work performance related to substance use; substance-related absences, suspensions, or expulsions from school; neglect of children or household
2. recurrent substance use in situations in which it is physically hazardous (e.g., driving an automobile or operating a machine when impaired by substance use)
3. recurrent substance-related legal problems (e.g., arrests for substance-related disorderly conduct)
4. continued substance use despite having persistent or recurrent social or interpersonal problems caused or exacerbated by the effects of the substance (e.g., arguments with spouse about consequences of intoxication, physical fights)

B. The symptoms have never met the criteria for Substance Dependence for this class of substance.

Note. From American Psychiatric Association (1994) with permission from author.

The distinction of dependence with or without physiological dependence is of some significance. Schuckit et al. (1998) report that the presence of physiological dependence as defined by withdrawal distinguishes between patients with different levels of symptom severity. Physiological dependence corresponds to what Jellinek (1960) called gamma alcoholism.

ACKNOWLEDGEMENTS

I appreciate the permission of the American Psychiatric Association to reproduce the DSM-IV criteria for alcohol dependence and abuse (Preface); the American Association for the Advancement of Science (AAAS) for Table 8.1 which appeared in *Science,* 1982, 217, 173; the AAAS and Dr. Philip Abelson for permission to quote his letter from the editor in *Science,* 1983, 220, 555-556; the Haight-Ashbury Publications to publish much of the material of my two articles from the *Journal of Psychoactive Drugs,* 1994, 26, 13-31; 1998, 30, 99-104 constituting portions of chapter 1 and chapter 2.

It is more than a quarter of a century since I embarked on an excursion into the field of alcohol studies and the sociology of science. It started in partnership with Mary Pendery. If she had lived, this book would have reflected her singular clinical ability. It would have provided a glimpse of the phenomenology of alcoholism. How alcoholism is "from within"; R.I.P., Mary. As it stands, this book is a reflection of my own more than half a century involvement in experimental psychology as an atomistic, elementaristic, reductionistic, mechanistic - behaviorist. One purpose of this book is to show what behaviorism is really about. It is not what psychologists with little understanding of its nature and history mistakenly say it is.

The adventure of the past quarter of a century has profited from the support and help of many individuals. My path was smoothed by caring people in the alcohol constituency. Thanks, John, Audrey, and Cliff. The battle would have been impossible without the legal assistance of Allan Charles, Esq., David Dorinson, Esq., Ken O'Rourke, Esq., Robert Vanderet, Esq., and the good works of O'Melveny and Myers. The encouragement as well as critical comments of my old friend Michael Myslobodsky were invaluable in producing this book. I am also indebted to Rock Ashton, Perry Jaster, Ken Justice, Robin Moulder and Bill Troyer for their help. Above all, I am indebted to my wife, children, and grandchildren for putting up with a nutty husband, father, father-in-law, and grandfather for so long. All my love, Diane, Ilaine, Kenny, Sara, Ing-Britt, Corinna, Josina, Lena, and Matthew.

I am also indebted to a great institution, UCLA, for providing resources, support, and freedom to pursue what I think is right.

EMES

1 WHY ALCOHOLISM IS A DISEASE

Introduction

"Hiyaaa, Irrrv". It was John calling out to me as he entered the rear of the lecture room in Tolman Hall. I was about to start my talk on the orienting reflex to some 100 faculty and graduate students from the Psychology Department at UC Berkeley. Invited by Leo Postman, Director of the Center on Human Learning at Berkeley to give the address on my current research (Maltzman & Raskin, 1968). I looked forward to the intellectual challenge and the opportunity to visit with John. I hadn't seen him for 10-12 years, since the last time I visited Berkeley, for a Western Psychological Association Convention. My most vivid memory of that occasion was of him driving me and two or three other old classmates from graduate school down the main drag of Berkeley at 2:00 AM in his battered old Plymouth after a night of convivial drinking and reminiscing about the bad good old days at the University of Iowa. John's car was noticeably drifting in and out of the traffic lane. We passed a patrol car at the curb behind a car it apparently had stopped with its flashing lights. Flashing lights appeared again a few minutes later - in our rear view mirror. We were pulled over. We were asked to step out of the car and John was asked to walk a straight line, the crack running down the sidewalk. He did fine until after about 15 paces when the police officer asked him to turn around and come back. Attempting to reverse his direction he stumbled. John was asked for his driver's license. On seeing it, the police officer said something to the effect, "Professor.... I had you for my psychology class... Would you please go to the luncheonette down the street and have a cup of coffee before you start driving again."

After my lecture John drove me to Postman's home for an informal reception. Hors d'oeuvres were served along with drinks. It was very pleasant. People started to leave after a few hours so it was time to go. We went pub crawling until closing time when we went to a liquor store to buy some whiskey to take home. It struck me as odd that every place we went the bar tender knew John by his first name. When we got to his home John opened the bottle and poured us drinks. His wife refused and we sat around and talked and drank and finally went to sleep, must have been about 4:00 AM. I had to be at Postman's Center at 10:00 AM for an informal talk and discussion of the research in progress at the Center. I was hung over, sleepy, head-splitting. My mouth felt filled with cotton but somehow I managed to survive the morning meeting.

About six months later I was talking on the phone to the chairman of the psychology department at Berkeley about a university policy matter when as best as I can recall, he remarked, "Did you know that John committed suicide? Everyone knew he eventually would do it. He was an alcoholic... His wife was too, but she started going to AA and quit drinking. John wouldn't go because he couldn't take the higher power crap." I was stunned. I had not heard the news. I could not understand how a group of highly intelligent psychologists would not intervene somehow, help a colleague suffering from alcoholism and prevent his suicide. The incident troubled me for a variety of reasons. I never thought of John as an alcoholic. We all drank a lot in graduate school, faculty and students. That was the norm. It was a small college town, not much to do at night except study and run rats; only two movie theaters in town. One showed cowboy movies; another showed the latest foreign movies, but the same show would play for weeks. On the other hand, the two main streets of the town were lined with beer parlors serving 3.2 beer and the places were packed wall to wall with college kids drinking. It was hazardous coming back to my rooming house at night, especially on a Friday or Saturday. A chair might fly out an open window in the summer; or someone may be falling down the stairs when I was half way up.

John wasn't much different than any other graduate student or faculty member among the "inner circle" which included the best students and the stars of the faculty. However, John apparently continued to drink after he graduated and more often and larger amounts. It eventually interfered with his performance at the university. John was an alcoholic; his colleagues at Berkeley knew it. He had not progressed up the academic ladder at the normal rate; didn't make full professor, and his research output had dwindled. He was depressed and talked about suicide, but no one helped him. I didn't even recognize that a problem existed. He simply went into his garage one day, stuffed the cracks under the door with rags, turned on the car's motor and died of carbon monoxide poisoning. He would not be listed statistically as a casualty of alcoholism but of carbon monoxide poisoning.

The whole business bothered me. I called a former Ph.D student of mine in experimental psychology, Mary Pendery, who at the time was married to a brilliant young psychiatrist. He had completed his residency in psychiatry at UCLA and had gone on to a position in the newly opened UC campus in Irvine and from there to the new UC campus in San Diego where he became the first chair of the psychiatry department. Mary in the meantime had received supervised internship training, taken clinical courses she needed, and passed the state licensing exam. She was now a qualified clinical psychologist. After working for a time with severely mentally retarded children she turned to alcoholism treatment. I described to her what had happened to John. She said it was not unusual. Alcoholics have a high suicide rate and most think about committing suicide some time or other during their drinking careers. I started to read a little about alcoholism. A year later I had an occasion to call her again about alcoholism. That story is described in chapter 4, the beginning of the Sobell odyssey. Several years into that adventure, when we knew we had to publish our findings we also agreed that we needed to write a book describing in depth our experience in trying to conduct the follow-up of the patients treated by the Sobells at Patton State Hospital. We never did write that book. Mary also became a victim of alcoholism. On April 16, 1994 she was shot to death by her fiancee who after drinking through the night killed himself as well.

John and Mary were wonderful people whose lives ended too soon, cut down by alcoholism. Neither would appear as statistical casualities of alcoholism adding to the already large number of deaths directly attributed to the disease. Statistics greatly underestimate the havoc produced by excessive alcohol consumption. I tell these stories, not to correct statistical tallies but to belie the stereotpe that alcoholics are unkempt street people living on skid row. Both victims, John and Mary were Ph.Ds with loving families. Mary's murderer was a successful businessman as well as an alcoholic.

Alcoholism is a well-kept middle class secret

Alcoholism snares people from all walks of life. It is a myth that alcoholics are derelicts living on skid row or members only of the lowest socioeconomic classes. Perpetuation of the stereotype of alcoholics as skid row bums appears in seemingly the strangest sources. A book designed to help problem drinkers, as distinguished from alcoholics, learn to control their drinking describes alcoholics, those chronic drinkers who do not fit the bill for moderation management (controlled drinking) as follows:

Chronic drinkers [alcoholics] usually lose more than their health, however. In many cases, they have lost the personal, economic, and social resources that people need in order to help themselves. They may not have a job or a place to live. They may have lost most of their friends and even their family. They often have poor problem-solving and coping skills. (Kishline, 1994, p.66).

Let's get rid of the stereotype of what alcoholics are like, a stereotype providing comfort to those who are in danger because of their excessive drinking. Kishline (1994) provides them with added ammunition for their denial, their rationalizations: they are not alcoholics despite the amount they drink and their difficulties in every-day living because they do have a family, job, and a place to live. On the contrary, it is estimated that the stereotypical skid row alcoholic constitutes less than 5% of alcoholics in the United States.

Alcoholism is a well-kept middle class secret unless such a person is hospitalized or enters a treatment program. Many are treated and return to productive fulfilling careers. I know some who recovered solely as a result of participating in AA and others who received formal treatment as well as participating in the AA fellowship.

Let's go beyond individual cases to review some statistics reflecting the scope of this major social problem, one of the most serious, noninfectious, preventable, diseases in the United States and all other industrialized nations. Keep in mind that these statistics are always approximations, may vary for many different reasons in addition to the ostensible one, for example the cause of death. Very often the cause is more complex than it seems.

It is estimated that 71% of men and 61% of women drink alcohol in the United States (Office of Applied Statistics, 1998). In the 1970s consumption leveled off and since 1978 it has declined somewhat. In 1987 apparent alcohol consumption reached its lowest level in 19 years. A majority of industrialized countries show a similar decline. In contrast, consumption of alcoholic beverages is increasing in developing countries. Consumption figures are averages and misleading, since they form a highly skewed distribution. One-third of Americans do not drink at all. The remaining two-thirds show a wide variation in use. Twenty-five percent of the drinkers consume approximately 90% of the alcohol; 5% drink 42% of all alcohol consumed (Greenfield & Rogers, 1999).

Between 1980 and 1984 percentage of fatal alcohol related automobile crashes decreased from 50% to 43%. In 1989 it decreased to 38%. In 1993 there was a rise; 44% of fatal crashes were alcohol related, 17,500 deaths and an additional 289,000 people injured. Alcohol is the fourth leading cause of accidental death in the United States, involved in falls, burns, fires as well as car crashes and other accidents. Alcohol was involved in approximately 38% of drownings and over 50% of home fires, usually due to smoking, drinking, and falling asleep with a lighted cigarette. Approximately half the successful suicides are by alcoholics or are alcohol related (Alcohol and Health, 1997).

These figures overlook accidental suicides or deaths such as Marilyn Monroe's and probably most heroin addicts thought to have overdosed on heroin. She presumably died from an overdose of sleeping pills, an unlikely occurrence. She had been drinking alcohol, a depressant, during the evening. Combining alcohol with sleeping pills, barbiturates, another depressant, has a synergistic, multiplicative, effect. It shuts down basic functions killing the person. Overdosing on heroin is not due to taking too much heroin, but taking a combination of two depressants, heroin and usually alcohol; the individual had been drinking and then injected heroin. Medical examiners see the syringe near the body and check it off as a heroin overdose. Wrong. People don't die from an OD of heroin. They die because of a synergistic effect with alcohol or another depressant (Brecher, 1972).

Before World War II death by heroin overdose was unheard of. Such deaths appeared during the war because the allies blockaded shipping out of Turkey, which was an ally of Germany and the major source of opium at the time which was shipped to Marseille for heroin production and distribution. Due to the shortage of heroin in the United States because of the blockade, heroin addicts started to drink to compensate for the lack of heroin. Combining heroin and other depressants such as alcohol or barbiturates became the deadly mixture that caused accidental overdoses (Brecher, 1972), another deadly tally for alcohol that has been overlooked. The toll continues. Drinking is implicated in over half of all homicides, especially between family members. Cirrhosis of the liver, mainly caused by excessive alcohol consumption, accounted for more than 25,000 deaths in 1991, the 11th leading cause of death in the United States.

What does all this human suffering translate into in terms of monetary costs in this time of concern for managed care and medical costs? The estimated bill in 1990 was 100 billion dollars (Rice, 1993). That was no mistake, 100 billion, not million. More than 10 billion of that amount went to health care costs, quite a nice size pie out of which psychologists would love to take a bigger bite. The cost of caring for infants born with the fetal alcohol syndrome (FAS) a major cause of mental retardation in the United States, was 2 billion dollars. More than 2,000 of these developmentally disabled infants are born each year and will need special care for the rest of their lives.

Make no mistake, however. There are benefits from alcohol consumption. It wouldn't be around since pre-biblical times if it did not lubricate social interactions and provide a feeling of gemütlichkeit. In moderation, not more than 2 drinks/day for men and 1/day for women, it may provide a reduction in cardiovascular diseases, although the same effects could probably be obtained by jogging a few miles a day. Economically, there are obvious benefits in terms of the employment it offers people involved in the production and distribution of alcohol beverages and the profits to the owners of the production and distribution systems. Let's not forget the sizeable tax benefits to federal and state governments. Sales of alcohol beverages in 1990 amounted to 73 billion dollars; 14 billion dollars generated in taxes, half going to the federal government and half to the state governments in which the sales occurred. An ugly side to the "benefits" is suggested by the disturbing revelations of the cigarette manufacturers' suppression of research reports concerning the addictive influence of nicotine, their enormous lobbying activities, and their power to influence federal and local governments (Kluger, 1997). It seems apparent that if such chicanery can go on over cigarette smoking, similar games may be played to manipulate alcohol consumption. Hidden and substantial influences of the alcohol beverage producers corresponding to what has been revealed concerning cigarette manufacturers is suggested when we examine the business connections of the alcohol beverage companies. In many cases they are part of multinational conglomerates owned by the big cigarette companies. Connections described below may no longer be entirely accurate, since little is static in big business, but they provide an indication of the intimate relationship between cigarette and alcohol beverage companies.

Phillip Morris owns Miller beer; Liggett (L & M cigarettes) owns J & B scotch, Grand Marnier liqueur, Bailey's Original Irish Cream, Bombay gin, and Absolute vodka; Brown and Forman tobacco company owns Jack Daniels bourbon, Canadian Mist, Early Times bourbon, and Southern Comfort; American Brands tobacco company (Lucky Strike, Pall Mall, Carlton,) owns Jim Beam Whisky; R.J. Reynolds tobacco company (Camel, Winston) owns Heublein, Smirnoff vodka, Black Velvet whiskey, Harvey's Bristol Cream sherry, Jose Cuervo tequila, and Popov vodka (Selvaggio, 1983).

More than 400,000 people die each year in the United States from cigarette smoking, 150,000 from alcohol use, and 100,000 from all other illicit drugs combined. Approximately 25,000 people had been dying each year from AIDS. Advances in treatment has reduced the number to approximately 16,000 in 1997-1998.

In 1997 federal funding for research, treatment, and prevention provided to the National Cancer Institute was the largest single health appropriation, $2,060,392,000; the National Institute on Alcohol Abuse and Alcoholism (NIAAA) received $212,079,000; the National Institute on Drug Abuse (NIDA) received more than twice as much, $487,341,000. In contrast, the Office of AIDS Research received $1,431,908,000, more than twice as much as NIAAA and NIDA combined (Burd, Mytelka, & Walker, 1996). How are the differences in the budgets for the three preventable diseases, drug addiction, alcoholism, and AIDS to be explained?

There still is much denial and stigma attached to alcoholism in the United States. There is not a great deal of activism by the recovery community. It is evident by the relative lack of funding for alcoholism as compared to the other preventable diseases. The difference in funding for AIDS compared to alcohol and other drugs reflects the effective lobbying activities and intense involvement by a well-educated intelligent group of gay advocates. They have successfully lobbied Congress and the President to fund research, treatment, and prevention efforts. They are actively involved as educated lay people in every aspect of AIDS from public policy to research. Their rallying call has been gay pride. They have shown it and are achieving their goals.

There are also well-educated intelligent and influential recovering alcoholics and their families, but they are not as activist and as a result do not have the clout that the gay community has developed. On the other hand, NIDA does relatively well in terms of their budget as compared to NIAAA because of the middle class concern about crime generated by addicts needing money for a fix. Furthermore, in the war against illicit drugs NIDA does not have to counter the lobbying pressure of an enormously wealthy and influential adversary- the alcohol (cigarette) industry. Recovering alcoholics, their families, friends and the treatment community must learn from the successes of the gay community. They too have a call to rally around and fight for funding for more research, treatment, and prevention. Alcoholics have been through hell and have made it back. Nothing should stop them in the fight to conquer alcohol misuse and alcoholism.

We have been writing about alcoholism but have not defined it, have not indicated what we mean by the term, how the usage developed, why it is a disease, and the powerful opposition to viewing alcoholism as a disease by - of all people - a particular group of clinical psychologists: behavior therapists. Let's now turn to a more formal consideration of these problems.

The Nature Of Disease

Whether alcoholism is a disease or not has been widely discussed in recent years. The conventional view that alcoholism is a disease was represented primarily by Jellinek (1952, 1960) who was one of the pioneers responsible for establishing alcoholism as a field of scientific research. Important commentaries and revisions from within the conventional view have been offered by Keller (1972, 1976) and others (e.g., Ludwig, Wikler, & Stark, 1974; Mann, 1950). Arguments of the numerous critics of the disease concept of alcoholism (e.g., Heather & Robertson, 1983; Marlatt, 1983; Pattison, Sobell, & Sobell, 1977) have been summarized and extended by Fingarette (1988b).

Despite the number and extent of the remarks concerning the disease concept of alcoholism such discussions have all suffered from the same shortcoming. None have examined the meaning of the concept of disease per se in any depth. They have not examined the notion of disease in the light of developments in biopsychosocial medicine (Dubos, 1968; Engel, 1977, 1980) and the philosophy of science and of medicine (Engelhardt, 1976; Fulford, 1989; King, 1954; Margolis, 1976; Reznek, 1987; Whitbeck, 1977) or its history (Cohen, 1961). A lack of conceptual progress or sharpening of the nature of the differences between proponents and opponents of the disease concept of alcoholism is not surprising when a crucial aspect of the problem remains largely unexamined. Not only has the concept of disease been left largely unanalyzed and its usage unspecified by both parties to these discussions but often the concept of alcoholism is also undefined or used in a manner different from the usage specified by the conventional view.

Much of the controversy centered around the question of whether alcoholism is a disease or not, has inappropriately treated this issue as though it is an empirical question that is in principle falsifiable. In fact, the controversy is largely over the description of the characteristic features of alcoholism and whether or not alcoholism shows a lawful pattern of signs and symptoms. These are empirical matters. However, there are two components of the notion of disease that have not been adequately differentiated in discussions of whether or not alcoholism is a disease, the evaluative and empirical. Whether the term 'disease' is applicable to alcoholism or not rests in part upon a convention based upon a volitional decision (Reichenbach, 1938). It rests in part upon a value judgment. There is general agreement that alcohol misuse is a serious social and individual problem (Alcohol and Health, 1997). Alcohol misuse is bad for the individual and for society. This value judgment is one of the two criteria that need to be met for classifying alcoholism as a disease. In dispute is the second aspect of diseases, the descriptive, the characteristic features of the condition labeled 'alcoholism', not the judgment that alcoholism is a serious deviation from commonly accepted standards of health.

Sifting through the research literature to arrive at an accurate depiction of the empirical characteristics of alcoholism requires that we overcome the selective filter of the ideology that has come to dominant the psychological literature in the field of alcohol studies since the 1970's.

Philosophers and historians of science have recognized the pervasive presence of ideology in science, including life sciences for generations (e.g., Canguilhem, 1988; Richards, 1992). Richards (1993) asserts:

During our century, the concept of ideology has speciated. In the social sciences and humanities, it has come to be applied with a variety of different assumptions and meanings. Historians and philosophers of science, however, have usually sustained the original presumption that a clear distinction can be made between true - or at least 'rationally sound' - and false ideas. Karl Popper for instance, conceives ideology as a pseudo-scientific system... that pretends to science but essentially lacks the requisite rational methodology. For Popper, of course, the rational method of science, by which it can be distinguished from its ideological counterfeit, is falsificationism. The uncritical and stubborn adherence to a position, protecting it from confuting evidence by developing ad hoc hypotheses, clearly indicates an ideological conception. (p. 103).

Bergmann (1954) has succinctly characterized ideology as follows:

As we survey man's history, we cannot, I believe, escape the following conclusion. The motive power of a value judgment is often greatly increased when it appears within the rationale of those who hold it not under its proper logical flag as a value judgment but in the disguise of a statement of fact. (p.310).

Ideology, value judgments in the guise of statements of fact, permeate the field of alcohol studies, determine what is published, the nature of the research conducted, the nature of the interpretation placed upon facts, and the very facts themselves. Our task is to sort out the value judgments from statements of fact surrounding the disease concept of alcoholism and related research.

Ideology has permeated discussions of alcoholism because classifying alcoholism as a disease or not has important and diverse consequences. Fingarette (1988a) states:

One may wonder why it is important whether or not alcoholism is a disease. To begin with, 'disease' is the word that triggers provision of health-insurance payments, employment benefits such as paid leave and workmen's compensation, and other government benefits. Civil law now often mandates leniency or complete absolution for the alcoholic from the rules, regulations, and moral norms to which non-diseased persons are held legally or morally accountable. Such is the thrust of a recent appeal to the U.S. Supreme Court by two veterans, who are claiming certain benefits in spite of their having failed to apply for them at any time during the legally specified ten-year period after discharge from the army. Their excuse: alcoholism, and the claim that their persistent heavy drinking was a disease entitling them to exemption from the regulations. The court's decision could be a bellwether. (pp.4-5).

The latter comment by Fingarette refers to Traynor v Turnage, No. 86-622. "At issue is a VA regulation that defines alcoholism as 'willful misconduct.' The regulation was used to deny... two former servicemen - and dozens of other alcoholic veterans each year - extensions of the 10-year deadline for using educational benefits provided to veterans in the GI Bill." (Neal, 1988, p. 58). Whether or not alcoholism qualifies for the classification of "disease" has enormous public policy, legal, and health care implications.

It is necessary in discussion of the disease concept, as noted above, to distinguish between the empirical aspects of 'disease' and the evaluative aspects (Fulford, 1987; Reznek, 1989; Whitbeck, 1977). Failure to distinguish between use of the term 'disease' in its descriptive and its explanatory sense as contrasted with its evaluative sense leads to considerable confusion and misunderstanding. We shall now turn to these different aspects of the meaning of 'disease'.

Criteria for use of the term 'disease'

A disease is a syndrome, a lawful pattern of recurrent observable signs and symptoms (Blakiston, 1979). There is no precondition that the etiology or cause(s) of the syndrome be known in order to classify the syndrome as a disease. Malaria was labelled a disease prior to knowledge that it was caused by a parasite transmitted by the bite of a mosquito. Tuberculosis was considered a disease for centuries prior to the discovery of the bacillus that caused the illness. Similarly for others such as infantile paralysis, Parkinson's disease, and cancer(s). It is also apparent that these syndromes were classified as diseases long before a cure was available. Neither the cause nor a cure for Parkinson's disease is known. But there is no dispute over whether or not it is a disease. Furthermore, there are enormous individual differences in the course of Parkinsonism. Its progression in different people may proceed at very different rates and with varying signs and symptoms. There is also great within-subject variability in some cases of Parkinsonism. Individual differences are striking but this is not taken as a reason for refusing to classify Parkinsonism as a disease. Despite the individual differences in the progression of the disease, it is diagnosable, classifiable as a distinct disease syndrome. Such is the case also for different cancers and for alcoholism or as it is called in DSM-IV, alcohol dependence as distinguished from alcohol abuse or problem drinking.

But not every syndrome is a disease. For example, if I get up every morning, shave, shower, and eat my corn flakes smothered with ketchup, this is a recurrent observable pattern of behavior. It is also a deviant pattern in a frequency sense. Few people smother their corn flakes with ketchup. However, deviance in the sense of uncommonness is not the basis for classifying a syndrome a disease, although this is a common, and mistaken, sociological position (Gove, 1980). There is a second essential feature of a disease as the term is used in medicine, and it is not infrequency.

A syndrome is classified as a disease if it represents a significant deviation from a norm or standard of health as judged by experts. For a syndrome to be classified as a disease it must be judged a serious threat to health.

This second essential feature of diseases is why deviant behavior per se, in a frequency sense, is not a criterion for use of the term "disease". It is why putting ketchup on my cereal may be aberrant and abhorent to some, but it is not a serious threat to health, neither for me nor for others. Therefore it is not a disease. On the other hand, dysentery is a disease regardless of its relative frequency of occurrence. The majority of children in third world countries may be dying of dysentery. It is a disease even though it is found in a majority of the population because it is a serious deviation from an accepted standard of health. Obviously, the standard of health may vary over time and in different cultures, and experts are members of a particular culture. As is true of other concepts, the definition of "disease" may be relative to a particular context, a culture in place and time. Classification of a syndrome as a disease or not is a value judgment, a comparison of a particular case against a norm or standard, in the case of diseases, a norm or standard of health. Classification of a disease is based on what the condition of the individual is relative to what he or she *ought* to be. Bio-behavioral science is replete with value judgments (Maltzman, unpublished e). The problem is to make them explicit not to eliminate them. Value judgments cannot be eliminated as science is practiced.

In none of the diseases mentioned, or any other, is there an assumption that the observable pattern of signs and symptoms is caused by some underlying disease state. Notions of an ontological state of disease, a process that exists independently of the observable signs and symptoms was rejected by Pyrrho the skeptic in approximately 300 B.C. (Cohen,1961). Disease is not some mysterious process underlying and causing cancer, AIDS, Parkinsonism, alcoholism, etc. The disease *is* the lawful pattern of recurring observable signs and symptoms.

Classifying a condition as a "disease" rests on meeting the conditions of a convention, an agreed upon set of criteria, a rule, for the use of the label "disease". The rule is that the condition must have two characteristics. It must be a syndrome, and it must be judged a significant deviation from a standard of health. Its classification is based upon a value judgement. Classifying alcoholism as a disease or as a form of dependence as defined by DSM-IV which merits the label "disease" is compatible with any number of so-called "models" of alcoholism. Such models are usually guesses at the etiology of the syndrome or suggestions for treatment. They are statements that are in principle falsifiable. The truth status of various models involves fundamentally different issues than the question, does a condition called alcoholism meet the criteria for the classification of "disease" or not? The latter requires a decision, a value judgment given the information at hand. One can accept alcoholism as a disease and hypothesize that the most important etiological factors are social learning in nature, bio-psychosocial, a consequence of self-medication for some more basic underlying condition, a moral fault, etc. An explanation for the presence of certain features of a syndrome involves empirical laws which permit the deduction of the phenomena in question. The alcoholism syndrome must be explained whether or not it is a disease. Labeling a condition a "disease" classifies it. This is the beginning of explanation, not the end. Such classification is a low order form of explanation in the sense that an individual's erratic behavior, injuries, personality change, social irresponsibility, etc., are deducible from the classification and its attendant low order empirical principles describing the characteristics of alcoholism. The apparently unrelated symptoms are part of a syndrome. An explanation of the syndrome and its etiology would permit more effective prevention, treatment, and the deduction of the characteristic signs and symptoms from more general principles. The difference between Aristotelian science and modern science is that for Aristotle explanation in science ended with classification. In modern science it is the beginning. Classification is not the same operation as the statement of etiology or the derivation of observable signs and symptoms from general principles.

Jellinek's formulation of the disease concept and its critics

Does alcoholism meet the above two conditions for classifying a condition as a disease, a syndrome and a significant deviation from a standard of health? Jellinek (1960), the leading modern exponent of the disease concept of alcoholism defined alcoholism as: "any use of alcoholic beverages that causes any damage to the individual or society or both." (p. 35). There is no question that there is enormous damage to self and society as a consequence of alcohol misuse (Alcohol and Health, 1997). The second of the two criteria is met. However, Jellinek notes that there are different kinds of alcoholics. They may be grouped as problem drinkers, alpha and beta in Jellinek's terms, and alcoholics, gamma and delta in his terms. The latter two qualify as a disease according to Jellinek. In North America and in countries other than wine drinking countries, gamma is the most common type of alcoholic. According to Jellinek the development or natural history of gamma alcoholism manifests a progressive pattern of observable signs and symptoms that are the negative biological, social, and psychological consequences of alcohol misuse. Alcoholism is a biopsychosocial disease because it is a lawful pattern of observable reoccurring signs and symptoms that is judged to be a significant deviation from a commonly accepted standard of health.

According to Jellinek most alcoholics probably start in the same fashion as everyone else. They are initally social, moderate, nonalcoholic drinkers. In contrast to most people who drink, however, their alcohol consumption becomes progressively greater. Problem drinkers and alcoholics before developing the disease enter a prodromal phase of alcoholism manifesting a series of characteristic symptoms. Frequent black outs is the marker for the initiation of this preclinical phase. Problem drinkers although they may drink very large amounts, may consume greater quantities of alcohol than many alcoholics, do not as a group progress into alcoholism, although some eventually may. If they do not progress or decrease their alcohol consumption they remain problem drinkers. Loss of control is the initial marker for the crucial phase of alcoholism. The final phase of chronic alcoholism is marked by frequent drinking bouts.

In the crucial phase of alcoholism gamma alcoholics display loss of control and signs and symptoms of pharmacological addiction: physical dependence. Objective indices of physical dependence are high tolerance and withdrawal symptoms such as frequent and severe seizures, hallucinations, and delirium tremens. Loss of control is a key behavioral sign and symptom. If it is a characteristic of alcoholism and not of problem drinking, as Jellinek asserts, it has two important implications. First, it implies that if loss of control characterizes alcoholics, then the treatment goal must be abstinence. Second, it implies that there is a qualitative difference between heavy drinkers. They are not all alike. Alcoholics and not problem drinkers show loss of control. It is therefore critical to distinguish between the two for theoretical reasons and for treatment planning.

Whereas the dominant position within the conventional view is that gamma alcoholism is a disease, there is no monolithic attitude towards this usage within the alcoholism constituency or among its critics (e.g., Marlatt et al., 1985; Peele, 1992). There are those who argue that the use of the disease concept is entirely pragmatic. It served its purpose in changing public and official attitudes. Other issues are now important and for pragmatic reasons the constituency is best served by considering gamma alcoholism as simply a severe form of problem drinking. Business and industry, traffic courts, and a host of other agencies including teenage crisis centers and public schools deal with the effects of excessive drinking that have not reached the stage of pharmacological addiction. Attention of the public and the constituency is primarily directed towards these problem drinkers just as much as clinical psychology is now directed towards problems of living rather than the profoundly disabling psychoses. Therefore, the argument goes, the conception of alcoholism as a disease is misleading and should be discarded. An alternative view is that the disease concept should be retained because it serves a very useful purpose in reducing the guilt of the alcoholic patient. Treatment may therefore proceed in a more effective manner.

Neither kind of argument, that it serves a useful purpose or that it does not, offers the grounds on which a decision may be reached concerning whether or not alcoholism may be labeled a disease. Within clinical practice and the science on which it is based the pragmatic argument for or against classifying a condition a disease is no more justifiable for alcoholism than it is for cancer.

Loss of control has been the focus of the attacks upon the disease concept because of the above two implications of Jellinek's description of alcoholism. Critics argue that heavy drinking, alcoholism, or problem drinking, whatever it is called, is on a continuum of drinking. It is a matter of degree of alcohol misuse. The same laws hold for all drinkers. There are no qualitative differences between or among subgroups of heterogenous heavy drinkers. According to Marlatt (1979):

All drinking behavior, from social drinking to alcohol abuse, is assumed to be governed by similar principles of learning and reinforcement. As such, it is assumed that there is no crucial difference that distinguishes the social drinker and the problem drinker, other than the amount of alcohol consumed. (p.32f).

Fingarette (1988b) argues that the notion of loss of control is either false or it is scientifically meaningless because it is not falsifiable. He insists that there have been two different versions of loss of control, the classic version formulated by Jellinek (1960) which is false and a revised version (Keller, 1972) formulated essentially in response to earlier criticisms. This latter formulation of loss of control is scientifically meaningless because it cannot be falsified. It cannot be falsified because it involves circular reasoning.

Fingarette is wrong on both counts. The classic version attributed to AA and presumably adopted at times by Jellinek is that once an alcoholic ingests alcohol an inexorable physiological process is initiated that will lead to loss of control over alcohol terminated only when the alcoholic drinks into an alcoholic stupor. Keller (1972) formulated a relative conception of loss of control. A variation of this "modified" formulation of loss of control is: "Given the opportunity to drink, the alcoholic cannot consistently refrain; once starting to drink, the alcoholic cannot consistently cease before drinking to a state of inebriation". Two features must be considered. The critical qualifier is "consistently". This formulation implies that upon occasion and for varying lengths of time, the alcoholic can and does drink moderately or can refrain from drinking entirely (see Schuckit, Tipp, Smith, & Bucholz, 1997). Second, there is an emphasis upon a loss of inhibition. The individual cannot consistently refrain from starting to drink, cannot consistently inhibit their initiating alcohol ingestion. Once started they cannot consistently inhibit further drinking. We emphasize inhibition to call attention to the critical role frontal lobe functions play in the self-regulation of alcohol consumption (Giancola & Moss, 1998; Lyvers, 1998, in press; Maltzman, 1991; Oscar-Berman & Hutner, 1993).

The "modified" version is not a revision of the classic version carried out in the face of contrary evidence. It was present from the outset. Mann (1950) describes the behavior of alcoholics and is quite explicit in indicating that loss of control over drinking is frequently not absolute and immediate. Alcoholics for varying periods of time at different times control their drinking. Such behavior, the uncertainty of their drinking, is one of the reasons for the great stress present in families of alcoholics. It also reinforces the rationalization that an alcoholic can quit or drink moderately if they so desire. Mann was sensitive to the nuances of the behavior of alcoholics and observed this temporary control over drinking in many alcoholics. The problem is that the control is inconsistent. "One drink away from a drunk" is a metaphor for the *eventual* loss of control that will occur if an alcoholic returns to drinking. As Keller (1972) points out, it was a mnemonic device devised by AA to help the alcoholic remember in a simple straightforward way what they must do in order to stay sober: refrain from drinking. The founders of AA had the insight to realize that alcoholics who are recently abstinent and struggling to remain sober have a limited working memory and a limited ability to engage in reasoning and rational problem solving. They suffer from a frontal lobe syndrome to varying degree.

Is Alcoholism a Syndrome?

Few would argue with the value judgment that a condition that may be labeled alcoholism is a significant deviation from a norm of health. Criticisms of the classification of alcoholism as a disease center around the empirical aspects of the concept: (a) whether alcoholism is a lawful pattern of signs and symptoms, whether it progresses through various phases as noted by Jellinek, and (b) whether loss of control is one of the features of this pattern.

Fingarette and other critics attack the description of (gamma) alcoholism as manifesting a lawful natural history, a progression, an orderly pattern, of signs and symptoms. According to Jellinek (1952) the syndrome consists of four phases, prealcoholic, prodromal, crucial, and chronic. Fingarette (1988b) states:

it was the inadequacy of Jellinek's data that caused much of his classic work to fail the test of later scientific scrutiny. For all of Jellinek's findings and hypotheses, all his charts, diagrams, and statistics were based on data obtained from A.A. members. Jellinek worked from questionnaires that A.A. had designed and distributed through its membership newsletter... Jellinek's own caution about the limitations of his data is reflected in his noting that the questions were not adequate and that 'essential categories' were lacking... In sum, Jellinek's highly influential articles were based on questionnaires completed by 98 male members of A.A. (p.20f).

In addition, Jellinek (1946) discarded the results from women because they were anomolous, discarded other results because the questionnaires were completed by more than one person, and so on. Results from such a biased sample are hardly an adequate basis for a theory of alcoholism. Fingarette asserts that a decade of work disconfirms the phaseology, the hypothesis of a lawful pattern of signs and symptoms. Furthermore, large national representative probability samples show that people misusing alcohol are a heterogeneous group who do not progressively develop more severe symptoms. Their drinking waxes and wanes, shows a variety of patterns (Cahalan & Room, 1974). There is no lawful pattern to the development of alcoholism.

Fingarette's account of Jellinek's formulation of the phases of alcoholism is misleading in its presentation of pertinent results. All of Fingarette's comments concerning the severe limitations of Jellinek's 1946 study are appropriate. They were criticisms that Jellinek (1946) himself made. However, Fingarette fails to report that Jellinek modified and added questions to the original questionnaire and then obtained results from a new sample of more than 2000 AA members (Jellinek, 1952). His formulation of a temporal progression is based on the latter report and not simply the 1946 study of 98 selected questionnaires from AA members. Schaler (1990) repeats Fingarette's error in a book review appearing ironically in the magazine, *Skeptical Inquirer*. He asserts that the entire formulation of the disease concept is based on a biased and inadequate sample of 98 male subjects. Lilienfeld (1995b) also makes this error as do Mendelson and Mello (1985) who probably are the source of the subsequent errors in the secondary literature.

Early studies of the phaseology (e.g., Chick & Duffy, 1979; Jackson, 1957; Orford & Hawker, 1974; Park, 1973) did not use all of the same questions employed by Jellinek. They changed questions, used different questions, or used different psychometric methods in the analysis of their data. Nevertheless, authors of the articles in question agree that even with different procedures and questions their results generally support Jellinek's formulation of phases in the development of alcoholism even if not the order of specific symptoms. Symptom clusters are not random in their appearance. The two most extensive and sophisticated studies published prior to Fingarette's book (Pokorny & Kanas, 1980; Pokorny, Kanas, & Overall, 1981) provide strong support for Jellinek's phaseology. They are not mentioned by Fingarette.

Pokorny and Kanas (1980) administered all of Jellinek's questions as well as additional questions used by other investigators to patients in a VA hospital rather than members of AA. A group of VA patients who drank but were not under treatment for alcoholism and with no history of alcoholism treatment served as a control group. A rank order correlation of 0.72 was obtained between the rank order of age of onset of symptoms and the ranks of Jellinek's symptom order. The control group showed many of the same psychosocial signs and symptoms as the alcoholics. They did not show the signs of physical dependence. Pokorny, Kanas, and Overall (1981) reanalyzed the data from the patients in alcoholism treatment using the method of paired comparisons to weight the order of symptom onset and correlated these weighted rank orders with ranks of age at symptom onset. A correlation of 0.84 was obtained, again confirming Jellinek's hypothesis and demonstrating that the progression although by no means perfect, is highly reliable. Piazza and colleagues (Piazza & Wise, 1988; Piazza, Vrbka, & Yeager, 1989; Piazza et al., 1986; Yeager, Piazza, & Yates, 1992) have conducted a series of studies with different populations including women, and consistently obtain high correlations in the ordering of symptoms, including a correlation of 0.81 between men and women. They thus extend the phaseology to women as well as men who are not AA members.

Schuckit et al. (1993) studied the progression of symptoms in 636 VA patients. Men above and below the median age of the sample showed an order of occurrence of 21 symptoms that correlated 0.89 between the two age groups. Other analyses of order of appearance of symptoms for family history positive vs. family history negative patients, comorbidity or not, etc., show correlations ranging from 0.89 to 0.92. Schuckit et al. used a structured personal interview to obtain symptom information rather than self-reports as in earlier studies, tried to limit the interview to objective symptoms, and obtained collateral confirmation of symptoms. They conclude that their results are in accord with earlier studies in showing a lawful progression in general agreement with Jellinek's results although differing in details of specific symptoms.

Ordering of symptoms within a phase for an alcoholic college professor who has little close supervision over his or her job performance will be different than for a worker on an assembly line, or a check-out clerk in a supermarket who is closely supervised and is directly interacting with the public. Errors, failure to report on time, unauthorized breaks are more obvious, likely to result in reprimands and dismissal in the case of a check-out clerk than in the case of an alcoholic professor who has tenure. Negative consequences are more apparent and come more quickly to the surface in the case of the assembly line worker or check-out clerk who provides a quantitative index of his or her performance in terms of the number of items fabricated/hour or the number of purchases processed/hour. A person unemployed because the company or store in which they worked has closed is in another position where negative consequences are different. There is a lack of opportunity for mistakes, inappropriate behavior, and failure to perform according to some standard. Appearance of one or another symptoms will vary to some extent as a function of specific circumstances. There may also be a threshold of severity for biobehavioral symptoms, blackouts, morning shakes, tolerance, etc., and these may show individual differences, determined by one or more biological, including genetic, factors interacting with experiential variables.

One of the more recent and extensive studies supporting the conception of an alcoholism phaseology as a progressive disease stems from a general populaton survey of more than 8000 people in a national stratified probability sample of noninstitutionalized adults in the continental United States (Nelson, Little, Heath, & Kessler, 1996). Nelson et al. (1996) set out to determine whether a corresponding progression of symptom groups, stages, or phases would appear in a sample from the general population, since previous studies usually employed hospital patients, members of AA or other convenience samples. Nelson et al. employed a national representative sample in an attempt to determine possible differences in rate of progression, onset of dependence, and possible differences in symptom progress as a function of variables such as comorbidity. Criteria for dependence were based on the DSM-III-R. Some of the findings reported by Nelson et al. (1996) are as follows: Gender differences were obtained where a larger percentage of men than women reported ever experiencing a symptom of alcohol dependence and men reported more symptoms of dependence than women. However, rank order of symptom prevalence for women and men correlated 0.97. Three clusters of symptoms were isolated. Cluster A consists of symptoms of abuse such as use in hazardous situations and use despite knowledge of problems. Cluster B is characterized by signs of tolerance and loss of control, unsuccessful attempts to reduce drinking, and increasing time spent drinking. Cluster C is characterized by withdrawal symptoms, drinking to avoid withdrawal, and restriction of activities due to drinking. An analysis of life time symptom profiles suggests that most people who have experienced alcohol dependence start with Cluster A and progress to Cluster B and then Cluster C.

The study by Nelson et al. (1996) extends the generality of the results obtained in prior research on clinical samples by finding a characteristic temporal progression of stages in alcohol dependence in the general population. It must be recognized, however, that as in all diseases, infectious as well as chronic noninfectious, there is variability. Not everyone shows the same progression.

Variability occurs even after the level of alcohol dependence has been reached. Periods of heavy consumption alternate with periods of lighter drinking and even abstinence. Schuckit, Tipp, Smith, & Bucholz (1997) studied periods of abstinence in a sample of more than 1000 participants diagnosed according to DSM-III-R as suffering from alcohol dependence for more than 10 years. One-third of the participants never receiving treatment showed at least one 3-month period of complete abstinence. Variability of this sort demands that studies evaluating treatment outcome use an extended evaluation window to avoid short-lived remissions reflecting the variability in drinking history.

Variability in onset and symptom progress of diseases

Revisionists underestimate the biological bases providing an "understanding" of alcoholism, and overestimate the precision with which disease entities are classified and "understood" in "organic medicine" (Evans,1993; Reznek, 1987). Explanation of the individual differences in the risk for developing alcoholism is a basic problem. However, alcoholism is no different from infectious and chronic noncontagious diseases in this respect. Individual differences in host response to an infection is the norm in most viral infections. For example, Evans (1993) describes a case where the hepatitis B virus contaminated the:

> yellow fever vaccine given to over 5000 healthy male soldiers of about the same age... Each received the same dose in the same arm on the same day... Of those inoculated, 1004 (20%) developed clinical jaundice, and the rest did not. The incubation period from injection to clinical illness varied from 60 to 154 days (mean 96.4 days). What 'third ingredient' influenced the variability in host response and incubation period among these soldiers? Unfortunately, we don't know the answer to this, since no studies were made to analyze this 'natural experiment,' and, even if they had been, the laboratory tools were not available at that time (1945) to identify susceptibility and immunity or to recognize subclinical infections. (p. 209).

It is noteworthy that variability in risk for developing an illness despite the presence of an infection, and lack of knowledge and understanding of the relevant biological mechanisms, did not result in the rejection of the classification of hepatitis as a disease. As in the case of alcoholism, common infectious diseases and especially chronic diseases are multidetermined (Evans, 1993). Etiology seems more evident and simpler in the case of infectious diseases because ordinarily the negative cases are not considered or determined. Negative instances are more obvious in the case of alcoholism where the number and per cent of people consuming alcohol without developing alcoholism can more readily be determined than in the case of infectious diseases. When the negative instances are apparent as in the above natural experiment described by Evans, the etiological picture is more like alcoholism. It is multidetermined, the etiology is by no means certain, an infection is necessary but not sufficient, and not all the risk factors are known. These limitations, however, do not prevent the classification of hepatitis as a disease or a virus as an etiological factor.

Phaseology: Dependence versus abuse

Contrary to claims of critics phaseology studies provide evidence supporting one of the two criteria that must be met for a condition to merit the classification of a disease; it is a syndrome. The second criterion, that alcoholism is an unhealthy condition is generally agreed upon.

Results obtained by Cahalan and Room (1974) purporting to contradict the description of an alcoholism syndrome, evidence that has repeatedly been cited by critics of the disease concept - does nothing of the sort. Their results do not contradict the notion that gamma alcoholism manifests a progression of symptoms, because Cahalan and Room provide no evidence that they were investigating gamma alcoholics or in current terms, alcohol dependence. They provide no evidence that the people in question suffered signs and symptoms of physical dependence. Since neither Fingarette nor Cahalan and Room demonstrate that they met the boundary conditions for an adequate test of the formulation of a progression of signs and symptoms for alcoholics - evidence of dependence, as distinguished from abuse, the results reported are irrelevant to the question of whether or not alcoholism can be classified as a distinct syndrome.

Hasin, Grant and Endicott (1990) used the extensive data base developed by Cahalan and Room (1974) to restructure dependent variables so that measures of abuse and dependence approximating those used in DSM-III-R for diagnoses of alcohol abuse, approximating Jellinek's problem drinking, and alcohol dependence, approximating alcoholism, could be derived. Reanalysis of the Cahalan and Room results obtained in a four-year longitudinal study in terms of the new variables showed that outcome at follow-up differed significantly from baseline for alcohol abuse as compared to alcohol dependence. Of the 71 men originally classified as alcohol abusers, four years later 46% were in remission, 17% were still alcohol abusers, and 30% progressed to alcohol dependence. Of the 109 men classified as alcohol dependent at baseline, four years later 15% were classified as alcohol abusers, 39% were in remission, and 46% were still alcohol dependent.

There are significant differences between outcomes for men diagnosed as suffering from alcohol abuse or alcohol dependence. According to Fingarette there should be no difference. There were an appreciable number of problem drinkers, 30%, who progressed into alcohol dependence, alcoholism, twice the percentage of men who shifted from alcohol dependence to alcohol abuse. Also, twice the percentage of men classified as alcohol dependent remained in that classification as those originally classified as alcohol abusers remained in the latter classification.

Hasin et al. (1990) conducted an interesting and important study, but it does have limitations. As the authors indicate, they did not capture all of the variables characterizing alcohol abuse and alcohol dependence as defined by DSM-III-R, since the study was not originally designed for this purpose (Cahalan & Room, 1974). Women were not participants in the study. Furthermore, generational changes, especially the increase in polydrug use since the time these data were collected by Cahalan and Room limit the generality of the reported results. The large age range, 21 - 59 years, requires a larger number of subjects permitting analyses within and between age levels, e.g., between 20-30 vs. above age 40, because of the differences in chronicity between age levels (Fillmore & Midanik, 1984). Very different variables may be at work determining shifts in drinking categories at these different age levels. They need to be examined in future studies designed explicitly to investigate the "natural history" of alcohol abuse and alcohol dependence. Furthermore, DSM-III-R itself does not adequately capture the characteristic signs and symptoms of physical dependence, pharmacological addiction, emphasized in Jellinek's classification of alcoholism. The important point of the study by Hasin et al.(1990) is that despite the apparent heterogeneity among heavy drinkers, it is possible to make reliable distinctions, classifications, among heavy drinkers that are meaningful, have important implications for theory and treatment (see also Hasin & Paykin, 1999; Hasin, Van Rossem, McCloud & Endicott, 1997; Langenbucher & Martin, 1996).

The most relevant evidence that alcoholism is a syndrome stems from studies of DSM-III-R and similar nosological systems (Beresford, 1991; Flavin & Morse, 1991). Thus, Williams et al. (1992) using the Structured Clinical Inventory (SCID) for DSM-III-R in a multisite multinational study showed that alcohol dependence and alcohol abuse can be diagnosed in a reliable manner and distinguished from other nosological categories. If alcoholism and problem drinking were not syndromes, they could not be reliably diagnosed. They are. Nonprofessionals can be trained to make reliable diagnoses of alcoholism as well (Helzer et al., 1981). Fingarette and other critics report on none of the important work over many years on diagnosis and classification, the nosology of alcoholism, conducted largely by members of the medical profession (e.g., Edwards & Gross, 1976). There are extensive reviews of this earlier work (e.g., Beresford, 1991; Flavin & Morse, 1991; Keller & Doria, 1991). These studies provide further evidence that alcoholism is a syndrome.

Perhaps, however, Fingarette is right for the wrong reasons. Even though alcoholism shows a progression and is reliably classifiable as a syndrome that causes damage, loss of control the critical marker for the crucial phase of alcoholism cannot be reliably measured in clinical cases. There is merely a quantitative difference in severity of alcoholism and a quantitative difference in the loss of self-control, relative or otherwise. It should be noted that DSM-III-R requires meeting any three of nine criteria for the classification of dependence, equivalent to alcoholic as distinguished from problem drinker or alcohol abuse. At least four, possibly five, of the criteria are indirect measures of loss of control. Remaining criteria refer to withdrawal symptoms and tolerance, all Jellinek's criteria for defining alcoholism as distinguished from problem drinking.

EVIDENCE PURPORTING TO CONTRADICT THE LOSS-OF-CONTROL HYPOTHESIS

Contrary to Fingarette (1988b) and other critics, the "revised" conception of loss of control is eminently testable. However, it requires certain boundary conditions, as does every hypothesis. These boundary conditions are ignored in so-called refutations of the loss of control hypothesis. A test of the hypothesis of loss of control requires a longer temporal window of evaluation than usually employed. It cannot be tested on any one drinking occasion. Gruenewald and his colleagues (Gruenewald, 1991; Gruenewald, Stewart, & Klitzner, 1990) have demonstrated, given repeated occasions for drinking, that measures of frequency of drinking and continuation of drinking can provide quantitative indices defining loss of control that predict severity of alcohol dependence. An indirect self-report questionnaire assessing loss of control has been developed by Heather and his colleagues with some success (Heather, Booth, & Luce, 1998; Heather, Tebbutt, Mattick, & Zmier, 1993).

Experimental studies

Fingarette (1988b) asserts that, "Loss of control is a confused notion that is contradicted by a bookshelf of experimental evidence." (p.48). This research is of two sorts. One are operant studies conducted on hospital wards indicating that drinking in alcoholics can be brought under the control of reinforcement contingencies. Alcoholics do not invariably drink themselves into a drunken stupor given the availability of alcohol. Given the high degree of tolerance of alcoholics, this should not be a common occurrence under any circumstance. However, one such study shows that the participants can become drunk, sick, throw-up, yet continue to work for alcohol (Funderburk & Allen, 1977).

Patients in hospital ward experiments may drink heavily, have high blood alcohol levels, and become intoxicated. It is a myth created by critics that alcoholics must drink themselves into a state of inebriation in order to demonstrate loss of control. Operant studies do show that the behavior of an alcoholic is manipulable and responsive to environmental contingencies. They can refrain from drinking at a high rate given the proper reinforcement contingencies. But these studies fail to demonstrate their generalizability to contexts outside the hospital where the physiological state of the individual and the reinforcement contingencies would be radically different. There is no evidence that with a different set and setting outside the hospital ward comparable results would be obtained, especially over the long term. There is no evidence that these laboratory demonstrations have ecological validity. There is no evidence that these experiments are relevant to the question of whether or not controlled drinking is a viable treatment goal for alcoholics or for problems drinkers in the world outside the hospital ward and to the hypothesis of loss of control manifest in drinking behavior outside the ward.

A second kind of study critical of the loss of control conception has attracted a great deal more attention than operant studies in recent years and has spawned a number of variations. Its impact in part is a consequence of its congruence with the current dominant approach in clinical psychology, cognitive behavior therapy, and the dominance of a cognitive approach in psychology as a whole. The study in question is the balanced-placebo experiment conducted by Marlatt, Demming, and Reid (1973) which purports to demonstrate that what is really important is not what you drink but what you think.

In a balanced-placebo design half the subjects are given alcohol and half are given tonic. Half of each of these two groups are told they are receiving tonic and half are told they are receiving alcohol. Will instructions have an effect regardless of what the subjects ingest or will what they ingest be more important than what they are instructed? Marlatt et al. 1973) conducted a double balanced placebo experiment. The 2 x 2 balanced placebo design was employed with a group of "alcoholics" and a group of social drinkers. Overall effects were the same. Instructions regarding the nature of the drink had a significant effect on the amount of alcohol consumed. What they were given did not have a significant effect on subsequent alcohol consumption. Participants who were instructed that they were given alcohol subsequently drank more alcohol than participants who were instructed that they were given tonic, regardless of what they actually ingested. Given alcohol groups did not drink more than given tonic groups. There was no interaction. These results were taken to mean that what you think is more important than what you drink.

There are a number of serious methodological shortcomings in this study which Fingarette (1988b) and other critics of the loss of control hypothesis overlook. Nor does Fingarette discuss the studies that contradict the results and implications of Marlatt et al. (1973) (Hodgson, Rankin, & Stockwell, 1979; Stockwell, Hodgson, Rankin, & Taylor, 1982) and still other studies which offer an alternative interpretation of the kinds of results obtained by Marlatt et al. (Knight, Barbaree, & Boland, 1986; Korytnyk & Perkins, 1983). None of this important literature is cited by Fingarette in connection with the interpretation of balanced-placebo experiments. Marlatt (1983) in his major defense of controlled drinking cites his own study, but fails to cite the studies available at that time that contradict his interpretation and fail to corroborate his results. Searles (1993) assumes that these contradictory results and others (Maltzman & Marinkovic, 1996) do not exist.

One difficulty with the study by Marlatt et al. (1973) and many other balanced-placebo studies is that the authors fail to distinguish between the independent experimental variable they are employing and the interpretation of the results obtained with this variable. The balanced placebo experiment is misleadingly called an expectancy experiment. Marlatt et al. purport to demonstrate that expectancies are more important than the actual beverage consumed. But it must be noted that expectancy is a theoretical interpretation, one of several possible interpretations, of the outcome following the manipulation of instructions. The balanced placebo design is an experiment on the effects of different instructions, one independent experimental variable, and the kind of beverage given, the other independent experimental variable. Expectancy is an interpretation of the results found when instructions concerning the nature of the beverage have a significant effect. There are alternative interpretations of the effects of instructions under the conditions of the balanced placebo experiment. This issue and other inadequacies in the Marlatt et al. (1973) experiment have been discussed at length elsewhere (Maltzman, 1987b; 1991; Maltzman & Marinkovic, 1996).

Most importantly, the study did not meet the boundary conditions for a test of the loss of control hypothesis. Marlatt et al. (1973) did not obtain measures of physical dependence, the benchmark of alcoholism as defined by Jellinek. Their measures of what they call "alcoholism", drunk driving arrests, membership in AA, etc., do not differentiate between problem drinkers and alcoholics.

An alternative interpretation for the obtained results is available in terms of demand characteristics (Orne, 1962). Fingarette, Marlatt, and other revisionists do not address this issue. According to Orne, the usual difference in status between the experimenter and subject in an experiment induces a tendency on the part of the subject to please the experimenter. Subjects try to produce the results ostensibly desired by the experimenter. An important difference in the implications of the expectancy and demand characteristic interpretations is that the latter suggests that the effect obtained by instructions is peculiar to the laboratory situation. It severely limits the generality of the instructions effect. In contrast, the expectancy interpretation has been generalized to the world outside the laboratory.

Studies that obtain independent measures of severity of dependence, differentiate between problem drinkers and alcoholics, contradict the results and interpretations of Marlatt et al. (1973). One such study was conducted by Hodgson et al. (1979) with inpatients of an alcoholism treatment program. Investigators provided no dose, a low dose or a high dose of alcohol in the morning and then made alcohol available to the participants three hours later. A within-subject design was employed where each subject participated in each of the conditions on different days. Qualitatively different effects were obtained for the moderately dependent problem drinkers and the severely dependent alcoholics. The larger the priming dose in the morning the less problem drinkers consumed and consumed more slowly in the afternoon. They showed a satiation effect. In contrast, the more the alcoholics drank in the morning the more and faster they drank three hours later. They showed a priming or appetizer effect. These behavioral effects contradict the continuum notion that social drinkers, heavy drinkers, and alcoholics all lie on the same continuum varying only in degree of alcohol consumption (Heather & Robertson, 1983; Marlatt, 1979). On the contrary, these results support Jellinek's conception that there is a qualitative difference between problem drinkers and alcoholics.

A second study by the same group of investigators (Stockwell et al., 1982) employed the balanced-placebo design with a new group of patients who were also independently assessed as either problem drinkers or alcoholics. Results for alcoholics showed that amount of alcohol ingested in the test situation was affected by the beverage given, not instructions. In contrast, problem drinkers were affected by instructions in the test situation not the beverage given. Results by Stockwell et al. (1982) thus contradict the expectancy interpretation as it is applied to alcoholics and support Jellinek's hypothesis that loss of control is a characteristic of alcoholics and not problem drinkers. Neither of the above two experiments are considered by Fingarette (1988b) and other revisionists (Searles, 1993). There is no "book shelf of research" contradicting the notion of loss of control.

Treatment outcome studies

Conditions for testing the loss of control hypothesis are most readily met in treatment outcome studies which have the ecological validity that laboratory experiments ordinarily do not possess. It is apparent, however, that the evaluation window for controlled drinking in treatment outcome studies must be at least two years (Pettinati et al., 1982; Miller et al.,1992). We shall discuss this issue further when we turn to clinical outcome studies in chapters 6 and 7.

There is a second condition for an adequate test of loss of control that Fingarette and other critics usually ignore. Its neglect is apparent in Fingarette's presentation of the initial cornerstone of the attack on the loss of control. Initial criticisms of the loss-of-control conception centered about clinical studies, such as Davies (1962) that claimed to show that 7 of 93 alcoholics returned to controlled drinking 7-11 years after treatment. Supporters of the disease concept argued that the participants who engaged in long term controlled drinking were not alcoholics. Critics, including Fingarette, in turn argue that such a criticism of Davies' study is circular. Any study of alcoholics that reports controlled drinking is said to have used problem drinkers rather than alcoholics and studies which show loss of control drinking used alcoholics. There is an inherent circularity in the conventional position. This argument of circularity is without merit because it fails to recognize that it is possible to specify whether or not alcoholics as distinguished from problem drinkers are employed in a study independently of any measure of loss of control.

As previously noted, characteristics of gamma alcoholism include objective signs of physical dependence including frequent and severe withdrawal symptoms. Individuals who have not experienced signs of withdrawal such as seizures are not usually alcoholics who would be expected to show loss of control. Who will show loss of control drinking and who will not, on the average, can be determined independently of measures of loss of control by evidence of withdrawal symptoms. Davies presented the case histories of the 7 who purportedly engaged in control drinking. Only one subject clearly experienced withdrawal, and a second possibly. Supporters of the disease concept were quite right. The majority of people purportedly engaging in controlled drinking in Davies' study were not alcoholics -

Results by Welte et al. (1983) and Küfner and Feuerlein (1989) are among several that call into question a major argument for controlled drinking, that it is effective with younger problem drinkers who have not been misusing alcohol for many years and are not severely dependent. Although it is now generally accepted by revisionists that controlled drinking is not a viable treatment goal for chronic alcoholics, they have promoted controlled drinking as a form of secondary prevention or harm reduction. It is purportedly ideally suited for younger problem drinkers who are not severely dependent despite the evidence by Welte and others (e.g., Pettinati et al., 1982) calling into question the truth status of this implication. A complexity ignored by Fingarette and others is the implication of the results obtained by Cloninger (1987) and his colleagues and their distinction between Type 1 and Type 2 alcoholics. Type 2 alcoholics are those who develop alcoholism before the age of 25 accompanied by anti-social personality characteristics. Because an alcoholic is youthful and has not been drinking for many years does not mean that they may not have a high degree of physical dependence. They are different in personality and biology than the Type 1 alcoholic. Fingarette and others (e.g., Marlatt, 1992) who promote controlled drinking as secondary prevention are misled by their continuity hypothesis which assumes that the only variable of consequence is the quantity and frequency of alcohol consumption. They fail to consider the profound import of individual differences, especially biological differences that enhance the risk of alcoholism and markedly influence severity of dependence and physiological vulnerability. Basically, in part, it is an issue of the effectiveness of assessment. Assessment of severity of dependence used by the facilities providing Rand with its data were relatively crude, as is still true of facilities in general.

The third pillar of controlled drinking presented by Fingarette is the Sobells' (1978) individualized behavior therapy study. In contrast to the Davies study and the Rand Reports which were evaluations of outcomes from traditional treatment programs, the Sobell and Sobell study was an experiment designed to compare abstinence and controlled drinking as treatment goals. It purportedly randomly assigned participants to an experimental group given training in controlled drinking and a control group receiving traditional abstinence treatment. It also is the only one of the three empirical cornerstone's of Fingarette's critique making the explicit claim that the participants were diagnosed gamma alcoholics. Fingarette (1988b) nevertheless declares, unsupported by evidence, that: "In over eighty studies in the past decade that report on alcoholics who return to some moderated form of drinking, at least half the subjects were diagnosed as gamma alcoholics." (p. 39). Fingarette mentions the follow-up study by Pendery et al. (1982) as failing to find successful controlled drinking years later and suggests the usual inappropriate criticism of the study: it failed to adequately address the issue of controlled drinking because it failed to compare the experimental and control groups. Pendery et al. only reported the failure to find successful outcomes in the experimental group. Perhaps the control group did equally poorly. This criticism echoes the reproof voiced by many others (e.g., Dickens et al., 1982; Heather & Robertson, 1983; Marlatt 1983). The criticism is inappropriate. It overlooks the fact that the two groups were compared by Pendery et al. (1982) and found to differ significantly in the order of their appearance for the study. There was a significant order effect, a violation of the assumption of random assignment, and therefore the two groups could not be compared further. This problem was discussed at some length in a later paper as well as the point that the order effect was not a trivial matter (Maltzman, 1984). Fingarette does not cite this rebuttal of the criticism of the Pendery et al. study.

Fingarette also fails to consider the best designed experiment of controlled drinking in chronic alcoholics that has been published (Foy, Nun, & Rychtarik, 1984; Rychtarik, Foy, Scott, Lokey, & Prue, 1987). It contradicts the notion that controlled drinking is a feasible treatment goal and fails to corroborate the Sobells' results. Patients in an alcoholism treatment unit in a VA Hospital were randomly assigned to traditional abstinence treatment or traditional abstinence treatment plus controlled drinking skills training. Follow-ups were conducted by a team of social workers blind to the group membership of the participants. At six months follow-up it was found that the experimental group, the participants who had received controlled drinking training in addition to traditional treatment, were significantly worse than the control group that received only the traditional treatment. A follow-up 5-6 years later found no significant difference between the two groups (Rychtarik et al., 1987). This means that controlled drinking training had no significant effect. An interesting aspect of the second study is that supporters of controlled drinking have consistently misinterpreted its results as indicating that traditional abstinence and controlled drinking skills training were equally effective (e.g., Graber & Miller, 1988; Institute of Medicine, 1990; Miller, Leckman, & Tinkcam, 1987; Peele, 1988; Sobell & Sobell, 1987a, 1987b, 1995a). This latter interpretation is incorrect. Both groups received abstinence training whereas the experimental group received controlled drinking skills training in addition to abstinence training. The addition had no effect. Basically, this is the same sort of "add on" design employed by Sobell and Sobell (1973b, 1978) - without the profound shortcomings of the Sobell study (see chapter 4 and 5; Maltzman, 1988, 1989).

Secondary prevention and controlled drinking

With the failure to sustain the three pillars of controlled drinking with chronic alcoholics the critics' emphasis on controlled drinking has shifted towards secondary prevention and harm reduction. Use controlled drinking with problem drinkers since it will be more attractive to them as a treatment goal than abstinence. Teaching such people moderation will prevent excessive misuse of alcohol with its attendant negative consequences.

A difficulty with the controlled drinking as secondary prevention approach is that its effectiveness depends on the effectiveness of assessment. How does one differentiate between two people who are problem drinkers one of whom if continuing to drink with moderation will remain at that level whereas the other may progress into alcoholism? Compounding the difficulty is the point previously noted that age is not a definitive variable. Young alcoholics may be dependent if they have the characteristics of Type 2 alcoholics and are not simply youths who are going through a stage which will pass, especially if they receive some guidance.

Miller (Miller & Hester, 1980) has been one of the strongest proponents of controlled drinking for problem drinkers and has claimed outstanding success for a program of moderation for socially stable problem drinkers. He notes that his behavioral self-control training (BSCT) methods have yielded success rates of 60%-

80% in his studies and others across the country. It was therefore with great interest that many of us waited for the complete report of the long term follow-up of controlled drinking participants in his studies. A preliminary report (Miller et al.,1986) of the follow-up of people 3.5, 5, 7, and 8 years after treatment did not support the enthusiasm with which the studies were originally presented and described in various places (e.g., Miller & Hester,1980).

The more extensive report of the long term follow-up (Miller et al., 1992) did nothing to change the pessimistic outcome. Depending on criteria used for dealing with attrition in the two reports, 10-14% of the participants were engaged in controlled drinking at follow-up and 23-31% of the people were judged abstinent. A considerably larger number of people were abstinent despite their training in controlled drinking skills designed to enable them to return to moderate drinking. These are not encouraging success rates for socially stable middle class people who were selected for treatment because they were problem drinkers, not alcoholics, who for the most part responded to media advertisements soliciting participants. Miller and Hester (1980) assert that 19% is the estimated spontaneous remission rate after one year. In other words the people presumably engaging in controlled drinking as a consequence of state of the art treatment by Miller et al. did no better than what would be expected if they were left to their own devices and received no treatment.

Follow-up assessments revealed that 66% of the people were either gamma or delta alcoholics, were physically dependent alcoholics. Yet they were initially screened and selected for the study because they were problem drinkers who were not pharmacologically dependent upon alcohol. It is apparent that the assessment was unsuccessful. Miller was unable to successfully differentiate the problem drinkers who would moderate their drinking from those who might progress on to pharmacological dependence. An obvious question is: what would have happened to these people if they had received traditional abstinence oriented treatment from the outset? What would have been the success rate then? The problem is not, as Miller and Hester (1980, p. 63) put it, for how many are moderation approaches a viable approach? The question is for whom is it appropriate and how do we know this?

Miller et al. (1992) found that engaging in controlled drinking at one year follow-up does not predict that the individual will be successfully engaged in controlled drinking at a later time. In contrast, abstinence at the end of one year post-treatment does predict successful abstinence at a later time. These results are in keeping with those reported by Pettinati et al. (1982) who found that controlled drinking after one year does not predict outcome four years later whereas abstinence does. An evaluation window of two years of controlled drinking is needed to predict controlled drinking outcomes in the long term. In other words the results obtained by Miller et al. (1992) and Pettinati et al. (1982) indicate that there is no good evidence that controlled drinking is a successful treatment modality for the long term even for socially stable people initially assessed as problem drinkers.

There is no good outcome evidence that controlled drinking is a viable treatment with ecological validity for problem drinkers, those misusing alcohol with no signs of physical dependence at the time they entered treatment. If they continue to drink in moderation the drinking in some cases progressively increases and these individuals ultimately become physically dependent upon alcohol. As previously noted, Hasin et al. (1990) reported that 30% progressed from problem drinking to alcoholism over a four year period.

Fingarette (1988b) and others (e.g., Heather, 1989; Peele & Brodsky, 1991) have cited a number of studies conducted abroad for the most part that report successful cases of controlled drinking (Elal-Lawrence, Slade, & Dewey, 1986; McCabe, 1986; Nordstrom & Berglund, 1987; Orford & Keddie, 1986). Contrary to the supporters of controlled drinking these studies provide no good evidence for the viability of controlled drinking as a treatment for alcoholics or problem drinkers. These more recent studies purporting to demonstrate the success of controlled drinking suffer from numerous shortcomings including unreliable brief follow-up intervals, small windows of evaluation, biased samples, and other forms of inadequate methodology (see chapter 6 and Wallace, 1989b).

Another aspect of revisionists' selective presentation of the treatment outcome literature is the failure to cite the striking outcome rates reported for a number of private inpatient treatment programs. For the most part these facilities treat socially stable middle class patients for whom the costs of treatment are usually defrayed by third party payments. They would be the same sort of socioeconomic status patients participating in the efficacy study conducted by Miller et al. (1992). Independent evaluation services such as *Benchmark* report 12-month abstinence outcomes of 58%, 55%, and 71% for samples of 2452, 398, and 390 cases, respectively (Maltzman, 1987a). An even higher success rate, 86%, for six months of continuous abstinence at one year follow-up is reported by Smith, Frawley, and Polissar (1991), which is significantly better than the 74% for matched comparison subjects from the CATOR registry. Each group in Smith et al. (1991) had approximately 200 participants. Both rates are considerably better than for controlled-drinking treatment outcomes reported by reasonably well-conducted studies. These kinds of outcome results obtained by independent evaluation services are not included in the usual reviews of treatment outcome studies (e.g., Miller & Hester, 1980, 1995) and are not cited by Fingarette (1988b) or other supporters of controlled drinking.

Smith et al. (1991) reported the results from a Schick Shadel Hospital which uses aversion conditioning therapy and sodium pentothal interviews as well as education and counseling in its program. Patients receive an educational program which emphasizes alcoholism as a disease. It is not a 12-step program although it recommends support groups including AA as after-care. Other treatment programs in the CATOR registry are characteristically 12-step oriented Minnesota Model programs. All of this suggests that there is considerable variation in treatment programs adopting a disease concept of alcoholism. Yet Fingarette propogates the myth of a monolithic rigid program of treatment based on a discredited classification of alcoholism as a disease. He is not alone in rewriting the professional literature.

Miller (1988) testifying before a Senate Government Affairs Committee stated that, "traditional U.S. alcoholism programs are based on treatment methods that are largely unsupported by current research evidence. In contrast, treatment modalities that appear promising from current scientific evidence are mostly unknown or unused outside of the (Veterans Administration treatment system) or research-supported programs." (p.3). Heather's (1980) position is clear concerning the current state of affairs in the alcoholism research and treatment field:

The treatment of alcohol abuse is now in a state of crisis and those involved in this treatment have a crucial choice to make. The choice is not between total abstinence and moderation, or between Alcoholics Anonymous and behavioural psychology. It is simply between dogma, prejudice and arbitrary authority, on the one hand, and openness, reason and a belief in the scientific method, on the other. (p. 258).

THE NEW LOOK IN ALCOHOLISM TREATMENT

Matching

Fingarette (1988b) has considered some of the purported innovative advantages of the new look in alcoholism treatment and theory in contrast to treatment based on a disease conception of alcoholism. One such new look, he claims, is the matching of patient and treatment.

There is a very extensive, varied, and complex literature on the general problem of matching patient and treatment (Lindstrom, 1992). Fingarette does not discuss the relevant issues or review the pertinent research. Instead, he emphasizes one of the first and most sophisticated matching studies, an investigation by McLachlan (1972), to illustrate advantages of the nontraditional approach to treatment. Participants in a residential treatment program were administered a test of conceptual level that assesses behavior related to locus of control, inner or outer directedness, the need for structure in the environment versus a need for independence, etc. Patients and therapists were administered the test. After-care programs were rated by McLachlan along a similar dimension. Fingarette erroneously states that McLachlan developed the measure of conceptual level himself; he did not. He states that it is a rating of the patient and therapist; it is not. It is a self-report scale.

McLachlan found that matching of patient and therapist and patient and aftercare environments had significant impact upon recovery. For those patients who were matched with therapist and environment, 77% were abstinent and functioning well at 12-to18- month follow-up as contrasted with only a 38% success rate for those who were mismatched with therapist and after-care environment. A recovery rate of 77% abstinence 12 to18 months following treatment is rather striking. Fingarette does not report this highly successful abstinence rate, which is contrary to the claims of critics that abstinence does not work. Instead, Fingarette emphasizes that the new look in alcoholism treatment is concerned with individual differences and the diverse patterns of alcoholism and is disposed to matching patients and treatments in contrast to the traditional treatment. The latter requires that everyone be treated in similar fashion because alcoholism unfolds inexorably in a manner common to all.

Fingarette's argument is false. This classic matching study by McLachlan (1972) was conducted at the Donwood Institute in Toronto, whose director at the time was R. Gordon Bell, author of *Escape from Addiction* (Bell, 1970). The Donwood Institute is a traditional treatment center that emphasizes the medical model with abstinence as the treatment goal. Matching is not an example of the advantages of the new look, but a demonstration of the flexibility and diversity of approaches employed by traditional treatment programs emphasizing abstinence and the disease concept of alcoholism (see chapter 7).

Classification of a syndrome as a disease does not entail any particular treatment. This is another myth promulgated by critics of the disease concept. Which treatments work is an empirical matter and is not entailed by labeling a syndrome a disease or not. Presence of biological correlates or having biological variables among the causes of alcoholism does not proscribe talk or behavior therapy as treatments. Baxter et al. (1992) found that behavior therapy, cue exposure and response prevention, significantly changed levels of serotonin in the caudate nucleus of people in treatment for obsessive-compulsive disorders and improved behavior, as did a serotonin re-uptake blocker. In like fashion, there is no logical reason why alcoholism could not have biological variables among its etiological factors yet have talk therapy change the biological state of alcoholics and so contribute to their recovery. This would be expected if alcoholism is a biopsychosocial disease. Striking preliminary results for treatment outcomes using naltrexone and different talk therapies provide further evidence of the biopsychosocial nature of alcoholism (O'Malley, et al., 1992; Volpicelli, et al., 1992). The burgeoning field of psychoneuroimmunology attests to the growing recognition and success in dealing with the biopsychosocial nature of a great variety of diseases (e.g., Ader, 1981; Glaser & Kiecolt-Glaser, 1994). Alcoholism is no exception (see chapter 7).

Relapse prevention

A great deal of attention has accrued to the issue of relapse prevention in recent years. Much of the attention and credit for this concern has been attributed to Marlatt (Cummings, Gordon, & Marlatt 1980; Marlatt & Gordon 1985). It is certainly true that for the treatment of a variety of problems, alcohol, nicotine dependence, narcotics, most relapses do not occur during treatment, whether inpatient or outpatient. Most relapses occur within the first three months following completion of treatment (Hunt, Barnett, & Branch, 1971). The problem is to prevent relapse following treatment and this prevention may represent a different problem than initiating cessation of misuse of a drug.

Attributing origins of an emphasis upon relapse prevention to the prescience of the new look in alcoholism is to rewrite history. Relapse prevention and methods for dealing with relapse, slips, what to do to prevent it in response to slips etc., have been part of AA teachings from the outset. After-care programs, even those that do not employ 12-step programs based upon AA teachings such as the Schick Shadel hospitals, make use of AA and other support groups as after-care programs to prevent relapse.

Fingarette limits his discussion to one kind of relapse prevention, Marlatt's approach, and presents it as though it is the original and principal approach to relapse prevention. It is obvious that the prevention of relapse is an important problem. But a critical examination of Marlatt's approach to relapse prevention is needed. This is not the place for the detailed critical examination of the formulation that Fingarette fails to offer. However, several issues will be commented upon here.

Marlatt's theory of relapse as originally formulated is a thinly veiled approach to controlled drinking and an attack on abstinence based on a caricature of traditional approaches to alcoholism treatment. His theory of relapse prevention (Cummings, Gordon, & Marlatt, 1980) is based on the notion of an AVE, the abstinence violation effect. An individual is likely to relapse when there is a slip, an isolated drinking episode that produces cognitive dissonance - a negative affective state or disequilibrium - induced because the drinking is incompatible with the self- image that person has of themselves as abstinent. Under such conditions two responses are possible as a consequence of the cognitive dissonance induced by a slip. Since drinking was a means of coping with stress in the past, it is resorted to once more in order to reduce the stress induced by cognitive dissonance. A second response is self-blame with the same consequence, excessive drinking. In either case cognitive dissonance is reduced by drinking to a state of inebriation. A relapse occurs. Marlatt argues that the loss of control is inevitable if a person who has tried to be abstinent takes a single drink. The drinker believes the mnemonic "one drink away from a drunk" and this rigid unrealistic image of themselves is responsible for the cognitive dissonance and subsequent loss of control and relapse. The solution is to train individuals in controlled drinking. Let them drink under supervision and they will see that they do not have an overwhelming desire to continue drinking after having a drink or two. Controlled drinking is the solution to relapse prevention.

A second aspect of relapse prevention is an emphasis upon problem solving skills. People must learn to avoid drinking when dysphoric, depressed, anxious, etc. They must learn to cope with these negative mood states constructively without resorting to drinking as an escape.

There are two major problems with Marlatt's theory of relapse prevention neither of which Fingarette considers. First, there are no good data supporting the theoretical formulation. Second, there are no good data demonstrating that this approach is more successful than other specific approaches to relapse prevention "based upon" the disease concept of alcoholism (e.g., Gorski & Miller, 1986). Furthermore, there is reliable evidence contradicting Marlatt's theoretical formulation. For example, studies have been conducted by Hall and her colleagues (Hall, Havassy, & Wasserman, 1990; Hall, Havassy, & Wasserman, 1991) demonstrating that the stronger the commitment to abstinence stated at the outset of treatment, the less likely the relapse from treatment for the misuse of opiates, alcohol, nicotine, and cocaine. Hall obtained prospective reports of mood and well-being as well as retrospective reports each week for three months, the critical relapse period. Prospective evidence showed no evidence of dysphoric mood immediately prior to a relapse. Only retrospective reports indicated relapse occurred because of dysphoria. The evidence is rather convincing that when a relapse occurs, the individual becomes depressed, anxious, dysphoric, etc., but when subsequently asked to report the event they attribute the relapse to the dysphoria rather than the dysphoria to the relapse (see also Shiffman et al., 1997 and chapter 7).

Alcoholism as a biopsychosocial disease

Fingarette's (1988b) notion of alcoholism as nothing but a central activity of life no different in principle than avid stamp collecting is based on the demonstrably false assumption that all alcoholics when sober are innocent of all structural and functional brain damage. If there is brain dysfunction, negative consequences of alcohol consumption, according to Fingarette it is only in the presence of alcohol - while under the influence. Any lingering dysfunction quickly disappears with sobriety.

His neglect of the evidence of structural and functional brain changes in the majority of chronic alcoholics when sober as well as when under the influence enables him to claim that the negative social consequences of alcoholism are the result of willful misconduct. An individual when sober and in full possession of his or her faculties decides to drink. An aftermath, a crime, an automobile crash, etc., is a consequence of that decision made when sober. Fingarette therefore argues that there is no basis for a claim of diminished capacity. Fingarette can make his argument of willful misconduct because of his omission of the very information he claims he will provide at the outset of his book and which he never does: major findings in mainstream biomedical science.

Relevant findings include, for example, the CT neuroimaging research by Cala (1987) that 95% of alcoholics studied showed brain atrophy. These are people who have been chronically drinking four or more ounces of alcohol a day, approximately 10 drinks/day or more. It is important to note that atrophy is not evenly distributed throughout the brain. There is a gradient of damage with the greatest amount in the frontal lobes and the least in the occipital lobes. Sixty-five percent to 85% of light and moderate drinkers also show brain atrophy. This is in people who regularly drink one to five drinks/day. Marked individual differences are evident. Some people who are heavy drinkers show less brain atrophy than light drinkers. Some heavy drinkers show no atrophy. Some light drinkers show greater atrophy than many heavy drinkers. Variables influencing the vulnerability and relative invulnerability to brain atrophy are unknown. Cala (1987) convinced some of the light and moderate drinkers to abstain for six months. There was a significant reversal of brain shrinkage in the abstinent sample. However, reversal of the atrophy was not complete in all people. Variables responsible for individual differences in atrophy and how and what variables facilitate or retard reversal of the atrophy with abstinence are not known. Continued alcohol consumption is related to continued and increased brain atrophy (Muuronen et al., 1989).

Harper and his colleagues (Harper & Kril, 1990; Harper, Kril, & Daly, 1987) conducted quantitative neuropathological studies on the brains of documented chronic alcoholics with and without cirrhosis and with no evidence of traumatic head injury. Control subjects matched for age with no history of alcoholism or of head injury were also studied. Approximately 30% of the neurons in the frontal lobes of alcoholics were dead as compared to the control group. There was no neuronal loss in the motor cortex. It was also observed that brain damage occurred prior to liver damage. When there was liver damage due to alcohol the brain damage was more severe. That there is a gradient of damage with the greatest amount occurring in the frontal lobes is of singular importance even though at present the reason for the differential damage is uncertain. A more recent study corroborates and extends previous findings (Kril, Halliday, Svoboda, & Cartwright, 1997).

The frontal lobes are known as the executive region of the brain (Lhermitte, 1986; Luria, 1980; Lyvers, 1998, in press; Maltzman, 1991; Oscar-Berman & Hutner,

1993; Stuss & Benson, 1984). They are responsible for planning, foresight, the anticipation of future events as well as the concomitant inhibition of other areas of the brain thus permitting the integration of behavior, requiring as it must initiation of some behaviors with inhibition of others. The frontal lobes also play an important role in emotions and moods and their integration into a consistent pattern of behavior, motivation and emotion (Stuss et al., 1992). It is apparent that dysfunctional frontal lobes could have enormous consequences for all aspects of integrated goal directed behavior, problem solving, planning, mood, and emotion. Diverse symptoms of alcoholics when sober as well as when under the influence of alcohol are influenced by frontal lobe function - and dysfunction. Diminished mental capacity, the inability to anticipate the consequences of one's actions, the absence of intent, are interpretable as a consequence of frontal lobe dysfunction, brain disease whether permanent or reversible in part or in whole. Alcoholism in part is a brain disease present when the typical alcoholic is sober as well as when under the influence of alcohol.

Volkow et al. (1992) used PET scans to examine regional brain glucose metabolism in a control group of social drinkers and a group of medically healthy neurologically intact men meeting DSM-III-R criteria for alcohol dependence. They were patients in a VA Hospital and had been detoxified 6-32 days earlier with no current signs or symptoms of withdrawal at initiation of the study. Despite the fact that patients were carefully screened medically and neuroradiologically, eliminating anyone with evidence of ventricular enlargement or cortical atrophy, the patients showed significant regional differences in brain glucose metabolism. They showed significant relative decreases in glucose metabolism in the left parietal and right frontal cortices. Physiological deficits were observed in the absence of structural damage. A long term prospective study is needed to determine whether the obtained differences were present prior to alcohol misuse and whether they would normalize after extended abstinence.

There is a large body of electrophysiological and neuroimaging research as well as neuropsychological research showing persistent brain dysfunction for extended periods following detoxification and continued sobriety that was in existence before publication of *Heavy Drinking*. These are mainstream findings in biomedicine. They are never considered by Fingarette or other critics of the disease concept (e.g., Heather & Robertson, 1983). These earlier studies show reversibility of dysfunction often occurs after varying amounts of sober time, although it is not always complete. Continued drinking usually results in continuing dysfunction (e.g., Begleiter, 1980; Eckardt et al., 1980; Goldman, 1983; Ron, 1984).

The above studies imply that before individuals are permitted to participate in controlled drinking treatment studies they should receive neuroimaging assessments demonstrating that there are no structural or functional brain dysfunctions present. Urgently needed are studies relating the dysfunctional brain physiology to behavior. Such studies have been conducted with schizophrenics (e.g., Berman, Illowsky, & Weinberger, 1988; Weinberger, Berman, & Zec, 1986). Similar studies and others are needed with alcoholics after varying periods of sobriety as well as alcoholics, problem and social drinkers, sober and while under the influence.

Conclusion

Much of the controversy in the field of alcohol studies stems from the failure to recognize that the classification of a condition as a disease is a value judgment that a lawful pattern of observable signs and symptoms is a significant deviation from a standard of health. This value judgment must be distinguished from the empirical issues of the descriptive features of the syndrome, its etiology, explanation, and treatment. Classifying alcoholism as a disease does not prescribe certain treatments, e.g., biological, and proscribe others, e.g., behavioral. It does not necessarily entail certain etiologies, e.g., biogenic and not others, e.g., psychosocial. Etiology and effective treatments are empirical issues not value judgments based on volitional decisions. A reasonable interpretation of the alcoholism syndrome as distinguished from problem and social drinking is that it is a consequence of brain dysfunction. Alcoholism is a brain disease. Its etiology and the biological processes involved in the disease will be considered in chapter 3.

2

Introduction

To adequately grasp the nature of the proposition that alcoholism is a disease entity we must put to rest misconceptions burdening many behavior therapists. We must consider what behaviorism is, not what behavior therapists in the alcohol studies field mistakenly say it is. We have to step back and briefly consider the history and philosophy of psychology, what behaviorism is -- and is not -- to adequately comprehend how many behavior therapists have misled themselves and others. Before we turn to the important issues of the etiology, treatment, and prevention of alcoholism we have to clear up some misunderstandings and resolve a fundamental controversy. Does the conception of alcoholism as a disease refer to nothing more than a bad habit following the same principles of learning as the acquisition of any other habit? Or, taxonomically does it "carve nature at its joints". In other words, is there a unique disease entity or bodily condition which we discover or is alcoholism an invention, merely the attribution of negative characteristics to the consequences of ordinary habit formation (Fingarette, 1988b, Szasz, 1972)? This aspect of the dispute concerning the status of the disease concept of alcoholism is in part a manifestation of the long standing controversy between nominalism and realism. Contributing to the unwillingness of many behavior therapists and other revisionists to accept the conception of alcoholism as a disease entity, a part of nature that is discovered in similar fashion as other disease entities such as malaria, diabetes, cancer and AIDS, are the ideological blinders forged by their misunderstanding of txhe fundamental nature of behaviorism.

Alcoholism is nothing but a bad habit

"the prevailing behavioral view is that the behavior of most alcoholics is learned."
(Nathan & Lipscomb, 1979, p. 306)

I want to talk today about the latest in behavioral approaches to alcoholism. Technically, this approach is now known as cognitive social learning theory and therapy. There are a variety of reasons for the name change. For several unfortunate reasons, behavior therapy has acquired an undeserved bad name, especially in the whole controversy over controlled drinking. We are now calling it cognitive social learning theory, and it is different in more than in name...What are the distinguishing characteristics of the cognitive social learning strategy as it applies to the treatment of alcoholism? ...the approach focuses on the observable characteristics of behavior, rather than, for example, on theory confirmation or the search for historical antecedents or unconscious determinants of behavior... Such variables are the amount, frequency and duration of drinking; the problems associated with excessive use; and situational and environmental factors in abusive drinking... Especially important are an individual's processes associated with drinking: expectations about the effect of drinking; expectations of its effects on behavior (it makes me more powerful, it makes me sexy, it makes me better). In a real sense, expectations exert their effect regardless of what alcohol actually does. (Nathan, 1985, p. 169).

Consider the assertion, "the approach focuses on the observable characteristics of behavior..." in relation to the claim that: "Especially important are an individual's processes associated with drinking: expectations about the effect of drinking; expectations of its effects on behavior... In a real sense, expectations exert their effect regardless of what alcohol actually does..." On the one hand these statements describe behaviorism as focused on observable characteristics of behavior and on the other Nathan affirms expectations as determiners of behavior. Undefined, unobservable expectancies replace undefined, unobservable unconscious psychodynamic processes. When it first evolved behavior therapy explicitly revolted against the latter kind of theorizing. How can an unobservable reified mental process given a label "expectancy" and nothing more, cause behavior? Expectancies in the hands of behavior therapists such as Nathan are a return to Cartesian ghosts. It is word magic.

Thombs (1994) tells us that:

The principal aims of 'behaviorism' are to elucidate the conditions of human learning and to develop a technology for behavior change. Behaviorists believe that most or all human behavior is learned; this includes not only adaptive but also maladaptive behavior (e.g., addiction). One of the major premises, then, is that certain fundamental laws (known and unknown) govern the initiation, maintenance, and cessation of human behavior. Alcohol or drug use is considered a behavior that is subject to the same principles of learning as driving a car, typing a letter, or building a house. (p.74).

Note the similarity in the statements of Nathan and of Thombs. Note also that the laws of learning in question are a promissory note. They cannot explain why approximately 90% of the people in the United States who consume alcohol do not become alcoholics. Behavior therapists cannot specify how male alcoholics may learn to beat their wives, may physically and sexually abuse their children, perhaps ruin their careers and health, etc. How are these deplorable kinds of behavior learned? Like taking tennis and driving lessons an alcoholic takes lessons in wife beating?

According to Marlatt (1985):

in recent years, a third approach has emerged as an alternative to the moral and disease modes [sic] of addiction. Derived from the principles of social-learning theory, cognitive psychology, and experimental social psychology, the addictive behavior model makes a number of assumptions that differ markedly from the disease and moral models. From a social-learning perspective addictive behaviors represent a category of 'bad habits' including such behaviors as problem drinking, smoking, substance abuse.... In terms of frequency of occurrence, addictive behaviors are presumed to lie along a continuum of use rather than being defined in terms of discrete or fixed categories such as excessive use (loss of control) or total abstinence. In contrast, *all* points along this continuum of frequency of occurrence, from very infrequent to 'normal' to excessive use, are assumed to be governed by similar processes of learning. (p.9).

If social drinking, problem drinking, and alcoholism are governed by the same processes of learning, once more, how is it that some people learn to drink excessively and others do not? How is it that given the same level of alcohol consumption some individuals may have serious social, personal, and biomedical problems and others have no such problems? Furthermore, behavior therapists ignore the variety of negative behaviors that appear in an alcoholic when sober as well as when they are under the influence. They may be unreliable, untrustworthy, unpredictable, and abusive, as well as anxious, moody, and depressed. Alcoholics are not always drunk. They may have days, weeks, months of abstinence or moderate drinking. Their dysfunction is that they cannot consistently refrain from drinking, for example, in important situations where sobriety is critical. How do they learn to be so unpredictable, inconsistent and inconsiderate? Social learning theory has no answer. It does not consider the multiple behavioral characteristics displayed by alcoholics in work, social, and family relations, in addition to their excessive alcohol consumption. Alcoholism in all its manifestations is not simply a matter of learning. It is matter of brain dysfunction. Behavior therapists argue that if alcoholism is simply a bad habit that is learned like any other habit, then alcoholism is not a disease entity. It is normal learning of bad habits. If alcoholism is learned, then psychologists can treat alcoholics, in fact, treat them more appropriately then psychiatrists, since the area of learning is in the domain of expertise of psychology not psychiatry.

Marlatt continues:

behavioral theorists define addiction as a powerful habit pattern, an acquired vicious cycle of self-destructive behavior that is locked in by the collective effects of classical conditioning (acquired tolerance mediated in part by classical conditioning compensatory responses to the deleterious effects of the addictive substance), and operant reinforcement (both the positive reinforcement of the high of the drug rush and the negative reinforcement associated with drug use as a means of escaping or avoiding dysphoric physical and/or mental states...). In addition to classical and operant conditioning factors, human drug use is also determined to a large extent by acquired expectancies and beliefs about drugs as an antidote to stress and anxiety. Social learning and modeling factors (observational learning) also exert a strong influence (e.g., drug use in the family and peer environment, along with the pervasive portrayal of drug use in advertising and the media). (p.11).

Marlatt assumes that tolerance is learned and involves conditioned compensatory responses, implying that since tolerance, a major symptom of alcoholism is learned, then alcoholism is not a disease. Marlatt fails to consider that there are at least three different kinds of tolerance, acute, rapid, and chronic and not all can be the result of learning and certainly not the kind envisaged by Marlatt (Kalant, 1996). There is good reason to believe that chronic tolerance is not due to classical conditioning of compensatory responses to the drinking situation but is an artifact of the experimental designs employed in its study. Factors responsible for the apparent role of compensatory conditioned responses are produced in the test situation. Novelty of the test situation elicits an organismic orienting-exploratory reflex which involves activation of more than half a dozen neurotransmitter systems including the dopaminergic system, the hypothalamic-pituitary-adrenal (HPA) axis, and the release of endogenous opioids. Chronic tolerance is not due to classical conditioning of compensatory responses. It only appears to be such an effect due to confounding with biological effects of situational novelty (Maltzman & Marincovic, 1996).

What does the term "expectancy" refer to in Marlatt's passage? It is not behavior. It is purportedly inferred from behavior, the very behavior it is supposed to explain. In the absence of a network of established laws and an independent measure, independent of the very behavior it is designed to explain, "expectancy" is circular. It is folk psychology where the meaning and explanatory value of the term are assumed to be self-evident. The difference between a behaviorist and a cognitive folk psychologist labelling themselves a behaviorial psychologist, is that the former if it is their want to use the term "expectancy", would define it by referring to a particular kind of behavior or its proximate physiology and the conditions under which it occurs. "Expectancy" for the mentalistic folk psychologist is a hypothetical process inferred from behavior whereas the behaviorist defines it in terms of observable behavior patterns (Tolman,1925a/1951).

Marlatt and other revisionist behavior therapists are behaviorists in name only, practicing poor science because their use of terms such as "expectancy" is ambiguous. Assertions containing such terms have been falsified and the contradictory evidence ignored (Korytnyk & Perkins, 1985; see Maltzman & Marincovic, 1996).

Before considering alcoholism as a disease entity it is necessary to correct the misunderstandings reflected in the above statements by Nathan, Marlatt, Thombs and others that characterize the "behavioral approach" to alcoholism promoted by clinical psychologists who initially called themselves behavior therapists or behavior modifiers and who now generally call themselves cognitive behavior therapists, social learning theorists, etc. Their distorted conception of behaviorism has for decades misdirected research and treatment and wasted vast sums of government funds.

A BRIEF HISTORY OF PSYCHOLOGY

Science is more than a body of verifiable knowledge, empirical generalizations, and abstract theories that integrate diverse sets of established generalizations forming a network of statements that have empirical content and are falsifiable. Such bodies of knowledge are influenced and set in one direction or another by value judgments, by volitional decisions that are neither true nor false, and by the conventions that are based on such decisions. Reichenbach (1938) observed that some volitional decisions lead to equivalent systems based on different conventions, e.g., different systems of measurement. They are equivalent in that for any unit in one system, e.g., Celsius, there is a unit in the alternative equivalent system, Fahrenheit, which can be substituted for it. Although based on conventions and logically equivalent, conventional differences are not necessarily trivial, as suggested by the enormous social resistance and costs encountered in an effort to switch from one conventional system of measurement to another, for example from meters and centimeters, etc., to feet and inches. Tool makers, the construction industry, automobile manufacturers, etc. must engage in major retooling in the United States if our measurement convention were to be changed.

Reichenbach (1938) suggests that there is another more fundamental kind of volitional decision in science. It is the volitional bifurcation, a volition decision to adopt what ought to be the fundamental aims and goals of science. Alternative systems of scientific thought diverge following such a decision because different problems, techniques, and related theories develop that are congruent only with one or with the other widely different aims of the divergent systems. For Wundt (1897), one of the founders of experimental psychology, the fundamental aim of psychology was the analysis of the contents of consciousness into its irreducible elements, the compounds formed by these elements, and the laws by which elements are synthesized into compounds. Watson (1913) proclaimed that the fundamental goal of behavioristic psychology ought to be the prediction and control of behavior. It is inconceivable, given these different aims that Wundt would invent the Skinner box - or use it.

The most fundamental volitional bifurcation in the history of science occurred in the 17th century with the appearance of the Galilean-Newtonian world view in which determinism replaced Aristotelian teleology. Classification became the beginning not the end of the scientific method. Added was the powerful method of experimentation exploited by Galileo, Harvey, and others. They studied how things happened, rather than reasoning why they happened, what was their purpose. Application of the experimental method in the cause of determinism produced a profound volitional bifucation, opened the opportunity for new methods and new knowledge.

Aristotle

Aristotle explained the occurrence of events as the result of the essential nature of a thing to behave in a given manner. An acorn grows into a mighty oak tree because that is its goal, end, determined by its inherent organization or soul. Explanation of things consists in classifying them according to the essential properties of the natural kind or class of things having identical characteristics. Aristotle's volitional decision was that explanation of natural events was teleological, in terms of their goals, and things were classified by their essential natures.

In the new deterministic framework of physical science every event has a cause, a prior event without which it would not occur, and with it, always occurs. Science was now concerned with predicting future events given their antecedent conditions and appropriate scientific laws. With the development of powerful laws of physics, science became able to postdict as well as predict. Cosmologists' "big bang" theory now postdicts when the universe began and what occurred within the first few minutes of its creation on the basis of present conditions and laws of physics.

Determinism, the principle of causality, must be distinguished from predictability. The latter presupposes determinism, but is not equivalent to it. We do not always know the causes of events until the event has occurred. An experience I had several years ago illustrates the difference between determinism and predictability and suggests that because we cannot predict an event does not mean that the event was not caused. I usually arrive at my office at UCLA every morning six days a week at the same time, plus or minus 15 minutes. I set out one morning at my usual time, turned on my car radio and entered the freeway. I immediately noticed something was wrong. Traffic was unusually heavy for that hour of the morning. A traffic bulletin informed me that an 18-wheeler had overturned between where I was and the next freeway off-ramp. Four of the five lanes were blocked. I was a half an hour late after a drive that covered approximately 8 miles from house to office. My tardiness was not predicted - or predictable. Nevertheless, it was caused. Behavioral science suffers from a similar problem. In contrast to a physics experiment or astronomical observations, behavioral science does not work within a closed system where all the relevant variables are generally controllable or known. This lack of control over critical variables makes prediction difficult. However, lack of predictability does not imply that events are not caused or that explanations, although after the fact, may not be forthcoming. It also suggests that our behavioral predictions would be more accurate when applied to aggregates or averaged over repeated sessions or people. However, the goal remains to predict the behavior of the individual. To attain this goal, there must be knowledge of the proximal conditions giving rise to behavior under particular conditions. Detailed knowledge of those proximal conditions can only come from behavioral neuroscience in all its branches, an area of knowledge essential to the prediction, control, and explanation of behavior, the basic goals of behaviorism. Nevertheless, this basic area of knowledge, behavioral neuroscience in all its ramifications has been spurned by revisionist behavior therapists.

Descartes

A volitional decision occurred in the 17th century that had a profound influence on the development of psychology for 300 years. Descartes reasoned that the new principle of determinism applies to living organisms including humans. Physiology and anatomy flourished under the cloak of the new science. However, Descartes also said, "I think therefore I am" and made a volitional decision that introduced a new vocabulary from "within". Mind, the soul, is not simply the complex organization of matter as Aristotle believed. It is an unextended substance equal to but qualitatively different from matter. Probably fearing the wrath of the Inquisition, Descartes stated that humans have free will, and a mind that is not subject to the same deterministic laws as the body. Furthermore, the two interact. Mind influences the body and vice versa. Descartes' volitional decision produced a volitional bifurcation. Anatomy and physiology, the study of structure and function of the body follows the same deterministic rule as physical science and can be studied by its methods. Mind does not. It must have its own method, looking inward. It led to the development of a consciousness centered psychology that dominated the field for 300 years, represented in the latter part of the 19th century by two preeminent figures. One, we already mentioned, Wundt, and a second, Brentano the grandfather of modern cognitive psychology.

Wundt

In keeping with the dominant philosophy of science at the time, Wundt (1897) found it necessary to carve out a unique subject matter for psychology, arguing that psychology studies immediate experience as dependent upon an experiencing individual whereas physical science studies mediate experience, concepts abstracted from experience. Experimental introspection is the special procedure used to study the unique subject matter of psychology. Observation may be used to study the products of immediate experience such as thinking which is too fleeting to capture in introspection.

According to   Wundt there are three basic problems facing the new experimental psychology: (a) discover and describe the basic, irrreducible, elements of experience; (b) describe the compounds into which the basic elements enter; (c) discover the laws by which the compounds are formed.

Brentano

Although both giants in the history of psychology are now largely forgotten, Brentano's view of the basic problem of psychology is still very much with us, although his contribution to modern psychology is not generally acknowledged. Problems Brentano addressed have reemerged and today distinguish cognitive psychology from other approaches in psychology. It must be recognized that cognitive psychology is not necessarily incompatible with behaviorism. Tolman, one of the founding fathers of behaviorism was a cognitive psychologist. However, not all cognitive psychologists are behaviorists and not all behaviorists are S-R psychologists (Maltzman, 1987b).

According to Brentano (1874/1973) consciousness is composed of two classes of phenomena, the physical and the mental:

Every idea or presentation which we acquire either through sense perception or imagination is an example of a mental phenomenon. By presentation I do not mean that which is presented, but rather the act of presentation. Thus, hearing a sound, seeing a colored object, feeling warmth or cold, as well as similar states of imagination are examples of what I mean by this term... every judgement, every recollection, every expectation, every inference, every conviction or opinion, every doubt, is a mental phenomenon. Also to be included under this term is every emotion: joy, sorrow, fear, hope... astonishment, admiration, contempt... Examples of physical phenomena, on the other hand, are a color, a figure, a landscape, which I see, a chord which I hear... odor which I sense. (p.78ff).

There is a unique characteristic of all of the above active verbs:

Every mental phenomenon is characterized by... the intentional (or mental) inexistence of an object, and what we might call, though not wholly unambiguously, reference to a content, direction toward an object (which is not to be understood here as meaning a thing), or immanent objectivity. Every mental phenomenon includes something as object within itself, although they do not all do so in the same way. In presentation something is presented, in judgement something is affirmed or denied, in love loved, in hate hated, in desire desired and so on... The intentional in-existence is characteristic exclusively of mental phenomena. No physical phenomenon exhibits anything like it. We can, therefore, define mental phenomena by saying that they are those phenomena which contain an object intentionally within themselves. (pp.88-89).

Brentano classified intentional terms or acts into three types: (a) presentations which refer to sensations, (b) judgments, (c) affects or feelings. For Brentano intentional psychology was entirely descriptive. Explanations for the acts or what are now called representations, would come from physiology. Acts do not explain the relevant processes; they are themselves to be explained. Brentano's psychology was descriptive, concerned with discursive analysis and classifications of different kinds. He believed that explanation must wait upon physiology which can detail their genesis, how these phenomena arise (Rancurello, 1968).

In contrast, many contemporary cognitive psychologists think they are explaining a process by labeling it a representation (act). They assert that they are inferring a representation (act) which is causing the behavior in question. For example, an expectancy inferred from a subject's behavior and the instructions they received causes their excessive drinking (Marlatt et al., 1973), causes the very same behavior from which the intention was "inferred" in the first place. Brentano never used such word magic: "X drinks excessively because he or she has a positive expectancy. How do you know they have a positive expectancy? Because they drink excessively". What was true in Brentano's time is true now. Proximal causes of behavior will be uncovered by tracing the physiological changes occurring in the brain interacting dialectically with the environment. This will also lead to explanations of behavior now said to be caused by cognitions, representations, mental processes, etc. The problem with much of current cognitive psychology including cognitive behavior therapy is that its theoretical terms are derived from the very same behaviors the terms are used to explain. To make matters worse, the acts or representations are reified, hypostatized, transformed into a real thing or process causing the very behavior taken as their marker. What they really are, is bad science.

BEHAVIORISM

Watson

Three hundred years after Descartes, Watson reached a different volitional decision, one that produced a major volitional bifucation, the one true revolution in the 2,000 year history of psychology. Watson (1913) stated that the goal of behaviorism *ought to be* the study of behavior - not consciousness. "Psychology as the behaviorist views it is a purely objective experimental branch of natural science. Its theoretical goal is the prediction and control of behavior." (Watson, 1913, p. 158). Note the interesting limitation of the fundamental goal of behaviorism to the prediction and control of behavior. No mention is made of explanation. We shall return to this point in our discussion of Lashley. Behaviorism as a systematic position resting upon a volitional decision is neither true nor false. The older consciousness centered mentalistic psychology such as the structural psychology of

Wundt, Titchener and their followers was not disproven. No critical experiment was conducted demonstrating its falsity. Behaviorism rests upon a volitional decision made, and adopted, by a large number of psychologists. It determined the future direction of psychology, because it was enthusiastically adopted by a large number of the younger psychologists.

The psychology which I would attempt to build up would take as a starting point, first, the observable fact that organisms, man and animal alike, do adjust themselves to their environment by means of hereditary and habit equipments. These adjustments may be very adequate or they may be so inadequate that the organism barely maintains its existence; secondly, that certain stimuli lead the organisms to make the responses. In a system of psychology completely worked out, given the response the stimuli can be predicted; given the stimuli the response can be predicted. Such a set of statements is crass and raw in the extreme, as all such generalizations must be. (Watson, 1913, pp.166-167).

It is important to consider the use of the term "control" in the above context. Knowing the stimulus that induces a particular response to occur, we can control that response, control the behavior, by withholding or changing the stimulus. This is the basis for disease prevention. If we know the stimuli or antecedent conditions, external and internal, that predict excessive drinking behavior, we can control that behavior, prevent excessive drinking by withholding or changing the stimuli that predict the response. If the absence of stimulation provided by human contact, especially contact from the mother, leads to the response of lowered levels of beta-endorphins and other neurotransmitters and subsequent increases in alcohol consumption, then this source of increased alcohol consumption can be controlled, avoided, by ensuring human attachments in infancy. Behaviorism by the nature of its basic volition decision as to what ought to be its goals, is concerned with behaviors' antecedent conditions in the external and internal environment. Knowledge of these antecedent conditions is a prerequisite for effective disease control and prevention.

Contemporary cognitive psychology suffers in comparison because it is interested primarily in inferring mental processes such as expectancies from behavior not what environmental events caused "the expectancy" and the behavior. Contemporary cognitive psychology is primarily concerned with changing hypothetical mediating variables. Effects obtained, when they are obtained, may be due to quite different variables such as a changed physiological state rather than the hypothetical mediating expectancy variable. Treatment would be greatly enhanced if the physiological state causing the behavior were treated directly or better yet, prevented entirely, controlled. Since cognitive behavior therapists treat the individual like an empty shell, treatments at the cutting edge of behavioral neuroscience are beyond their ken.

Behaviorism's goal is to predict, control, and an essential function added by Lashley (1923), explain, the behavior in question. Theoretical concepts that refer to events that are not directly observable are legitimate, provided that they are adequately defined. Behaviorism can take advantage of all natural science knowledge, genetics, molecular biology, neurochemistry, physiology, etc., as well as objective social science knowledge, epidemiology, and the social context at the moment. There is no methodological reason for behaviorism to be limited to muscle twitches, or molar behavior, gross behavioral changes, or the products of gross behavior changes such as bar presses, or check marks on a questionnaire. We must distinguish empirical hypotheses of behaviorists from stylistic decisions and judgments about which research direction would be fruitful, and fundamental decisions concerning the goals of the science of psychology. Methodological (Watson, 1913), physiological or "molecular" (Lashley, 1923), molar (Tolman, 1925a/1951, 1932) and radical behaviorism (Skinner, 1938) are variations in behaviorism based on relatively specific decisions as to how one ought to best proceed in reaching the common goal of predicting and controlling behavior. These stylistic decisions were in large part a function of the state of scientific knowledge at the time.

Watson, Tolman and Skinner were not anti-physiological, anti-biological, or anti-genetic. Their judgment was that given the meager base of pertinent physiological information, the most fruitful approach would be to develop reliable behavioral principles. Lashley (1923), in contrast, insisted that behaviorism as an explanatory science must be based on knowledge of the central nervous system, brain science. These founders of behaviorism differed in their individual decisions as to how behavioristic experimental psychology ought best proceed. Tolman felt that a truly molar behaviorism was possible and that Watson was too much of a "muscle twitch" behaviorist, emphasizing movement rather than goal directed actions. Lashley (1923) believed Watson did not adequately appreciate the importance of the central nervous system in explaining behavior and consciousness. Explanations of behavior must ultimately come from physiological principles. In this sense and by his later research, Lashley was the father of modern behavioral neuroscience. Both Dewey (1918) and Lashley (1923) emphasized that Watson's methodological behaviorism, the decision to ignore conciousness did not go far enough. Consciousness must also be examined, and Lashley, trained as a biologist, insisted that the study of integrative brain activity was the approach behaviorism ought to take in studying consciousness. Behavioral neuroscience does not put radical behaviorism out of business. See for example, the successful combination of the two by Brady (1972) a leading Skinnerian radical behaviorist. Reliable principles ranging from operant contingencies to questionnaire results are needed as dependent measures in the examination of the relationships between neuroscience and behavior as they occur in given social and physical environments.

Decisions, which are neither true nor false, must be distinguished from hypotheses with empirical content, assertions that are in principle falsifiable. Watson, who made the revolutionary decision to change the goal of psychology from the study of immediate experience, for practical purposes the average normal adult human mind, to the study of behavior, also formulated a number of empirical hypotheses. Any one or all of them could be rejected, falsified, or accepted, confirmed, and one would still remain a behaviorist. These or any other falsifiable hypotheses do not characterize behaviorism per se. They characterize Watson the theorist. He held a frequency theory of learning, a motor theory of thinking, a particular theory of emotions, and generally, nurture rather than nature as the major determiner of behavior. The truth status of these hypotheses is irrelevant to the volitional decision concerning the basic goals that distinguishes behaviorism from all prior psychologies. One can adopt a drive reduction theory of learning, a drive induction, or a contiguity theory, etc., and still remain a behaviorist. Neither a particular theory of learning nor a position on the question of nature versus nurture constitutes a criterion for being classified a behaviorist. These are not "postulates" of behaviorism. Behaviorism is not anti-heredity, an empirical problem. It is not anti-physiological. Early behaviorists with one exception, Lashley, did not adopt physiological methods and theory because at the time physiology had little to offer in the way of attaining the goals of behaviorism, prediction, control, and the explanation of behavior.

Tolman (1935/51), the first cognitive behaviorist, included heredity among the intervening variables he assumed determine behavior:

behaviorism... may take either of two courses. On the one hand, it may seek to develop a set of what may be called molecular or microscopic concepts. These are essentially physiological. This form of behaviorism attempts a complete neural, glandular and visceral picture... there is also... a second type of behaviorism which seeks rather to develop a set of molar or macroscopic concepts concerning what I shall designate as 'behavior readinesses.' This second form of behaviorism seeks to describe and explain behavior in terms of such 'readiness variables.' And these latter it fashions directly from the more surface facts of behavior itself. This molar form of behaviorism does not deny the possibility and need of neural and glandular concepts but it prefers to leave the latter to the adequately trained physiologist... Both types of behaviorism begin by listing four independent or causal variables, as follows: (1) the environmental stimulus set-up... (2) the specific heredity of the given organism... (3) the specific past training of the organism...(4) a releasing internal condition of physiological appetite or aversion. (pp.101-102).

Tolman (1925b/1951) also recognized that, "physiological concepts will ultimately prove the more comprehensive and accurate." (p. 47). He showed that there is no fundamental contradiction between behaviorism and cognitive psychology, as long as one properly defines the theoretical terms employed:

orthodox psychology maintains that... mind exhibits 'purpose,' whereas body does not. Purpose is held to be essentially a mentalistic category... it will be the thesis of the present paper that a behaviorism... finds it just as easy and just as necessary to include the descriptive phenomena of 'purpose' as does a mentalism. Purpose, adequately conceived... is itself but an objective aspect of behavior. When an animal is learning a maze, or escaping from a puzzle box, or merely going about his daily business of eating, nest building, sleeping, and the like, it will be noted that in all such performances a certain *persistence until* character is to be found. Now it is just this *persistence until* character which we will define as purpose... upon further analysis, we discover that such a description appears whenever in order merely to *identify* the given behavior a reference to some 'end object' or 'situation' is found necessary. (Tolman, 1925a/1951, pp. 32-33).

Tolman discusses the relationship of cognitive, intentional, concepts to physiology, noting:

Eventually we will undoubtedly have to reduce and explain our more immediate categories of goal seeking and object adjustment in terms of physiological categories. But the date at which this last will be possible is far distant... the above discussion, in spite of its use of the terms *purpose* and *cognition,* is *behavioristic.* For in no place in using these concepts have we defined them 'mentalistically'. We have not in some mysterious fashion 'looked within' and so discovered them. Rather have we looked without at the rat in the maze and merely proceeded to describe the behavior which we saw. And the animal's cognitions (object adjustments) and his purposes (goal seekings) as we have observed them have been described and defined in purely objective terms. (1925b/1951, p. 47).

At the time Watson formulated his position and for almost half a century more the volitional decision to ignore consciousness or to redefine it in terms of behavioral dispositions (Ryle, 1949) seemed a reasonable one, since there was little evidence available to the behaviorist other than overt behavior. Physiology had not advanced to a stage where it could be helpful in the areas of primary interest to the new behavioristic psychology, learning and motivation.

A few behaviorist psychologists and philosophers refused to halt at the barrier created by the volitional decision to limit behaviorism to the prediction and control of molar behavior. Just as Watson's interest in animal problems and the methods of dealing with them could not be limited by fiat, there were behaviorists who would not be limited by the confines imposed by Watson's volitional decision to ignore consciousness and brain science. One of these was a former volunteer assistant of Watson's at Johns Hopkins University, Karl Lashley (1923) who initiated "molecular" as distinguished from "molar" behavorism. The other dissident behaviorist was a philosopher considered a founder of the Chicago school of functional psychology (Boring, 1950) who self-consciously (that is a pun!) considered himself a behaviorist. We will first note Dewey's criticisms of Watson and then turn to Lashley's more extensive arguments opposing Watson's volitional decision limiting behaviorism to methodological behaviorism.

Dewey

Dewey (1918) was one of the first calling for an addition to Watson's "postulates" of behaviorism: do not exclude any realm of investigation from study. Dewey addressed his criticism of Watson within a broader context concerned with the unfortunate influences of the traditional conception of consciousness in philosophy and psychology and the assumption of a unique method, introspection, providing privileged access to inner states of consciousness. He argued that the naive use of consciousness as a tool by the physicist and lay observe alike must be studied from a behavioristic point of view. Dewey (1918) asserts:

there is no more reason for supposing that personal events have a nature or meaning which is one with their happening, and hence open to immediate infallible inspection, than is the case with impersonal events. In each case the event only sets a problem to knowledge, namely, the discovery of its connections. Secondly, it is desirable and possible that we should observe and understand observation and understanding and allied phenomena themselves. Such a study would be a study of 'consciousness' in the naive sense mentioned. Thirdly, such a study, with a recognition of 'consciousness' in this sense, is quite compatible with a behavioristic standpoint, whether or no the technique exists at a given time for its successful accomplishment. (p. 35).

Lashley

In a two-part article entitled, "The behavioristic interpretation of consciousness", Lashley (1923), like Dewey, rejects Watson's formulation of methodological behaviorism as not going far enough. It is not enough to simply ignore consciousness as recommended by Watson or to redefine it, as in Tolman's variation of methodological behaviorism.

Methodological behaviorism has serious disadvantages and Dewey (1918) has already called attention to one of them. According to Lashley, methodological behaviorism:

puts the behaviorist in the position of the dog in the manger... Simply because he can make nothing of the facts of consciousness (which he admits are facts) in his system of physical causation, the methodological behaviorist refuses to believe that any other system can be devised which will permit the development of a science of pure psychics. And so long as he admits the existence of a universe of consciousness he lays open to attack his major premise, that behaviorism can account for all human activities. For the psychophysical dualist is constantly finding mental facts which he holds to be inexplicable in any mechanistic terms and by refusing to discuss such data the behaviorist prohibits himself from answering arguments based upon them. Moreover, so long as he admits the existence of entities in human existence which behaviorism disregards, he can not deny to others the right to try to study those entities and reduce them to a science by any means whatever. (pp. 239-240).

Lashley's (1923) principal argument is as follows:

if behaviorism is to become a complete science, if it is to avoid becoming merely a coordinate system with subjectivism, it must subordinate questions of method, of objectivity, to the application of mechanistic or physiological principles to the whole of psychology. This point is emphasized by Dewey... to whom the facts of consciousness appear as an experimental behavioristic problem...

Let me cast off the lion's skin. My quarrel with behaviorism is not that it has gone too far, but that it has hesitated, that it has been diverted by details of experimental method, when more fundamental issues are at stake; that it has failed to develop its premises to their logical conclusion. To me the essence of behaviorism is the belief that the study of man will reveal nothing except what is adequately describable in the concepts of mechanics and chemistry, and this far outweighs the question of the method by which the study is conducted. I believe that it is possible to construct a physiological psychology which will meet the dualist on his own ground, will accept the data which he advances and show that those data can be embodied in a mechanistic system. A behaviorism will thus develop which will be an adequate substitute for the older psychology. Its physiological account of behavior will also be a complete and adequate account of all the phenomena of consciousness. It will be methodological only in insisting that the concepts of the physical sciences are the only ones which can serve as the basis for a science, and in demanding that all psychological data, however obtained, shall be subjected to physical or physiological interpretation....

The key to the development of behaviorism lies here. When the behaviorist denies that consciousness exists, he denies, not the existence of the phenomena upon which the conception is based, but only the inference that these data constitute a unique mode of existence or that they are not amenable to analysis and description of the same sort as are 'physical' data. Unfortunately, the psychological terminology current today involves not only an enumeration of phenomena but also a definite theory of reality. It is this theory which behaviorism repudiates. (pp. 244-245).

Lashley turns to more general implications of the volitional decision to consider behaviorism a branch of natural science:

The acceptance of the postulates of physical science, whether we regard them as the attributes of a real objective world or merely as explanatory hypotheses, brings with it an avalanche of consequences which has not always been foreseen or enjoyed by the unwary adventurer in science. Once they are accepted, we cannot arbitrarily set a limit to their application and reserve a favored corner of our experience for consideration in other ways. Only empirical evidence of such limits can justify the claim to their existence. I have attempted to show that the so-called phenomena of consciousness do not constitute such a limit. Physical postulates are as fully applicable to mind as to the material world and there are no subjectively definable attributes of mind which distinguish it from other physical processes. The acceptance of a physical world seems to me therefore to involve as a corollary a behavioristic psychology. (pp.343-344).

Finally, after a brilliant analysis of a series of issues still plaguing psychology, philosophy of science, and philosophy of mind, Lashley turns to the behaviorist's program. He initiates his discussion by a description of a current textbook in psychology:

The behaviorist is interested to discover the wells of human action: how does the individual meet the complex situations in which he finds himself, how solve his problems, how acquire social conventions, whence come his interests, prejudices, ambitions, what is the source of his genius or commonplaceness? These are not the problems of the introspectionist... Only a vision grown myopic by long introversion could behold sensory physiology as twelve times more important than [relative amounts of space in a current textbook] all the problems of human personality combined.

It is by this demand for change of emphasis in psychology that behaviorism has broken most completely from the traditions of the older psychology, which is willing to leave the problems of every-day life to the 'applied sciences' of sociology, education, and psychiatry. The behaviorist holds that the greater part of introspective psychology is only a poorly devised physiology of the sense-organs and that its minor importance as such should be generally recognized. He would make of psychology a true science of human conduct.

By what means? From physiology we inherit reflexes, conditioned reflexes, and glands; from animal psychology, habit, trial and error, and instinct; from psychiatry, emotional complexes and conflicts; from subjective psychology, a horrible example. With this meager equipment we must begin our task. The task is first to define more clearly the behavior, to analyze the behavior components in specific human activities; second, to state these in terms of the physiological mechanisms involved. Without physiology behaviorism can make but little progress, for its explanatory principles are physiological and no sharp line can be drawn between the two sciences. For the present, if we are to deal with complex human activities, we must be content with the pseudo-explanations offered by such conceptions as 'set,' 'habit,' 'gestural reaction,' 'drive,' 'conflict,' 'dominant stimulus,' and the like, but our task is not completed until we can show something more definite than these as the foundation of the science. (pp. 348-349).

Skinner

Skinner's variation of behaviorism developed in somewhat different form but with the same thrust as Dewey and Lashley: leave no area of behavior unexplored. It is a radical behaviorism, differing from Watson's methodological behaviorism in that it pursued Dewey's instrumentalism by providing a functional analysis of behavior and by examining how the verbal behavior of the individual may come under the control of singular events via reinforcement from the community. Skinner's radical behaviorism differs from methodological behaviorism by proposing an experimental philosophy of mind through the analysis of verbal behavior.

Radical behaviorism... takes a different line [from methodological behaviorism]. It does not deny the possibility of self-observation or self-knowledge or its possible usefulness, but it questions the nature of what is felt or observed and hence known. It restores introspection but not what philosophers and introspective psychologists had believed they were 'specting,' and it raises the question of how much of one's body one can actually observe... It does not insist upon truth by agreement and can therefore consider events taking place in the private world within the skin. It does not call these events unobservable, and it does not dismiss them as subjective. It simply questions the nature of the object observed and the reliability of the observations... what is felt or introspectively observed is not some nonphysical world of consciousness, mind, or mental life but the observer's own body. This does not mean, as I shall show later, that introspection is a kind of physiological research, nor does it mean (and this is the heart of the argument) that what are felt or introspectively observed are the causes of behavior. An organism behaves as it does because of its current structure, but most of this is out of reach of introspection. At the moment we must content ourselves, as the methodological behaviorist insists, with a person's genetic and environmental histories. What are introspectively observed are certain collateral products of those histories. (Skinner, 1976, pp.18-19).

There is a common misunderstanding among people who call themselves behaviorists, behavior therapists, or behavioralists, that Skinner was anti-physiological. To be a real behaviorist means that one must assume that behavior is primarily learned and that one must eschew physiological processes. Skinner did not study physiological processes. Neither did Tolman, Hull, Guthrie, and other molar behaviorists because at the time they came into prominence, the 1920s and

1930s, physiology had little to offer the behaviorist whose primary interest was in learning and motivation. Skinner's position concerning physiology and behaviorism is indicated in the following remarks:

New instruments and methods will continue to be devised, and we shall eventually know much more about the *kinds* of physiological processes, chemical or electrical, which take place when a person behaves. The physiologist of the future will tell us all that can be known about what is happening inside the behaving organism. His account will be an important advance over a behavioral analysis, because the latter is necessarily 'historical'- that is to say, it is confined to functional relations showing temporal gaps. Something is done today which affects the behavior of an organism tomorrow. No matter how clearly that fact can be established, a step is missing, and we must wait for the physiologist to supply it. He will be able to show how an organism is changed when exposed to contingencies of reinforcement and why the changed organism then behaves in a different way, possibly at a much later date. What he discovers cannot invalidate the laws of a science of behavior, but it will make the picture of human action more nearly complete. (Skinner, 1976, pp. 236-237).

Two decades after this passage was written, Skinner's predictions are being confirmed by neuroimaging, single cell recording, in vivo microdialysis, radioimmunoassays, and other methods of behavioral neuroscience. They illustrate what distinguishes leaders of a movement from followers. The former are creative, questioning, and farsighted. Followers, foot soldiers, are none of these. That is why they are followers.

There is no conflict between physiology and behaviorism or heredity and behaviorism. The success of behavorial neuroscience depends as much upon securing reliable behavioral laws as it does reliable neurochemical principles. On the other hand, Skinner fails to consider that in real life very often the environmental contingencies that contributed to a person's developing a dependency upon alcohol or other drugs cannot be reconstructed in detail. The state of their nervous system can be examined. From the present state it may be possible to predict the behavior, relapse or recovery as a function of behavioral treatment and pharmacotherapy, to the extent that there is control or the ability to predict the environment in which the individual is located. As in physics, it may be possible to postdict from the present abnormal state of the nervous system what happened in the past to bring about the present state (Bracha, Torrey, Gottesman, Bigelow, & Cunniff, 1992; Suddath, Christison, Torrey, Casanova, & Weinberger, 1990). Neuroimaging studies of the brains of identical twins discordant for schizophrenia have shown that there are significant differences in brain morphology absent in identical twins without schizophrenia. Differences in fingerprints of identical twins discordant for schizophrenia indicate that prenatal insult occurred during the second trimester. Growing evidence suggests that such insults may stem from a viral infection such as influenza (Barr, Mednick, & Munk-Jorgensen, 1990). Evidence also indicates that prenatal famine may be another nongenetic biological risk factor for schizophrenia (Susser et al., 1996). An obvious implication, one in need of detailed study is that alcoholism, another noninfectious chronic disease may be a consequence of similar prenatal risk factors as well as others, particularly low levels of prenatal alcohol exposure (Baer, Barr, Bookstein, Sampson, & Streissguth, 1998; Griesler & Kandel, 1998).

Another misconception concerning Skinner and behaviorism in general is the insistence by behavior therapists such as those cited earlier, that behaviorism deemphasizes or does not recognize the influence of genetics. Skinner's (1976) comments on "nature and nurture" are revealing:

It is hard to understand why it is so often said that behaviorism neglects innate endowment. Watson's careless remark that he could take any healthy infant and convert him into a doctor, lawyer, artist, merchant chief, and, yes, even beggarman or thief can scarcely be responsible, because Watson himself repeatedly referred to the 'hereditary and habit equipment' of people...

Social and political issues have probably played a greater role than has been apparent, and some have recently come into the open... But the roles of heredity and environment are to be discovered through observation, not assigned in conformity with political beliefs. Species differ in the speeds with which they can be conditioned and in the nature and size of the repertoires they can maintain, and it is probably that people show similar inherited differences. Nevertheless, the topography or form of behavior is only rarely affected. To say that intelligence or some other ability or trait is twenty percent a matter of the environment and eighty percent a matter of genetics is not to say that twenty percent of a person's behavior is due to contingencies of reinforcement and eighty percent to genetic endowment. Raise one identical twin in China and the other in France and their verbal behavior will be completely different. (pp. 243-244).

One accepts the evidence that there is a genetic component in some forms of schizophrenia or not, and remains a behaviorist. One can accept the evidence that there is a genetic component accounting for some of the variance in alcoholism, as I do, or not, and remain a behaviorist. In the latter case, I believe, it is a mistaken behaviorist, but still a behaviorist. Behaviorism as a philosophy of psychology based on a set of fundamental value judgments does not require that alcoholism be learned or must be a genetically determined disease, whatever the meaning placed upon such vague and ambiguous positions. Value judgments concerning the basic goals of their science distinguish behaviorism from all other schools of psychology, not falsifiable hypotheses. Revisionist behavior therapists fail to distinguish between the essential volitional bifurcation forming behaviorism and a falsifiable hypothesis held by Watson who held it at a time when very little was known about herredity in relation to behavior.

What is evident in reading the founders of behaviorism, including Watson, is their critical approach to problems, their skepticism, and concern for evidence. Watson (1930) in his most current textbook, reviews in detail research on heredity and emphasizes that the possible influence of early learning was neglected, showing that cases of identical twins reared apart manifest marked differences in intelligence test performance and achievement in keeping with their different experiences. He is not opposed to the influence of heredity per se, he is opposed to overgeneralizing from an inadequate data base. He also was obviously unaware of evidence which is now extensive, of the continuous dialectical relationship between environmental influences and brain development. Biology and environment are in continuous interaction and development of the brain is dependent upon such environmental interactions (Gottlieb, 1997, 1998; Schore, 1996). Reading Watson (1930), Tolman (1925a, 1925b,1935/1951) or Skinner (1976) should convince one that none of these founders of behaviorism would conclude that the behaviorist position on alcoholism is that it is learned no more than the behaviorist position is that learning is the result of drive reduction. There is no behaviorist position on such issues because they are empirical matters to be resolved by research. The behaviorist position, like that of any good scientist, is to be critical of the evidential basis for generalizations and at the same time open to generalizations counter to one's own hypotheses.

Why behavior therapists misunderstand behaviorism

Insistence that behaviorism demands that alcoholism is learned reveals a lack of understanding of the nature of behaviorism and a failure to study the founders of behaviorism. Aside from the lack of scholarship the motivation underlying behavior therapists' denial that alcoholism is a disease entity with a physiological basis is obvious. They reason, incorrectly, that if alcoholism is learned it is in the domain of the psychologist whereas if alcoholism is a disease it is in the treatment domain of the MD. It is a battle over turf reflecting a naive view that fails to adequately recognize the nature of diseases, all diseases, as biopsychosocial conditions (Glaser & Kiecolt-Glaser, 1994; Maier & Watkins, 1998; Maier, Watkins, & Fleshner, 1994).

Conclusion

Observable clinical signs and symptoms of a disease are accompanied by pathophysiological processes. These latter must be examined along with the behavioral signs and symptoms which are obvious to the eye. Studies of the phases of alcoholism must go beyond verbal response data, self-reports and the results of structured interviews. Measures of concomitant changes in physiological processes and anatomy must be obtained. Laboratory tests and magnetic resonance imaging (MRI) and other forms of neuroimaging including multiple lead event related potentials (ERPs) need to be repeatedly administered. These measures must be obtained repeatedly to map the progression in the pathophysiological and morphological changes accompanying the changes in overt behavioral signs and symptoms. They are all part of the disease syndrome of alcoholism, the disease entity.

A more adequate understanding of the disease and its variable course in different people would accrue, understanding which could facilitate treatment, the course of recovery, relapse prevention, prognosis, and possibly prevention. Progress in the explanation, treatment and prevention of alcoholism would be accelerated if it were treated as any other disease. This would be research in the historically behavioristic manner foreseen by Lashley and by Skinner, not the pseudo-behaviorism of behavior therapists' search for "expectancies" as a "cause" of excessive drinking. Can you imagine the diagnosis, assessment, and treatment, of cancer, cardiovascular disease, or AIDs limited to the verbal report of the patient? Of course not. Neither should the diagnosis assessment, and treatment of alcoholism be limited in such a manner.

about the hypothesis that the dopaminergic system is the final common path for all drug reinforcement and that is its unique function. Research suggests that all neurotransmitter systems constituting the reticular-thalamic-cortical activating system underlying the OR are reinforcing to varying degree (Beluzzi & Stein, 1977; Hubbell et al., 1991).

Contrary to the assumption that dopamine is the final common path of reinforcement for all drugs, it is more likely that dopamine is part of the initial orienting elicited by drugs as well as other biologically significant stimuli, aversive as well as positively rewarding, and novelty. Dopamine is activated by innocuous novel stimuli, stimulus change, as well as innately rewarding biologically significant stimuli and stimuli signaling their presence (Horvitz, Stewart, & Jacobs, 1997; Mirenowicz & Schultz, 1994).

Dopaminergic neurons show the same basic characteristics of the OR as peripheral SCR measures to novelty, stimulus change, and to stimuli that have acquired significance or that are innately biologically significant (Maltzman, Weissbluth, & Wolff, 1978; Maltzman, Gould, Barnett, Raskin, & Wolff, 1977; Pendery & Maltzman, 1977). Other research indicates that dopaminergic neurons in the nucleus accumbens make a unique contribution to orienting-exploratory behavior. Injection of dopamine directly into the nucleus accumbens of rats produces exploratory behavior. Injections of norepinephrine, saline, or serotonin into the nucleus accumbens do not produce such an effect. In contrast, dopamine injected into the caudate nucleus produces stereotypical behavior (Makanjuola, Dow, & Ashcroft, 1980).

Dopamine has an important role in the development of alcoholism and the misuse of other drugs because it is a component of the OR, the initial organismic response to stimulus change, novelty, and biologically significant stimul that the organism would ordinarily approach or avoid. Dopamine contributes to sensitization and selective orienting to alcohol, the "salience" of alcohol and related cues (Robinson, & Berridge, 1993). In addition to stimulation from dopamine which occurs with the OR to innocuous novel stimuli, a more powerful reinforcement occurs with positive and negative biologically significant stimuli, including alcohol. Biologically significant stimuli in addition to stimulating the amygdala also activate the HPA axis resulting in the release of beta-endorphins and glucocorticoids such as cortisol. Most people who consume alcohol remain at a moderate level of consumption. An occasional drink with friends before a meal, some wine with dinner, a beer watching Monday night football, etc. That's it. For some 10% of the population in the United States that drink alcohol it is a different story. Alcohol consumption increases with the frequency of drinking occasions. A number of adaptive and, basically, maladaptive physiological changes occur. Tolerance to the positive reinforcing effects as well as the negative consequences of alcohol develop. An individual finds that they have to drink increasing amounts to get high (Kalant, 1996).

Increasingly large amounts of alcohol circulating in the bloodstream become an increasingly powerful and chronic stressor releasing larger amounts of cortisol. The heavy drinker is in an internal state of chronic stress in the operational sense of increased activation of the HPA axis. The blood alcohol level decreases during the night. They wake up with the cold sweats, tremulous and scared, mild withdrawal symptoms. A drink or two in the morning straightens things out - except for one problem. The minor withdrawal they went through is not really minor. It causes further brain damage. Such damage is not indiscriminately dispersed throughout the brain. It is concentrated in certain areas, those concerned with working memory, problem solving, and planning, the so-called executive functions of the brain concentrated in the prefrontral cortex (Giancola & Moss, 1998; Kril, Halliday, Svobvoda, & Cartwright, 1997; Lhermitte, 1986; Luria, 1980) as well as damage to the neurons of the hippocampus and cerebellum.

Two processes are simultaneously occurring. Both contribute to the development of the pathognomic sign of alcoholism, loss of control over alcohol consumption. One is sensitization of neural pathways in the amygdala and elsewhere and the establishment of a sensitized dominant focus concentrated on consumption of alcohol. The other on-going process is brain damage.

JANUS I. ALCOHOL AS A POSITIVE REINFORCER

Once alcohol is consumed, a new variable comes into play, reinforcement, the verbally expressed "high" (Tiihonen et al., 1994). An obvious source of the "high" is the release of beta-endorphins, but is beta-endorphin a behavioral reinforcer? Does the release of beta-endorphins increase the probability of occurrence of behavior?

This critical question was answered in experiments by Belluzzi and Stein (1977) using the intracranial self-stimulation (ICSS) technique. They demonstrated that endorphins injected into brain ventricles each time a lever in a Skinner box was pressed produced a slightly higher rate of lever pressing than morphine and a significantly higher rate than placebo injections. In another study a group of rats received electrical brain stimulation in the central grey area each time they pressed a lever until they reached a steady high rate of lever pressing. Injections of naloxone produced a dose related decrease in self-stimulation, indicating that reinforcement had been provided by endorphins. Since the central grey area is also rich in norepinephrine-producing neurons, an antagonist of norepinephrine was administered to rats following attainment of a steady rate of lever pressing to brain stimulation. A decrease in response rate again occurred, suggesting that self-stimulation of the central gray area stimulates norepinephrine as well as endorphin-containing neurons providing positive reinforcement. Since the areas stimulated are also rich in dopamine neurons, all three may be involved in reinforcement, suggesting that reinforcement involves the interaction of endorphins, dopamine and norepinephrine, among other neurotransmitters (Belluzzi & Stein, 1977).

A series of 10 experiments by Hubbell et al. (1991) using consumption of a sweetened alcohol-water solution versus water as dependent variables, clarified some of the questions concerning the source(s) of reinforcement for alcohol consumption. Rats deprived of water and provided with a sweetened alcohol cocktail were exposed to varying dosages of antagonists and in some cases agonists of endorphins, serotonin, and dopamine. Effectiveness of the agonists and antagonists in different dosages was also determined by their impact on ICSS. Results indicated that of the three neurotransmitters studied, the greatest reinforcement from alcohol consumption was opioidergic as shown by the extent to which an opiate antagonist reduced consumption of a sweetened alcohol cocktail as compared to water consumption. A serotonin uptake inhibitor which increased the level of circulating serotonin also decreased consumption of a sweetened alcohol solution. Manipulations of dopamine on the other hand had relatively slight effects, indicating that dopamine is not the final common path for reinforcement from alcohol consumption. Alcohol consumption appears to be reinforced primarily by release of beta-endorphins. Dopamine has a critical role in the development of alcoholism, the acquisition of alcohol seeking or wanting (Robinson & Berridge, 1993). It is not the primary source of reinforcement maintaining excessive alcohol consumption. Dopamine is primarily a "forcer" rather than a "reinforcer" of alcohol consumption. Dopamine affects orienting to alcohol and related cues whereas beta-endorphins primarily reinforce consummatory behavior and the behavior instrumental in attaining the reinforcement.

Although a major source of reinforcement, beta-endorphins are not necessary as mediators of alcohol reinforcement. Other neurotransmitters including norephinephrine and possibly other endorphins also may reinforce alcohol consumption. Beta-endorphin deficient mice acquire a differential operant response for alcohol when completely lacking this endogenous opioid (Grahame, Low, & Cunnigham, 1998).

Norepinephrine and dopamine as reinforcers of alcohol consumption were studied by allowing rats to lever-press for intragastric doses of alcohol following establishment of a base-line of responding and then extinguishing the response with saline substituted for alcohol as a reinforcer. Reacquisition of lever-pressing for alcohol was preceded by administration of saline as a control solution for antagonists of norephinephrine and dopamine. Results indicated that blocking the dopaminergic system did not prevent reacquisition of bar-pressing. Blocking the noradrenergic system reduced bar-pressing significantly. Norepinephrine therefore appears to be a more important source of reinforcement for alcohol consumption then dopamine. Activation of the dopaminergic system is important as a "forcer" rather than a reinforcer of instrumental behavior (Davis, Smith, & Werner, 1978) because it is a sensitizer of perception (Robinson & Berridge, 1993) and learning as part of the OR to alcohol and other biologically significant events as well as innocuous stimulus change and novelty.

Further support for the hypothesis that dopamine plays its role as a "forcer", directing attention and instrumental behavior differentially to alcohol and other significant stimuli, rather than a reinforcer maintaining the instrumental goal directed behavior, stems from research by Ikemoto, McBride, Murphy, Lumeng, & Li (1997). Two groups of experimental animals from an alcohol-preferring line of rats were employed in the study. One received a chemical lesion designed to decrease dopamine innervation to the nucleus accumbens. A second group received a sham lesion. Half the animals in the two groups were alcohol naive and half had previous experience consuming alcohol. Testing for the acquisition of alcohol choice behavior occurred in the individual home cages where animals were provided a choice between a 10% solution of alcohol with water versus tap water. Animals were offered a choice of an alcohol cocktail or water for the first time following recovery from surgery. Acquisition of alcohol drinking behavior was significantly retarded in the lesioned animals lacking dopamine. Alcohol consumption in the lesioned experimental animals was 60% lower than the controls

AUGUSTANA UNIVERSITY COLLEGE
LIBRARY

after one week and 30% lower after three weeks. There was no difference in alcohol consummatory behavior in the two groups of animals when lesioned after they had learned to consume alcohol despite the fact that dopamine levels in the nucleus accumbens was 60% lower in the experimental than control animals.

Results by Ikemoto et al. (1997) demonstrate that dopamine is an important component of the physiological processes facilitating acquisition of alcohol consummatory behavior but not the maintenance of that differential behavior once acquired. Further evidence that dopamine does not play a critical role in reinforcing alcohol consumption has been obtained by analyzing the behavior of strains of alcohol preferring and alcohol avoiding rats. Kiianmaa, Nurmi, Nykänen, and Sinclair (1995) found that an intraperitoneal injection of alcohol increased extracellular levels of dopamine equally in alcohol preferring and avoiding rats, suggesting that differences in levels of dopamine are not the critical variable determining the differences in alcohol preference between the two strains of animals.

Blum, Futterman, Wallace, & Schwertner (1977) were among the first obtaining evidence for the role of endorphins in the development of alcohol dependence by demonstrating that naloxone blocked the occurrence of alcohol withdrawal symptoms in animals. Blum et al. (1977) demonstrated a commonality between alcohol and morphine and support for the hypothesis that a common biological mechanism is shared by opiates and alcohol (Blum, 1991; Myers, 1990; Myers & Melchior, 1977).

Human studies

Additional early indirect evidence suggesting that alcohol stimulates the release of endorphins is the finding that alcohol has an analgesic effect in alcoholics and people at risk for alcoholism whereas alcohol does not produce an analgesic effect in nonalcoholics (Cutter & O'Farrell, 1987; Brown & Cutter, 1977; Cutter, 1986; Cutter, Jones, Maloof, & Kurtz, 1979; Cutter, Maloof, Kurtz, & Jones; 1976).

Gianoulakis and her colleagues (Gianoulakis, Krishnan, & Thavundayil, 1996; Gianoulakis et al., 1989) have demonstrated that alcohol increases plasma levels of beta-endorphins in humans. In addition, Gianoulakis' research demonstrates that individuals with positive or negative family histories of alcoholism differ in their basal levels of circulating endorphins and their reaction to alcohol. In an initial study Gianoulakis et al. (1989) compared the responses of the HPA axis to a placebo and a moderate dose of alcohol. Cortisol released by the adrenal cortex and beta-endorphin released by the pituitary gland were selected for study.

Three groups of participants were employed, a high risk group of men and women who had a three generation history of alcoholism in their family (FH+) and a low risk group with no history of alcoholism in their family for three generations (FH-). A third group consisted of alcoholics who had been abstinent for six months and had a strong positive family history (FH+). All members of the first two groups were social drinkers as diagnosed by the Michigan Alcoholism Screening Test (MAST) and the DSM-III. Participants were required to remain abstinent for 48 hours prior to each of two testing situations. In one session they received a moderate dose of alcohol mixed in orange juice and in the other an orange juice and tonic placebo. Abstinent alcoholics participated only in the placebo test. To control for the circadian rhythm of hormones all subjects started the experiments at 8:00 AM with a light breakfast. Testing began at 9:00 AM with drawing of a blood sample followed by ingestion of alcohol or placebo. Additional blood samples were taken at 15, 45, and 120 minutes after administration of the drink.

Results showed that the FH+ group of social drinkers had significantly lower plasma endorphin levels than the FH- group for all 120 minutes following consumption of the placebo. Cortisol levels did not differ significantly among the three groups. Following alcohol consumption quite different results were observed. An initial increase in plasma endorphins occurred in the FH+ group followed by a gradual decline. In contrast there was a monotonic decline in endorphin levels for the FH- group but at a slower rate than in response to placebo. A comparison of the two groups shows that although the FH+ group had a much lower resting level of plasma endorphins prior to consumption of alcohol, following consumption their increase in endorphins approximated the level of the FH- group. Alcohol had no effect on the plasma cortisol level of the FH- group. In the FH+ group the plasma cortisol level showed approximately a 20% increase 15 minutes after alcohol consumption returning to baseline by 120 minutes.

These results suggest that FH+ people at risk for alcoholism have lower basal levels of plasma endorphins than FH- participants. Alcohol produces a greater increase in endorphins in FH+ than in FH- people suggesting that alcohol may be more reinforcing for the FH+ group and temporarily compensates for their lower resting level of beta- endorphins. Blood alcohol concentrations did not differ for the FH+ and FH- groups.

Gianoulakis et al. (1996) conducted a second study this time varying the alcohol dose on different test days. High and low risk participants had either two generations of alcoholic relatives (FH+) or two generations free of alcoholic relatives (FH-), respectively. None of the participants were diagnosed as alcoholic. Ten women and 10 men participated in each of the two groups. Each subject received one placebo session and three alcohol test sessions in different prearranged orders. Amount of alcohol in each of four different sessions was 0, 1, 2, and 3, drinks, respectively. As in the previous study, participants arrived in the laboratory at 8:00 AM. A catheter was placed in their arm to draw blood; at 8:30 they received a light breakfast; at 9:00 AM a blood sample was drawn and the participant received either a placebo or one of the alcohol drinks. Blood samples were drawn after 15, 45, 120, and 180 minutes. Blood alcohol concentrations did not differ as a function of risk status or gender. Statistical analyses indicated no difference between genders in either cortisol levels or plasma endorphins. Gender was therefore combined within each risk group.

Analyses of plasma endorphins following the placebo indicated no overall differences between the two groups but a significant risk x time interaction reflecting a slight increase in endorphins for the high risk group and an increase then decrease in the low risk group. The two groups did not differ significantly. There was no main effect for groups, but their trends differed over time. Levels of endorphins following alcohol consumption were a different matter. In all three test sessions the level of endorphins was lower in the FH+ than FH- group before alcohol was consumed. In all three test sessions an abrupt increase in endorphin level occurred between the pre-alcohol level and post-drink endorphin level. Endorphin levels increased systematically with increases in alcohol dose for the FH+ but not the FH- subjects. Under all three alcohol conditions high risk subjects showed a significant increase in their endorphin levels over time and an interaction with amount of alcohol. Following the low dose the trend for the FH- low risk group was essentially a horizontal straight line whereas the FH+ high risk group showed an increase in endorphin level which then remained constant. Following the large alcohol dose the endorphin level of the FH+ group was significantly higher than the FH- group. An analysis of the relationship between endorphin and blood alcohol levels indicated a significant correlation of 0.91 in the FH+ group and a nonsignificant correlation of 0.26 in the FH- group. Significant results were obtained reflecting a dose response curve selectively occurring in high risk participants. Alcohol consumption did not significantly affect plasma cortisol levels, a result not in keeping with the effect obtained in the prior study. It is possible that greater control over situational stress in the present study was responsible for the lack of cortisol reactivity or the within-subject design permitted habituation to the stress as a result of the repeated testing situations. If so, there should be a session effect, cortisol level decreasing as a function of the number of preceding sessions. Such an effect was not assessed.

Gianoulakis and her colleagues acknowledge the need to systematically vary starting time of experiments to examine the possible effects of circadian rhythms. It is possible that the lower initial plasma endorphin levels consistently found in FH+ groups and their greater increase following alcohol consumption may reflect different circadian rhythms in the two groups. It can be argued in rebuttal to the circadian rhythm hypothesis that the pain tolerance study by Cutter and Farrell (1987) was conducted in the afternoon yet they found evidence of greater endorphin response in FH+ than FH- subjects. Admittedly, the assessment of endorphin increases was indirect, using an opiate antagonist, and risk was assessed in a different manner. The combined outcomes of Cutter and Farrell and Gianoulakis and her colleagues suggest that a robust phenomenon is at work that is more than an expression of different circadian rhythms found in high and low risk people.

An additional necessary assumption of the endorphin compensation hypothesis is that the endorphin levels circulating in the blood are correlated with levels of endorphins circulating in the central nervous system directly affecting the brain. Evidence suggests that endorphins in the brain can cross the blood brain barrier and that alcohol increases the permeability of the blood brain barrier facilitating such crossings (Banks & Kastin, 1993).

Additional evidence that a family history of alcoholism is related to hypothalamic opioidergic activity is provided by Wand, Mangold, El Deiry, McCaul, & Hoover (1998). They found significant differences between FH+ and FH- participants in their response to low doses of nalaxone. Both groups showed greater cortisol responses to high doses of naloxone than to low doses and to a placebo. However, FH+ participants showed greater sensitivity to naloxone reaching their maximal cortisol response at a lower level than FH- participants.

Research by Gianoulakis and her colleagues suggests that individuals with a family history of alcoholism may be at risk because alcohol may have greater reinforcement value for them than individuals without such a history. A disproportionately greater positive reinforcement effect is obtained with consumption of relatively large amounts of alcohol.

JANUS II: BRAIN DYSFUNCTION

Animal models

Brain atrophy may occur in moderate drinkers long before they reach the criteria for diagnosis as an alcoholic or alcohol abuser (Cala, 1987). Brain damage is not merely the end-result of the bad habit of alcoholism. It is a cause. However, the causes of brain damage in human consumers of alcohol may be difficult to determine. Diet and physical health of study participants cannot be continuously monitored much less controlled over the period of time extending from their initiating alcohol consumption to the first signs of alcohol dependence. Here again, animal models are of value. They permit monitoring and control of diet throughout the life of animals and enable the investigator to maintain the animals on a balanced nutritional diet. Neuronal damage under such conditions, if it occurs, can be attributed to alcohol, its metabolites, and glucocorticoids rather than nutritional and vitamin deficiencies. Under carefully controlled nutritional conditions animal studies show that chronic alcohol consumption (CAC) and its withdrawal have neurotoxic effects causing neuronal degeneration and cell loss in the cerebral cortex, cerebellum, and hippocampus (Phillips & Cragg, 1984; Walker, Barnes, Zornetzer, Hunter, & Kubanis, 1980; Sapolsky, 1993).

One controlled study (Paula-Barbosa, Brandão, Madeira, & Cadete-Leite, 1993) compared eight groups of rats under three different conditions: (a) three different groups of animals were given a 20% ethanol solution as part of their liquid diet for 6, 12, or 18 months, (b) matched control animals received the same diet except that sucrose replaced the alcohol, and (c) two withdrawal groups received alcohol for 6 or 12 months and were then gradually switched to the nonalcoholic liquid diet for 6 months.

Quantitative analyses revealed a significant reduction in brain cells in the hippocampus in alcohol fed rats as compared to the matched nonalcohol fed control animals. Magnitude of the effect was related to the length of alcohol treatment. Animals in the withdrawal groups showed significantly greater neuronal loss than the alcohol fed rats who did not suffer withdrawal from alcohol. Earlier research by the same group using the same experimental design examined the medial prefrontal cortex and found a significant loss of brain cells in that region as a function of duration of alcohol treatment with additional loss of cell density following withdrawal (Cadete-Leite, Alves, Tavares, & Paula-Barbosa, 1990).

Degeneration of the cholinergic afferentation of the cerebral cortex found in humans can be reproduced in rats. Animals receiving a 20% alcohol solution showed a time dependent degeneration of the thalamocortical system and decreased release of acetylcholine in the cerebral cortex. Experimental animals also showed a progressive loss of memory for maze learning. In humans cholinergic cell lose in the cerebral cortex is accompanied by a loss of semantic memory and a decrease in attention (Arendt, 1993).

Human studies

A study conducted in Spain used a broad array of laboratory tests and medical examinations to ensure that the only disease present in the participants was alcoholism (Nicolás et al., 1993). Forty male patients met DSM-III-R criteria for alcoholism. Participants were carefully selected following a battery of laboratory and medical examinations ensuring that they were free from other diseases, were not suffering from nutritional and vitamin deficiencies, were nonindigent, and came from a stable work environment. Participants were matched with 20 male friends and relatives who had no history of alcohol problems. Cerebral structure and function were assessed by means of single photon emission computed tomography (SPECT) providing regional cerebral blood flow (rCBF), a measure of brain function, and a neuroradiological CT scan providing measures of cerebral atrophy. Neuropsychological functioning was assessed with a battery of tests including measures of memory, IQ, and frontal lobe executive functions. Average age of the patients was 44 years. Their average daily alcohol consumption was approximately 6 drinks/day over a period of more than 20 years. They could be controlled drinkers according to the Rand Report I and the Sobells' criteria (Armor et al., 1976; Sobell & Sobell, 1978). Eighty percent of the participants, patients and controls, smoked at least one pack of cigarettes a day for 20 years. No other drugs were used.

Average significant SPECT scan analyses, qualitative and semiquantitative, showed diminished rCBF in all brain lobes of the patients as compared to the matched control subjects. Thirty of the 40 patients showed significant reductions in rCBF. Frontal lobes were most frequently found to be hypoperfused (65%), followed by the temporal (40%), parietal (30%) and occipital (20%) lobes. SPECT scans taken after two months of complete abstinence showed normal rCBF in eight patients without frontal lobe atrophy. Patients who continued to have frontal atrophy continued to show hypoperfusion but less than on treatment entrance. Patients with and without diminished rCBF did not differ in mean age, duration of alcoholism or nutritional status. Alcoholics with diminished rCBF had significantly higher alcohol intake during the month prior to admission. A significant correlation was obtained between the amount of alcohol consumed in the month prior to admission and rCBF in the anterior frontal lobes, -0.64.

Eleven of the 40 patients showed significant frontal lobe atrophy. Eight of these 11 also showed reduced rCBF. The majority of patients showing significant functional deficits, diminished rCBF, did not show structural damage, cerebral atrophy. Patients with cerebral atrophy were older and had a higher lifetime intake of alcohol. Frontal lobe atrophy and lifetime intake of alcohol were significantly correlated, 0.64.

Neuropsychological assessments showed that none of the patients suffered diminished IQ as defined by measures of the Wechsler Adult Intelligence Scale. They did show significant deficits in measures of frontal lobe executive functions, performance on the Trail making tests, the Weigl card sorting task, and visual memory. Patients with significantly reduced rCBF in the anterior frontal lobes showed significantly greater deficits in the neuropsychological tests assessing frontal lobe function than those with normal rCBF. Patients with frontal lobe atrophy also showed significant impairment on the neuropsychological tests of frontal lobe function. Seventeen of 18 patients with diminished rCBF of the anterior frontal lobes but with no evidence of atrophy showed significant neuropsychological deficits whereas only one of the 11 patients with no evidence of cerebral atrophy and with normal rCBF showed such a deficit. Deficits in brain function reflected in brain metabolism especially in the prefrontal cortex, and neuropsychological deficits in executive functions may be present in the apparent absence of brain atrophy in asymptomatic and otherwise healthy alcoholics (Nicolás et al., 1993; see also Hunt & Nixon, 1993; Kril et al., 1997; Lyons, Whitlow, Smith, & Porrino, 1998; Schmahmann, 1997).

As described in chapter 1 CT results by Cala (1987) showed evidence of brain atrophy in 65% to 85% of light and moderate drinkers. Such high rates of brain dysfunction in social drinkers cannot be dismissed as the consequence of chronic alcoholism. Physiological and anatomical changes are apparent before the stage of alcoholism is reached. Brain dysfunction may develop in the majority of light to moderate drinkers. Continued drinking leads to persistence of dysfunction and its exacerbation (Eckardt et al., 1980; Shear et al., 1994). Brain dysfunction is not merely an end result sometimes found in alcoholics. In a majority of individuals it can be produced by as "little" as five drinks a day (Cala, 1987), a level below that which the Rand Report (Armor et al., 1976, 1978) and the Sobells (1978) considered a return to controlled, moderate, drinking.

Sensitization

Not only is there brain atrophy and cell loss with chronic drinking and withdrawal, changes in neuronal excitability also occur. Infrahuman and human studies suggest that withdrawal from alcohol after heavy drinking, which is inevitable since the human drinker will eventually go to sleep, jail, or stop for lack of supply, results in neuronal sensitization (Adinoff, O'Neill, & Ballenger, 1995; Linnoila, Mefford, Nutt, & Adinoff, 1987). Recordings of brain wave activity (EEG) in rats during withdrawal from alcohol show a marked increase in excitability, especially in the hippocampus, during the second as compared to the first withdrawal (Poldrugo & Snead, 1984) and varies as a function of length of alcohol exposure (Veatch & Gonzalez, 1996). Clinical studies suggest that "kindling" may be a determiner of the frequency and severity of withdrawal (Brown, Anton, Malcolm, & Ballenger, 1988; Lechtenberg & Worner, 1991; Weisman, 1994).

Kindling theory (Adinoff et al., 1995; Ballenger & Post, 1978) suggests that changes in limbic neuronal excitability is a factor influencing the characteristic behavior of the alcoholic when sober as well as when under the influence. The enormous stress produced in withdrawal from alcohol following a long period of chronic alcoholic consumption activates and sensitizes the HPA axis and the noradrenergic locus coereleus branch of the sympathetic nervous system. The best predictor of withdrawal symptoms is having had a withdrawal experience in the past. Increased sensitization of the limbic system may also be the basis at least in part for craving (Blum, 1991; Childress et al., 1999; Robinson & Berridge, 1993). It mediates the correlation between reported withdrawal experiences and verbal reports of craving (Ludwig et al., 1974). The fact that both an endorphin antagonist (O'Malley et al., 1992) and a dopamine antagonist (Modell, Mountz, Glaser, & Lee,

1993) reduces craving in alcoholics suggests that sensitized endorphin and dopamine circuits contribute to reported craving and alcohol seeking behavior. The implication is that pharmacotherapy should employ a package of haloperidol and naltrexone to reduce orienting to alcohol and its cues, craving, and the reinforcement from a slip.

Elements in our account of the sociobiobehavioral bases for alcoholism will become more readily apparent in our consideration of the etiology of alcoholism. A critical factor remains to be elucidated in the evolution of the Janus effect. Why does it occur in only a small minority of people who ingest alcohol and not others? We must now turn to the etiology of alcoholism and the critical role of individual differences which was only touched upon in the preceding section.

ETIOLOGY OF ALCOHOLISM

Three major sociobiobehavioral classes of risks for alcoholism will be considered in our analysis of the etiology of alcoholism.
(1) Two kinds of biological predispositions will be described, (a) genetically determined risk factors and family history as indicated in adoption studies, and (b) teratogenic effects to the fetus.
(2) Two kinds of severe stress will be examined, (a) filial separation and, (b) traumatic experiences.
(3) Environmental situations that promote and reinforce heavy drinking will be appraised. Such situations may lead to alcoholism in the absence of evident high risks from biological dispositions or severe stress. All three factors, as well as others, may interact in varying degree to increase the risk of alcoholism.

Biological predispositions

It is unlikely that alcoholism, a complex sociobiobehavioral disorder, is the result of an anomaly in a single gene. Alcoholism(s) is genetically heterogeneous. Different people may become alcoholic because of different genetic variations and in any given individual there may be multiple genetic anomalies placing them at risk for alcoholism. Such complexities may be reduced in part if markers of genetic risks could be obtained from young people who do not as yet show the manifest symptoms of alcoholism but do show specific behavioral or biological responses that predict future alcohol dependence. Such markers would aid in the search for relevant genetic material that have a possible causal connection with the disease. Examination of genetic material in diagnosed alcoholics always raises the problem of possible confounds. The expressed genetic anomaly may be an effect along with the alcoholism rather than its cause.

One of the first markers studied is the event related positive potential (ERP) in the electrical activity of the brain recorded approximately 300 msec (P3) following a stimulus (Begleiter, Porjesz, Bihari, & Kissin, (1984). Other behavioral (Schandler, Brannock, Cohen, & Mendez, 1993) and psychophysiological markers (Iacono, 1998) have been studied with reliable results. A difficulty with such biological and behavioral markers is their lack of specificity of cause. A biological marker such as P3 may be present in many different disorders behaviorally manifest as a deficit in attention. It may be caused by many different factors and is less predictive of the disease of alcoholism than a specific response to an alcohol challenge such as body sway (Schuckit, 1994). The problems are complex but the rewards may be great if the pattern of genetic anomalies influencing the development of alcoholism in different people can be mapped. A hope is that the Collaborative Study on the Genetics of Alcoholism (COGA) project will make real progress in unraveling some of the complexity of the problem of genetic factors influencing the development of alcoholism. Research on the human genotype and its implications for alcoholism as well as other evidences of genetic influences are occurring at an accelerated rate. We will review a small sample of that research including some of the classic studies on so-called nature versus nurture in the pages that follow.

GENETIC INFLUENCES

Among the many possible genetic influences on the development of alcoholism, three types will be considered varying in the specificity of inheritance (Goldman & Bergen, 1998), (a) differences in the metabolism of alcoholism, (b) differences in neurotransmitters, and (c) adoption studies.

Metabolism of alcohol: genes for lowered risk

Some of the most interesting and important research on genetic variables affecting the risk for alcoholism have been studies of individual differences in the metabolism of alcohol. Most of the alcohol we consume is catalyzed or broken down into simpler products in the liver. Alcohol dehydrogenase enzymes (ADH) change alcohol into acetaldehyde in the first stage of alcohol catalysis. A second enzyme, acetaldehyde hydrogenase (ALDH) transforms acetaldehyde into acetate in the second stage of the catalysis. Acetate is eventually transformed into energy. Acetaldehyde the product of the first stage is highly toxic. Disulfiram or antabuse as it is known under its trade name, serves as a deterrent to drinking alcohol because it inhibits the activity of ALDH permitting an accumulation of acetaldehyde as a consequence which stimulates excessive sympathetic nervous system activity producing nausea, vomiting, rapid heartbeat and lowered blood pressure. Obviously, acetaldehyde may produce a very unpleasant reaction serving as a punishment and deterrent against future drinking.

Everyone has five different classes of alcohol dehydrogenase enzymes, ADHs, but only class I ADH has a strong affinity for alcohol. It has three classes of subunits that are encoded by ADH1, ADH2, and ADH3 genes. Genes for ADH2 and ADH3 are polymorphic, have more than one form or allele. The ADH2 gene has three alleles; ADH3 has two alleles, and the ADH1 gene has only one form. Different forms or alleles are written in a text preceded by an asterisk. Thus, the three alleles for the ADH2 gene are written, ADH2*1, ADH2*2, and ADH2*3, respectively. Everyone has two copies of each gene. Both copies of the gene for ADH1 are identical. For the others, the forms may be identical, homozygous, or different, heterozygous (Thomasson & Li, 1993).

There are also several different forms of ALDH with the ALDH2 having the greatest affinity for acetaldehyde. The well-known facial flush experienced by many Asian people is produced by elevated levels of acetaldehyde in the blood. They have their own endogenous antabuse. A deficiency or absence of the ALDH2 enzyme is responsible at least in part for the facial blush and the elevated levels of acetaldehyde. The deficiency in the ALDH2 enzyme is due to the inheritance of a mutated variation of the ALDH2*2 allele of which there may be several kinds. Behavioral geneticists attempt to relate these variations in genes producing the enyzmes metabolizing alcohol to variations in drinking behavior and other consequences of alcohol consumption. The greatest advances in genetic typing for protection against alcoholism has been made in studying differences in alcoholism and alcohol consumption among Asian people, primarily Japanese, Chinese, and Korean. Studies have shown that approximately half of Chinese, Japanese, and Koreans experience facial flushing along with other unpleasant symptoms. It has the tendency to reduce drinking and the risk for alcoholism (Higuchi, Matsushita, Murayama, Takagi, & Haytashida, 1995; Thomasson & Li, 1993; Wall, Thomasson, Schuckit, & Ehlers, 1992; Wolff, 1973).

Genotyping suggests that the greatest facial flushing and toxic buildup of acetaldehyde is due to a relatively inactive ALDH2 gene which allows the accumulation of heightened levels of acetaldehyde. Also contributing to the deterrent effect of excessive acetaldehyde is an efficient form of the ADH enzyme which converts alcohol to acetaldehyde very quickly. Studying genotype frequencies in more than 600 alcoholic patients and 400 controls, Higuchi et al. (1995) found highly significant differences in the frequencies of ADH2 and ALDH2 genotypes in the alcoholic and control groups. Among other effects, it was found that a homozygous ALDH2*2 genotype regardless of the ADH2 genotype produces very severe flushing and completely inhibits the development of alcoholism. Different combinations of genetic variations influencing the rate of conversion of alcohol to acetaldeyde and how quickly the toxin is removed by ALDH determines the odds of developing alcoholism among the Japanese people studied.

A study of self-reported flushing and genotypes of ALDH and ADH2 and ADH3 among Taiwanese Han people suggests that certain people are at risk for alcoholism because they fail to show flushing following alcohol consumption (Chen, Chen, Yu, & Cheng, 1998). Subjects genotyped as ALDH2*1/*1 and ADH2*1/*1 all failed to show flushing. Lacking the heightened sensitivity to the alcohol, they are at greater risk for alcoholism than those who show flushing and other sympathetic responses induced by the rate of production and elimination of acetaldehyde. A long term prospective study is needed to determine whether in fact there is a difference in the rate of development of alcoholism in the different genotypes. Such evidence would be more convincing than cross sectional studies which may reflect the result of alcohol and other chemical changes on gene expression.

Evidence of a high prevalence of alcohol consumption but a low incidence of alcohol problems and alcoholism among Jews has been studied and discussed for many years (Keller, 1979; McCready, Greeley, & Thiesen, 1983). The phenomenon has usually received some form of psychosociocultural interpretation. Alcohol has a ceremonial significance; it is part of religious rituals; sobriety distinguishes the

Jewish minority from the heavy drinking majority, etc. Recent evidence suggests that there may be a difference in metabolism that makes Jewish people from Eastern Europe more sensitive to the effects of alcohol consumption, an effect similar to one experienced by Asian people, but of a lesser degree.

Monteiro, Klein, & Schuckit (1991) studied a sample of Jewish men matched with the men in Schuckit's (1988) longitudinal study of level of response to an alcohol challenge. A higher level of response, greater sensitivity, to the alcohol challenge was shown by the Jewish men than the men in the longitudinal sample. Significantly greater unpleasant subjective effects were reported by the Jewish men and greater, although not significant, body sway to the alcohol challenge. A lack of power due to the relatively small sample may be responsible for the latter statistically nonsignificant result.

More recently a study obtained genotypes from a representative sample of Jewish men in Jerusalem who are light drinkers and a group in treatment for heroin dependence with a history of heavy drinking. Neumark, Friedlander, Thomnasson, & Li (1998) report that the ADH2*2 allele which is extremely rare in Blacks, rare in Whites, and common in Asians was significantly related to a reduced peak alcohol consumption and to infrequent drinking in both groups of Jewish men. Neumark et al. suggest that the high frequency of the ADH2*2 allele which is four times higher in Jewish men than that reported for other white ethnic groups serves as a protective factor. It functions in a similar but less obvious manner as the aversive experience observed in Asian people with the ALDH2*2 allele. The ADH2*2 allele seems to stimulate the ADH enzyme to more rapidly transform alcohol to acetaldehyde leaving for a time a larger than normal amount of the toxin which must be transformed to acetate by the ALDH enzyme. This subtle excess of acetaldehyde may be sufficient to discourage drinking.

Protective effects of specific genetic influences on the rate of production of acetaldehyde and its elimination suggest that people at risk may have genetic variations of ADH and ALDH which stimulate unusually rapid elimination of acetaldehyde, reducing negative consequences of alcohol while leaving the positive reinforcing effects. Mapping the genome in individuals at risk for alcoholism may shed considerable light on the role of genetic variations in the two principle enzymes involved in the metabolism of alcohol. Genetic variations in another kind of metabolism provides a provocative problem in need of further study.

First pass metabolism

A striking experiment conducted in the Bronx VA Medical Center and the University of Trieste demonstrated that under normal conditions some 20% of alcohol is metabolized by ADH in the gastric mucosa, the lining of the stomach, before reaching the liver (Frezza et al., 1990). Most interesting is that there are highly significant gender differences. As much as 30% more alcohol is subject to "first pass metabolism" in men than women. One drink for a woman may have as much effect as two for men, because so much more of the alcohol is metabolized in the stomach in men than women before it gets into the blood stream. This difference in first pass metabolism helps explain the perplexing gender differences showing women at greater risk for the negative consequences of alcohol than men.

Initially two subgroups formed the control group. In one subgroup none of the biological parents had been hospitalized for a psychiatric condition. In the second control group one biological parent had been hospitalized for a psychiatric condition other than alcoholism, primarily depression or a character disorder. Since the outcomes for the two subgroups were quite similar their results were combined to form a single control group, FH-. These results are important because they indicate a degree of causal specificity. Alcoholism and not psychiatric disorders such as depression in a biological parent is a risk factor for alcoholism in adopted out offspring. Both groups of adoptees received detailed interviews as adults. A variety of demographic and personal characteristics were assessed including their history of drinking and drinking related consequences. A significant association between a positive family history of alcoholism (FH+) and alcoholism was obtained in that significantly more of these men were judged to be alcoholic as adults, 18%, than the men with a negative family history (FH-), 5%.

It is noteworthy that the effect obtained by Goodwin for the FH+ group was specific to alcoholism and its symptoms of dependence (Jellinek, 1960) as distinguished from problem drinking determined by raters blind to the participants' group membership. Groups FH+ and FH- did not differ in incidence of problem drinking, heavy drinking, or personality characteristics. They differed only in the severest form of alcohol misuse, the incidence of alcoholism, a finding contradicting the assumption emphasized by revisionists that alcoholism lies on a continuum with social drinking. An implication of their continuity assumption is that FH+ and FH- men should overlap in all categories of drinking.

Only the severest symptoms characteristic of alcoholism such as hallucinations and loss of control were reported significantly more often by FH+ men. No significant difference was obtained between FH+ and FH- groups in the incidence of drunk driving arrests. Specificity of effect is dependent upon the number and kind of measures obtained as well as sample size. A larger sample and a larger number of measures of potential effects might change the picture by increasing the number and variety of significant differences between the two groups. Specificity of effect must be distinguished from specificity of cause. Although specificity of effect enhances the judgment that there is a causal relation between cause and effect, lack of specificity of effect does not negate causality. Specificity of effect does not necessarily imply specificity of cause. Alcoholism may have many causes, may be multidetermined. Evidence for a biological predisposition, including a genetic one, does not prohibit other determinants of alcoholism in combination with biological predispositions. Absence of a difference between the two FH- subgroups indicates some specificity in cause. Not any psychiatric disorder in a biological parent is a risk factor for alcoholism in their offspring; treatment for alcoholism as defined by physicians at the time was such a risk.

Goodwin's results indicated that 5% of the FH- men developed alcoholism presumably in the absence of a genetic effect. Other predisposing biological effects are possible (Baer et al., 1998; Griesler & Kandel, 1998; Yates, Cadoret, Troughton, Stewart, & Giunta, 1998), although they remain to be clearly established as risk factors. Men with a negative family history of alcoholism may become alcoholic in the absence of a genetic effect, but at a lower probability than FH+ men. It is also apparent that a positive family history is not sufficient to cause alcoholism. Most FH+ men, 82%, did not become alcoholic.

Alcoholism is multidetermined and is a function of the culture and historical period in which the study was conducted. Goodwin and his colleagues found no effect of family history on the development of alcoholism in women. An important consideration is that the incidence of alcoholism among Scandinavian women was much lower than men at the time, approximately 0.1%-1% versus 3%-5% (Goodwin et al.,1977a), suggesting considerably more cultural pressure against women drinking.

Additional results obtained by Goodwin and his colleagues (1974) are of considerable importance yet are rarely cited. Despite the ambiguities inherent in the social learning theory of alcohol dependence (Marlatt, 1979, 1985b; Nathan, 1985) it has been disconfirmed in striking manner by Goodwin and his colleagues. Male siblings with alcoholic biological parents where one was put up for adoption within the first six weeks of life and the other not, did not differ in their incidence of alcoholism as adults. Being raised in an alcoholic family did not increase the rate of alcoholism as compared to siblings raised by foster parents. If modeling or expectancies were a risk factor for alcoholism, there should have been significantly more alcoholics among male siblings raised in the alcoholic family than those raised by nonblood related foster parents. There was no such statistically significant difference.

Cloninger (1987) and his colleagues conducted another adoption study, this time in Sweden rather than Denmark, and with a different procedure. Data consisted of official records from hospital registers, and local temperance and insurance boards, etc. There were no personal interviews. This kind of study was possible because it was conducted in a relatively small country with a relatively homogeneous and stable population with a long-standing centralized medical and social care system. A larger sample was obtained than in Goodwin's study permitting more analytical examination of types of alcoholism and their environmental interactions. Criteria used for classifying individuals as alcoholics were not the same as those employed by Goodwin and his colleagues and were not, of course, based on current DSM criteria.

Detailed analyses of alcoholism in women as well as men were made possible by the larger sample size obtained by Cloninger and his colleagues. Goodwin's finding that FH+ increased the risk of alcoholism in men was replicated in Cloninger's study with the additional finding of an alcoholism increase in FH+ women, as well as distinctions among risk factors for the type and severity of alcoholism.

Additional information on the interaction between environment and family history as risk factors was also obtained. Cloninger and his colleagues obtained evidence for two types of alcoholics. Type 1 alcoholism occurred in adulthood after the age of 25 and was not accompanied by criminality, occurred in women as well as men, and could be severe or relatively mild as a function of the early environment. Type 2 alcoholism occurred before the age of 25. Onset was accompanied by repeated social and legal problems. Severity was moderate, did not interact with the environment and was limited to males.

A replication of the procedures and measuring instruments on a new sample obtained in a different Swedish city than the source of the original study participants obtained similar overall results for the males. A relatively small number of women, lack of sample size, was probably responsible for failing to replicate results for women (Sigvardsson, Bohman, & Cloninger, 1996).

The obtained results are limited to a particular culture and historical period, infants born between 1930 and 1949 to unwed mothers. Incidence of early onset alcoholism among females is not unknown in the United States (Hill, 1995; Maltzman & Schweiger, 1991, Office of Applied Studies, 1998). Whether alcoholism among teenage females would be more common today in Denmark and Sweden I do not know; I suspect it is. Another variable absent in these early studies because of the historical period, is the prevalence of polydrug use that is so common today in young people, exacerbating problems with the social, educational, and justice systems. Despite these complexities, the evidence suggests the presence of a biological predisposition including a genetic risk factor, a determinant which is neither a necessary nor a sufficient condition for alcoholism but does increase the probability of developing alcoholism.

Adoption studies such as those by Goodwin and Cloninger have not been without their critics. One difficulty is that the criteria used for classifying individuals as alcoholics in these studies is idiosyncratic. They did not use standardized widely available criteria such as DSM-IV. An obvious reason is that there were no generally accepted criteria other than those suggested by Jellinek (1960) at the time some of these studies were conducted. Procedures in Cloninger's studies did not permit assessments during a personal structured interview. Subsequent studies using criteria such as DSM-IV indicate that there are specific biological predispositions increasing the risk for alcoholism in humans. Whether these biological dispositions are all inherited or in part confounded with prenatal teratogenic effects or stress in the mother must await long-term prospective studies carefully assessing prenatal and perinatal maternal drinking and stress. That genetic factors increase the risk for alcohol dependence has been established beyond a reasonable doubt in infrahuman animal models bred to prefer or not prefer alcohol and other infrahuman animal and human studies (see Begleiter & Kissin, 1995).

Specific biological predispositions

Research by Schuckit and his colleagues (Schuckit, 1994, 1998; Schuckit & Smith, 1996) has examined family history as a risk for alcoholism in terms of the level of response to an alcohol challenge. Specific effects examined include the level of behavioral response to alcohol measured by body sway, self-reported level of intoxication, and biological measures of the HPA axis, cortisol (Schuckit, Gold, & Rish, 1987) and ACTH (Schuckit, Rish, & Gold, 1988). All measures show a lower level of response by nonalcoholic FH+ than FH- college age men and nonfaculty staff. Level of response results have essentially been replicated in an independent sample taken from a larger collaborative study on the genetics of alcoholism (COGA) (Schuckit, Tsuang, Anthenelli, Tipp, & Nurnberger, 1996).

Schuckit hypothesizes that low response level men need to drink more to get "high" or they can drink more and get high with less negative behavioral consequences. In a heavy drinking subculture as found at many universities, such low response level men would be encouraged to drink as a sign of toughness or sophistication. They can hold their liquor. One now sees a devastating combination: greater positive reinforcement from beta-endorphins in FH+ men reported by Gianoulakis (1989; 1996) and her colleagues and less negative reinforcement shown by Schuckit and his research team.

As part of an ongoing longitudinal prospective study Schuckit (1994) followed-up his original sample approximately 8 years after initial testing. Significantly more men with a low as compared to a high level of response at base level had become dependent on alcohol. Within the FH+ group and within the FH- group level of response to alcohol approximately 8 years earlier differentiated between those who developed alcohol dependence and those who did not. Thus, FH- men who showed a low response level to alcohol at the initial assessment, base level, were more likely to develop alcoholism 8 years later than FH- men who showed greater sensitivity to intoxication and body sway in response to an alcohol challenge. Level of response to alcohol was not significantly related to other forms of psychiatric disorder or dependence on other drugs as determined by DSM-III-R criteria.

The approximately 8-year follow-up involved 192 FH+ and 166 FH- men (Schuckit, 1998). Approximately 14% of the FH+ men were diagnosed as meeting DSM-III-R criteria for alcohol abuse and 29% met the criteria for alcohol dependence. In contrast, 7% met criteria for alcohol abuse and 11% met criteria for alcohol dependence within the FH- group. Both categories of alcohol misuse were significantly greater in the FH+ than FH- men. An interesting note is the greater incidence of dependence as compared to abuse in the combined groups. These results contradict the argument of harm reduction advocates that their promotion of controlled drinking meets the treatment needs of the much larger pool of people in need of treatment, alcohol abusers compared to people suffering from alcohol dependence (see chapters 8, 10).

The FH+ and FH- men did not differ significantly in marijuana or stimulant abuse/dependence, or in the relative frequency of anxiety and mood disorders. The significant correlation between level of response and alcohol abuse/dependence approximately 8 years later is significant, -0.37 and although slightly reduced, remains significant controlling for family history. The significant correlation between family history and alcohol abuse/ dependence, -0.27, does not remain significant when level of response to alcohol is controlled. Level of response remains a significant predictor of alcohol abuse/dependence approximately 8 years later following multiple regression of a variety of paper and pencil questionnaires that account for additional variance in alcohol abuse and dependence in a subsample of the original group.

Schuckit notes that his longitudinal study necessarily has limitations. To avoid heterogeneity in a sample of limited size, the sample is restricted to white males. It does not sample antisocial personality, a common personality risk factor, although the questionnaires sample some of its characteristics. Another shortcoming is that detailed information on the drinking patterns of the mothers of the men in the original sample is absent. Although FH+ history excluded alcoholic mothers, the problem remains of possible teratogenic effects, especially "social" drinking in the mothers, a risk factor that cannot be ignored. Since "birds of a feather flock together", the chances are that an alcoholic or heavy drinking male will be married to a woman who is not abstinent. It is also unfortunate that beta-endorphin measures were not among those selected for study as one of the biological indices of level of response to alcohol challenges.

Schuckit's (1998) prospective study has many positive features including the care exercised in obtaining FH+ and FH- young men matched for drinking history and patterns. Another positive feature of Schuckit's longitudinal project is that the children of the men in the original sample and their wives will be followed-up in future phases of the project. At that time females as well as males will be studied and personality characteristics will be examined. Another salutary feature of the project is that the COGA sample in which level of response variables have been used will be subject to genotyping. It may then be possible to search for the genes linked to level of response measures. I suspect that a good place to look would be the genes programming ADH and ALDH enzymes.

There may be multiple genetic and other biological influences affecting the response to alcohol at different levels of biological organization. Schuckit's research suggests that one such inherited influence is a high level of initial tolerance, a lack of sensitivity to alcohol which may increase the risk for alcoholism in subcultures that promote heavy drinking. The other side of the coin is that a high degree of sensitivity to alcoholism may serve as a protective factor against alcoholism (Monteiro et al., 1991; Neumark et al., 1998). Caution must be exercised in attributing to heredity the entire effect of low response level to alcohol. There remains the possibility that fetal alcohol exposure may have affected the level of response in FH+ men and in FH- men at a lower rate.

Disconfirmation of a theory stating that alcoholism is learned does not mean that the environment plays no role in the development of alcoholism, that alcoholism is due solely to heredity. Absolutely not. The social learning formulation by behavior therapists is simplistic and false (e.g., Goodwin et al., 1974). However, environmental influences are enormously important at every level of biological organization. At the molecular level they may affect the expression of DNA (Gottlieb, 1997,1998). Experience may change brain function and morphology. Levels and interactions among systems of neurotransmitters as well as behavioral patterns of drinking may be affected by experience and the social environment at the moment. An adequate theory of alcoholism must be in part a neurobiological developmental theory, one that considers the role of the environment in continuous interaction with the neurobiological development of the individual which in turn is determining behavior continuously interacting and influencing the environment. There is a continuous dialectical relationship among the environment, brain, and behavior from the molecular to the cultural level (Gottlieb, 1997, 1998). Learning is part of that dialectical interaction.

TERATOGENIC EFFECTS

Two general classes of biological predispositions serve as risk factors. One we have considered above, the genetic. The second is environmental insults or teratogenic factors of different kinds. These have been inadequately and insufficiently studied (Smith, 1994) except for the extreme case of the fetal alcohol syndrome and fetal alcohol effect (Abel, 1984; Hutchings, 1989) produced by excessive maternal drinking. Fetal alcohol syndrome and effects have not been studied as risk factors for alcoholism but as profound consequences to the fetus of maternal heavy drinking. Studies of fetal alcohol exposure to smaller amounts of alcohol consumed by pregnant women has only recently appeared and with important results and implications (Baer et al., 1998; Griesler & Kandel, 1998).

Environmental influences on the mother, her fetus, and infant cannot be ignored. A woman in a difficult marriage with an alcoholic is likely to be under considerable stress. If she is pregnant, it is possible that the stress she experiences will affect her fetus, modify its gene expression, influence its brain development, and may increase the risk for alcoholism. A familial influence may be a biological one, but need not be an inherited one. Detailed information is necessary in adoption studies specifying during which phase of the male alcoholic's career his spouse was pregnant and the infant reared. Did the alcoholism develop in the father or mother after the offspring was born and put out to adoption, before, or during an active alcoholic phase of a parent? Detailed information on the perinatal period, measures of maternal alcohol consumption, cigarette smoking, and other drug use is critical. It is important to assess the degree of stress under which the mother found herself, medical complications during these periods, viral infections, nutrition, and family living arrangements. Measures of all these are essential if the role of environment and heredity and their interaction in creating a risk for alcoholism are to be adequately determined. Animal models help to clarify the problem of control over extraneous sources of variables. We shall see that they provide striking evidence of the interaction of environment and neurobiology in determining excessive alcohol consumption. Careful prospective studies also help. Evidence from such studies are beginning to appear (Baer et al., 1998; Griesler & Kandel, 1998) as well as retrospective studies (Yates, Cadoret, Treoughton, Stewart, & Giunta, 1998). We will now turn to these studies.

Low level prenatal alcohol exposure

It is often assumed that biological risk factors refer to heredity expressed as various genetic contributions to the development of alcoholism. There are, however, biological risk factors that are not genetically transmitted. These are environmental insults that may contribute to anatomical or functional teratogenicity. Alcohol is one of the worst when consumed during pregnancy. Others are still in need of study. These include environmental pollutants and pesticides, viral infections, poor maternal nutrition, difficult childbirth, and severe maternal stress. Some of these have been found to be risk factors for schizophrenia, conduct disorders, and criminal behavior (Raines, 1993; Susser, 1989; Venables, 1998). Prospective studies are needed to investigate their possible role as etiological risk factors for alcoholism.

Two long-term prospective projects, the Seattle Longitudinal Study and the New York State Cohort Study, have now demonstrated that prenatal exposure to maternal alcohol consumption at the level of "social" drinking predicts levels of adolescent drinking (Baer et al., 1998; Griesler & Kandel, 1998). A retrospective study (Yates et al., 1998) shows that prenatal alcohol exposure significantly affected adult rates of nicotine, alcohol, and drug dependence. An infant's attachment to its mother may also be affected by light social drinking during pregnancy (O'Connor, Sigman, & Brill, 1987). Studies by Baer et al. (1998) and Greisler and Kandel (1998) demonstrate that alcohol consumption by pregnant women far below clinical levels of alcoholism may affect the alcohol consumption of their adolescent offspring some 14 years later. On the basis of their current results it cannot be asserted that moderate maternal drinking produces alcoholism in their affected offspring. Prospective projects need to continue following these adolescents for another 20 years to adequately ascertain whether indeed prenatal exposure to moderate maternal drinking is a significant risk factor for alcoholism. Such prospective studies may indicate whether or not a significant percentage of the familial influence in adoption studies ordinarily attributed to heredity may be due instead to a teratogenic effect of maternal drinking.

Streissguth et. al. (1994) demonstrated that 14-year old adolescents exposed to prenatal maternal drinking at moderate levels suffer brain damage manifest as significant deficits in attention and memory. The Seattle project subsequently analyzed the contribution of family history of alcoholism and prenatal exposure to moderate maternal drinking as predictors of the alcohol consumption of these 14 year old adolescents.

Baer et al. (1998) report results from 439 families over a 14-year period beginning with self-reports of drinking by the biological mother receiving prenatal care. At an average age of 14 years the adolescents and their mothers provided detailed information concerning the adolescents' alcohol consumption, demographic information and a family drinking history. Twenty percent of the women abstained from alcohol during their entire pregnancy. Prior to discovery of their pregnancy women who drank alcohol averaged about 11 drinks/week; after discovery of their pregnancy they averaged 4 drinks/week. Average drinks/occasion prior to pregnancy discovery was 2.5 drinks and during pregnancy, 2.2 drinks. Maximum number of drinks for the two periods averaged 4.0 and 3.6, respectively. Three mothers had a history of alcohol problems.

Baer et al. (1998) found that 57% of the adolescents had consumed alcohol at some time in their lives and 25% had done so during the past month. The usual number of drinks/occasion was 1-2; 21% of those who ever had a drink usually had three or more/occasion and 31% had been intoxicated. Six of the adolescents had already been in treatment programs. Three of the four measures of the mothers' drinking during pregnancy correlated significantly with measures of their child's alcohol consumption. Mothers' episodic drinking, the number of drinks/occasion and the maximum number of drinks/occasion were the best predictors of adolescents' alcohol use and problems. A combination of the prenatal alcohol measures correlated 0.27 with a combination of the adolescent drinking variables. A combination of the family history of alcoholism measures correlated 0.18 with the same combination of adolescent variables. Regression analyses show that the prenatal alcohol exposure measures account for more of the variance in adolescent alcohol consumption than do the family history measures. There were no gender differences.

Griesler & Kandel (1998) conducted a longitudinal study of 185 mothers followed for 19 years, since the women were 15-16 years old. They were a representative sample of adolescents enrolled in New York State high schools.

During pregnancy their average age was 21. Their first-born child was interviewed at ages ranging from 9-17 years. Assessment of prenatal drinking was retrospective, approximately 3.3 years after birth of the first born child. Among drinking pregnant women, alcohol consumption ranged from 0.01 to a maximum of 3.5 drinks/day with a mean of 0.33 drinks.

Griesler and Kandel (1998) did not obtain detailed family histories or detailed drinking histories of the father. Their analyses were limited to the effects of maternal alcohol use and smoking as well as other demographic and family characteristics, the kinds of measures also obtained and controlled by Baer et al. (1998). Griesler & Kandel found that maternal drinking during pregnancy was significantly related to their adolescent daughter's current year, $r = 0.34$, and life time, $r = 0.25$, alcohol consumption. Maternal alcohol consumption was not related to their adolescent sons' alcohol use. Maternal smoking was significantly correlated with life-time and current drinking in females and current drinking in male adolescents.

Baer et al. (1998) and Griesler and Kandel (1998) leave several unanswered questions. Some may be answered with continued longitudinal study of the two samples. Most importantly, will the relatively low levels of prenatal alcohol exposure found in these studies increase the risk for alcoholism among the adolescents when they reach adulthood? The great majority of offspring in both samples are still below the age of heaviest drinking and risk for alcoholism. Continued follow-up of their sample by Griesler and Kandel (1998) may shed further light on the gender difference they found. Once they reach adulthood will males be as affected as much by their mothers' alcohol consumption as females? Baer et al. (1998) found no gender difference, but the mothers in their study were drinking somewhat greater amounts/occasion than the mothers studied by Griesler and Kandel (1998). More detailed information on drug use of the offspring is needed, since drug use may play a synergistic role interacting with alcohol. Information is also needed on postpartum drinking by mothers, especially if they nurse their babies. Even one drink affects lactation in the human female (Mennella, 1998). Effects of postpartum alcohol consumption on neurobiological development, attachment, and subsequent behavior of offspring including alcohol use are areas in need of further careful study.

Longitudinal studies of the effects of maternal drinking need to integrate all of the information available on their offspring. Maternal drinking at "moderate" levels of "social" drinking during pregnancy not only affects alcohol consumption in the offspring they also affect basic neuropsychological processes such as attention and memory. Adolescent deficits in attention and memory have already been demonstrated in the Seattle sample (Streissguth et al., 1994). It is important to relate these intellectual deficits to the adolescents' alcohol consumption and success in school. Prenatal alcohol exposure need not be directly affecting alcohol consumption by sensitization of the HPA axis or some other biological mechanism (Weinberg, Taylor, & Gianoulakis, 1996). It may be affecting adolscent alcohol consumption indirectly as the result of stress produced as a consequence of difficulty in adapting to school and social life as a result of diminished intellectual capacity. Multivariate analyses of alcohol consumption should include measures of neuropsychological functioning.

It is apparent that the results obtained by Baer et al. (1998), Griesler and Kandel (1998), and Yates et al. (1998) challenge future studies of hereditability to carefully evaluate the influence of prenatal alcohol exposure as a contributor to the risk for developing alcohol problems in adolescence and adulthood. Excluding alcoholic mothers from a study sample does not avoid the influence of prenatal alcohol exposure, since the levels of maternal alcohol consumption that appear to have had a significant impact on alcohol consumption in adolescence are on the average below clinical levels.

Granted that adoption studies may suffer from confounding teratogenic effects, there still is overwhelming evidence of important genetic and other biological influences interacting with the environment to generate increased risks for alcoholism. Whatever the latter are, they are not social learning, operant conditioning, or expectancies.

Animal models

Some of the best evidence for a genetic risk factor comes from animal studies. Such experiments avoid the sloppiness inherent in human studies where complete control over the participants is impossible, permitting maternal alcohol consumption thereby confounding heredity and teratogenic effects. Selective breeding has developed strains of alcohol preferring and nonpreferring rats and mice. Studies with these animal models not only demonstrate a genetic influence on alcohol consumption and dependence, they permit neurobiological studies of the differences present in animals from the preferring and nonpreferring strains prior to exposure to alcohol. Such animal models promote the development of possible behavioral and pharmacological techniques for reducing alcohol consumption (Hyytiä & Sinclair, 1993). More extensive and detailed reviews of twins, adoption studies, and behavioral genetics may be found in Heath (1995) and McGue (1993). A range of current genetic investigations, infrahuman as well as human, may be found in the book edited by Begleiter and Kissin (1995).

Expectancy and biological predispositions

In recent years behavior therapists have increasingly fallen back on cognitive folk psychology in attempts to provide a learning interpretation of the enormously complex behavior of alcoholics and alcohol use in general. They argue that alcoholism and alcohol use are determined by expectancy, attitudes toward alcohol and beliefs about the effects of alcohol. These conceptions are assessed - defined by - responses to questionnaires as well as balanced placebo design experiments. We have already seen (chapter 1, Maltzman & Marinkovic, 1996) that these balanced-placebo studies suffer from a variety of problems including inconsistent results and alternative interpretations. An implicit assumption of cognitive social learning behavior therapists is that attitudes, beliefs, expectancies, etc., are entirely learned dispositions.

Significant correlations are frequently obtained between questionnaire self-reports of positive expectancies and self-reports of the amount of alcohol consumed. It is therefore of considerable interest to learn that there may be a biological predisposition, possibly an inherited component, in attitudes toward alcohol. Perry (1973) assessed attitudes toward alcohol, cigarettes, and coffee of monozygotic-identical (MZ) and dyzygotic-fraternal (DZ) adult same sex twins. He found that the correlation in attitudes toward alcohol was significantly greater for MZ than DZ twins. There were no significant differences for cigarettes and coffee. These results suggest that "expectancies" toward alcohol are influenced by teratogenic or genetic factors, a possibility not considered by behavior therapists.

Directionality in Perry's study cannot support a simple learning interpretation. Can a coherent hereditary conception be offered? One hypothesis is that heredity influences levels of monoamine oxidase (MAO) which serves as a mediator between the genotype and attitudes towards use of alcohol and other drugs. Research indicates that MAO is genetically determined, moderates central monamine turnover, and its levels are inversely related to sensation seeking, risk taking, and excessive use of alcohol and other drugs (von Knorring et al., 1991; Sullivan et al., 1990). An obvious implication of the MAO mediator hypothesis is that similar effects would be obtained in twin studies investigating attitudes towards other commonly used illicit drugs such as marijuana, cocaine, and amphetamines. Amount and frequency of use should also be assessed. Additional research with larger samples using different designs is needed to more fully explore the relation between heredity and attitudes, beliefs, expectancy, as defined by questionnaires and drinking behavior.

At the very least, it is apparent that a correlation between questionnaire defined expectancies, attitudes, and the like and alcohol consumption is not evidence that expectancies have a causal influence in the determination of alcoholism. Correlation is not causation. An obvious implication of the above argument is that verbal reports of expectancy of positive consequences from alcohol consumption would be positively correlated with alcohol consumption and that sensation and novelty seeking are correlated with both verbal reports of positive expectancies and verbal reports of alcohol consumption. Our hypothesis is that sensation seeking scores are mediating the correlation between questionnaire responses of expectancy and alcohol consumption. There would be an inconsequential correlation between the latter two if sensation seeking were controlled. The latter in turn is determined by levels of dopamine and serotonin. If measures of their metabolites were obtained, they should predict verbal reports of expectancy of positive consequences.

Further evidence that the correlation between verbal reports of expectancy and reported alcohol consumption is mediated by a common biological variable(s) comes from a study by Deckel, Hesselbrock, and Bauer (1995). They demonstrated that neuropsychological tests designed to assess frontal lobe functioning and an EEG measure of power from frontal leads predicted scores on an alcoholism expectancy questionnaire in men with sociopathic tendencies at risk for alcoholism. Their results further suggest that strong positive expectancies are not causal factors but are expressions of frontal lobe dysfunctions which place individuals at heightened risk for alcohol and other drug misuse. Causal directionality between verbal reports of expectancy and alcohol use cannot be sustained.

STRESS

We have considered one of the three classes of risk factors for alcoholism, biological predispositions. The two other classes of risk factors for alcoholism are (a) severe stress, and (b) social environments that promote heavy drinking such as particular occupations. Various combinations of these three risk factors, biological predispositions, stress and occupational risk may interact in different patterns to set the individual on the path toward alcoholism. Which particular path taken may depend on the biological state of the individual, their temperament and the social environment. Although we use the singular "alcoholism", there may be different subtypes yet to be discovered as well as those that have been proposed (Anthenelli, Smith, Irwin, & Schuckit, 1994; Babor et al., 1992; Cloninger, 1987; Jellinek, 1960; Sannibale & Hall, 1998). We will now examine risk factors in the etiology of alcoholism in which the environment, experience, plays a critical role in influencing neurobiology. There are a variety of subtypes of chronic severe stress and trauma. One source of stress that will be considered here is the disruption of familial attachments.

Disruption of attachments

One particular area of biobehavioral research has converged on a fundamental risk factor for alcoholism and other drug misuse, infant attachment and separation stress. Its origins are in the research of ethologists and biobehavioral scientists interested in imprinting and attachment (Hinde, 1970), the creative research of Harlow (1958) and his students, colleagues, other primatologists and behavioral neuroscientists and a psychoanalyst (Bowlby, 1982). Schore (1994) has traced in exquisite detail the dialectical relationship between the human infant and its mother necessary for the infant's normal neurobiological development. Plasticity of the human brain is molded by critical physical and social interactions with the mother and peers during infancy and early childhood and may continue into adulthood (Karni, 1997). Failure to have these interactive experiences results in fundamental biological disorganizations in brain function and structure (Greenough, 1977; Carlson & Earls, 1997) which may serve as risk factors for alcoholism, other drug misuse and behavior problems in adolescence and adulthood (Werner, 1986). What follows is a presentation of some of the research showing how certain experiences are part of the woof and warf of nature, nurture, and chance which may produce risks for alcoholism by producing persisting changes in brain function. Heredity as a risk factor is only one thread in the yarn. More weight is given to one variable, heredity, in the adoption studies described in the previous section, whereas more weight is given to another variable, experience, in the attachment and separation studies that will be described in the present section. Each, heredity and experience, is part of the yarn in which nature and nurture are inextricably woven to produce the growth of the brain and behavior, including alcohol misuse.

This second pathway toward a risk factor for alcoholism depends on experiences of severe stress. Social separation early in life is one such stressor. It is not learning in the usual sense of classical or operant conditioning - or social learning or modeling. When I was a student many years ago, the general belief among learning theorists was that an infant becomes attached to its mother because she is a secondary reinforcer. Mother is associated with satisfaction of her infant's basic needs, milk when hungry, warmth when cold. She becomes a secondary or conditioned reinforcer because she, a previously neutral cue, is associated with primary reinforcers. This conditioning interpretation was considered a sophisticated advance over Watson who believed that infant love is the consequence of tactual stimulation of their erogenous zones. The learning theory view was overturned by the work of ethologists, Hinde, Lorenz, Tinbergen, and a comparative psychologist, Harlow, who demonstrated that attachment of an infant to its mother is based on primary reinforcement, is unlearned and innate. Mom is a primary reinforcer (Harlow, 1958; Hoffman, 1996; Hoffman & Ratner, 1973).

Years ago when ethological research was gaining popularity, I saw a film in which Eckardt Hess, one of the first psychologists in the United States to investigate imprinting, showed a group of ducklings waddling down a path following a Hoover vacuum cleaner in the same fashion as other ducklings followed their mother. If their mother, real or surrogate - duck or vacuum- was removed, they became agitated and emitted distress vocalizations, they cried. A wide range of stimuli characterized by movement, change, evoke an unconditioned, innate, orienting reflex (OR), and a filial response of approach and attachment; imprinting occurs. Cessation or removal of the stimulus elicits distress vocalizations and agitation which cease with return of the mother or surrogate. Such filial behavior is not peculiar to birds. Similar kinds of innate unconditioned responses occur in puppies, nonhuman primates, and humans, among other species. There is a biological preparedness for a filial attachment. Movement and auditory stimuli elicit orienting and attachment in ducklings and goslings. Tactile and auditory stimulation are significant stimuli evoking the basic filial OR in puppies, nonhuman primates, and humans. Attachment occurs because movement, novelty, tactile stimuli, and species specific auditory calls are innately reinforcing for the infant. They have biological significance. The problem is to unravel the biological nature of that significance and its implications. A major contribution of behavioristic biobehavioral science is the demonstration that attachment and separation stress can be independently manipulated by changing the proximal neurochemical bases of the filial behavior.

A biological basis for attachments

Based on similarities between social attachments and their disruption and opiate addiction and withdrawal, Panksepp and his colleagues (Herman & Panksepp, 1978; Panksepp, Herman, Conner, Bishop, & Scott, 1978) hypothesize that endorphins mediate bonding of infant and mother and other social attachments. Crying in the human infant when separated from its mother and separation distress vocalizations in infrahuman animals are analogous to the distress of opiate withdrawal in the addict.

In one series of studies (Herman & Panksepp, 1978) infant guinea pigs were studied under two experimental conditions: (a) separated physically from the mother by a wire mesh cage, but visible, and (b) socially isolated, mother not present. On different days the infants were administered an injection of either a placebo, morphine, or naloxone. Separation distress vocalizations were present under both separation conditions, more so when the infant was socially isolated. Distress vocalizations were significantly decreased by morphine as compared to the placebo control treatment under both conditions of separation, mother present but in a separate cage, and social isolation. Naloxone increased distress vocalizations over the placebo control condition in both kinds of separation, even in the condition where the mother was visible. Morphine produced highly significant dose dependent decreases in distress vocalization in both the mother present and the mother absent groups with the greatest influence in the mother absent group. Under placebo the animals in the mother present group emitted significantly less distress vocalizations than the animals in the mother absent group. Sight of the mother despite the absence of physical contact resulted in significantly less distress. Opposite effects of naloxone and morphine on distress vocalizations suggest that the attachment of infant to the mother is based on endorphins stimulated in the infant by presence of the mother. Decreasing the levels of endorphins either by naloxone or by isolation from the mother produces signs of withdrawal and stress (Herman & Panksepp, 1978). Similar results were obtained with litters of puppies (Panksepp et al., 1978).

Panksepp's interpretation of separation stress in terms of a reduction in the level of endorphins is based on an inference from the opposite effects of naloxone and morphine on distress vocalizations. More direct evidence of the role of endorphins in separation stress and the interaction between behavior, brain chemistry and the social environment is now available. Keverne, Martensz, & Tuite (1989) conducted a series of experiments examining the role of beta-endorphins assayed from cerebrospinal fluid (CSF) in relation to sociality, attachment, and bonding between same sex adult monkeys.

Monkeys living in isolation cages were permitted social interactions with a same sex neighbor on alternate days. Social interactions involved grooming the neighbor, characteristic behavioral overtures soliciting grooming, and occasional aggressive behavior. Closed circuit TV cameras taped the behavior which was later analyzed by observers blind to the experimental treatments. Samples of CSF were obtained when animals were in isolation and within three minutes after grooming behavior in a test period.

Highly significant increases in concentration of CSF endorphins occurred following grooming and when animals were permitted to interact with another same sex monkey following isolation. All animals showed the increase in endorphins following grooming behavior except one female whose concentration of endorphins in isolation was very high. This animal made no overtures for grooming but intensely groomed her neighbor during the test period.

A second experiment studied pairs of same sex monkeys permanently living together. Frequency of grooming was low. Half the partners were then given naltrexone and half were given a placebo. Grooming invitations and time spent grooming their cage mate increased significantly in animals receiving naltrexone. Comparable behavior occurred following isolation and following administration of an opiate antagonist. In both cases the experimental treatment, isolation or naltrexone, lowered endorphin levels which were significantly increased following grooming, suggesting that animals living in groups maintained high levels of endorphins as a result of their social interactions.

A low dose of morphine was administered to half the cage mates following isolation and a placebo to the other cage mates in a third experiment. There was no sign of sedation from the small dose of morphine administered. It resulted in a significant decrease in overtures for grooming and the amount of time spent in grooming, the same effect seen in the monkey with a high level of circulating endorphins.

Social behavior in the form of grooming, touching, physical contact, increased markedly following social isolation. Social affiliation changed the neurochemical brain state of these animals, significantly increasing the concentration of endorphins and positive affect obtained from social contacts. Administration of morphine significantly decreased grooming of cage mates and the sociality it represents. Loss of interest in social affiliations also characterizes the behavior of addicts high on exogenous opiates.

A fundamental dialectical relationship is apparent between behavior, social affiliation, and the neurochemical brain state of the animal. Grooming, touching, close physical contact, raise the level of endorphins, are reinforcing, and for that reason bond social relationships. A high level of sociality maintains a high level of endorphins. The neurochemical brain state in part determines behavior which reciprocally modifies the brain state along with the social environment. What does all this have to do with the etiology of alcoholism, its prevention and treatment? Let's see.

Separation stress and alcohol consumption

One study combined features of the previous experiments and added an important longitudinal dimension as well as a critical dependent variable: effects of separation stress on alcohol consumption in rhesus monkeys (Higley, Hasert, Suomi, & Linnoila, 1991). Two sources of stress served as independent variables: (a) separation from the mother in infancy and, (b) separation from peers in adulthood. Alcohol consumption was the dependent variable. Effects of stress on social interactions with cage mates, including aggression, affiliation, and social dominance were also studied. Metabolites of neurotransmitters in CSF served as the proximal measures of stress.

Rhesus monkeys were randomly assigned at birth to a mother-rearing (MR) or a peer-rearing (PR) condition. In the MR condition infants were raised by their mothers for approximately 7 months at which time they were weaned. They were then placed in a peer group and raised with other monkeys. Peer-reared monkeys were separated from their mothers at birth, raised with other monkeys and fed Similac by human caretakers until the age of weaning. From the age of 7 months the two groups were treated in identical fashion.

At the age of 50 months, adulthood, monkeys in both groups were given access to a red-colored sweetened solution of water containing 7% alcohol for 1 hour a day, 4 days a week for 8 consecutive weeks. The first two weeks served as a baseline, control phase. The final two weeks served as a post-separation phase. During the intervening social separation phase monkeys were housed in individual plexiglass cages where they could hear but not see their cage mates. Sweetened green-colored water as well as the red-colored sweetened water-ethanol solution was available during the separation phase and the pre- and post-separation phases.

Alcohol consumption was affected by the two kinds of stress, separation from the mother in infancy and social separation from peers as adults. Peer-reared monkeys consumed significantly more alcohol than the MR animals during the pre-separation baseline and post-separation recovery phases. Mother-reared animals significantly increased their alcohol consumption during the social separation phase of the experiment occurring in adulthood, matching the PR animals during this phase. Mother-rearing did not provide protection when the offspring encountered a different and very stressful separation from peers in adulthood. As the animals matured, stress induced by social separation decreased, an effect that could be the result of physical maturity, habituation to separation, or both. It is unfortunate that the experimenters did not employ a third group that received MR and PR from birth, the usual social situation in the natural environment. Such a group should have significantly less alcohol consumption following social separation in adulthood than MR and PR animals.

Amount of alcohol consumed in many cases was equivalent to the amount producing a legally drunk blood alcohol concentration in the average adult human male. Some monkeys consumed enough alcohol to fall, vomit, or lapse into unconsciousness despite having available a choice of sweetened water. In addition to consuming more alcohol during the baseline periods, Higley et al. (1991) found that PR monkeys exhibited more behavioral and physiological signs of anxiety and fearful behaviors during their home-cage interactions. An early rearing experience of separation from the mother produced increased neurochemical signs of stress and behavioral signs of anxiety as well as significant increases in alcohol consumption during the pre-social separation baseline phase. Average peak plasma cortisol concentration was positively correlated with the average alcohol consumption and Peer- as compared to Mother-reared monkeys showed significantly higher plasma cortisol and corticotropin concentrations indicating greater activation of the HPA axis and stress in the PR monkeys.

There were no significant gender differences in alcohol consumption. During year 5 norepinephrine as well as serotonin metabolites were negatively correlated with alcohol consumption during the social separation phases. A significant negative correlation between time in social affiliation and alcohol consumption was also found. The greater the amount of time engaged in affiliative behavior the lower the alcohol consumption. Infantile behavior such as ventral clinging was positively correlated with alcohol consumption. Serotonin deficits were correlated with increased alcohol consumption during separation stress. Norepinephrine deficits were correlated with high levels of alcohol consumption during nonstress as well as separation stress periods.

Reliable, stable, individual differences in alcohol consumption were apparent independent of rearing conditions and social separation. These stable individual differences in alcohol consumption were related to heredity. Infant monkeys having no contact with their father and nurtured by foster mothers showed significant correlations with parents in terms of metabolites of norepinephrine, dopamine, and serotonin, as well as the stress hormones cortisol and corticotropin.

Higley et al. (1996a) also observe that the stability of individual differences in serotonin level over time and the correlation of serotonin level with impulsive aggressive behavior suggests that the stability of such forms of aggression may be determined in part by the stability of low levels of serotonin. Although serotonin levels appear sensitive to stress from infancy to adulthood, as the animals matured they were less disturbed by separation as indicated by the decreased affect on dopamine and norepinephrine levels.

Animals with low levels of serotonin are at risk for impulsive aggressiveness and lack of social competence. Peer-reared as compared to MR animals engaged in more violent aggressive behavior and more infant-like ventral clinging. Serotonin level was positively correlated with social competence and negatively correlated with excessive aggression, a relationship repeatedly obtained in human studies. Men who engage in impulsive unplanned acts of violence or arson, also have a lower CSF concentration of metabolites of serotonin than the population average (Virkkunen et al., 1994). In monkeys serotonin metabolites were negatively correlated with spontaneous aggression in the home cage, chases and assaults. Low serotonin levels were also related to aggression induced injuries requiring removal from a cage. The negative correlation between serotonin level and impulsive violent aggression was obtained in female rhesus monkeys as well as males (Higley et al., 1996c).

A positive correlation between serotonin level and social dominance ranking was found by Higley et al., a result obtained by other investigators and with different species of monkeys (Raleigh et al., 1991). A causal relation is suggested in that concentrations of serotonin obtained from monkeys living alone predicted social dominance after they joined a group. A low level of serotonin predicted low social dominance whereas a high level of serotonin obtained during the time the monkey lived in isolation predicted high social dominance after joining a group.

Further evidence that serotonin level is a causal factor related to social dominance is reported by Raleigh et al. (1991). They increased or decreased serotonin levels in nondominant males by administering serotonin agonists or antagonists and removing the dominant male from the group. Increasing or decreasing serotonin levels by pharmacological intervention increased or decreased social dominance of the affected male by increasing or decreasing their affiliative behavior.

These results do not imply that social dominance and affiliative behavior are determined solely by serotonin levels. Affiliative behavior also increases levels of plasma endorphins. Both serotonin and endorphins along with norephinephrine and dopamine need to be studied in the same social situations to fully assess their contributions individually and in combination. Hormones such as testosterone also need to be studied in conjunction with neurotransmitter levels because of their well-known relation to dominance (Bernhardt, 1997; Kemper, 1990).

Despite the striking implications of the research by Higley and his colleagues for the understanding of an experiential risk factor of separation stress for alcoholism, it must be kept in mind that the implications are basically correlational in nature. Separation stress, from mother or peers, is clearly followed by heightened alcohol consumption and lower levels of serotonin. However, it cannot be concluded that low levels of serotonin caused the increase in drinking. More complex causality may be at work. Separation stress induces lower levels of serotonin, but stress also activates the HPA axis, producing a momentary increase in beta-endorphin levels, the release of stress hormones, and a heightened level of orienting. Persistent stress results in lowered levels of endorphins and serotonin which interacts with and modulates dopamine in reaction to alcohol ingestion (Olauuson et al., 1998). Consumption of alcohol under these circumstances may produce a disproportionately greater reinforcement from endorphins than normal. A similar effect may be obtained as a consequence of a positive family history of alcohlism (Gianoulakis et al., 1989).

Trauma

One of the more surprising results we obtained some years ago in a study of 280 middle class adolescents in treatment for chemical dependency was the high rate of physical and sexual abuse they had experienced (Maltzman & Schweiger, 1991). Approximately 75% of the females and 43% of the males had experienced abuse. Sexual abuse was more commonly reported by the females and physical abuse by the males. Differences between abused and nonabused adolescents were observed on a number of measures. Abused adolescents were significantly lower in self-esteem, higher in neuroticism, and performed more poorly than the nonabused adolescents on an educational achievment scale. They were more severely dependent on alcohol and other drugs, less socialized, and reported greater anger than the nonabused adolescents in treatment. Abused adolescents also reported significantly less organization in their family environment than nonabused adolescent patients.

A high rate of sexual and physical abuse among the adolescent patients suggests that abuse, especially sexual abuse of females, may be a risk factor for alcoholism. Our study had not been designed with the specific purpose of examining sexual and physical abuse in adolescents. As a result, severity of abuse was not evaluated using DSM criteria. We could not determine whether or not instances of abuse met the criteria for posttraumatic stress disorder (PTSD). We also failed to measure frequency and severity of abuse. Information identifying the adolescents who had experienced abuse was obtained from alcoholism counselor reports. Incidence of abuse in our comparison group of adolescents could not be determined for ethical and legal reasons.

A review of the relevant literature indicates that the incidence of physical and sexual abuse, especially among children and adolescents, may vary considerably depending on the method of assessment. Adults as well as adolescents are ashamed, embarrassed, and afraid to report their experience to an unfamiliar interviewer. A variety of variables may influence reporting sexual abuse in children as well as adults. One reason the rate of abuse appears to be high in our study is that the information was obtained by a trusted counselor in a supportive environment. Research suggests that surveys attempting to obtain information of a personal nature such as sexual abuse, drug use or other kinds of stigmatized behavior, may not obtain accurate information unless special efforts are made to assure privacy and trust (Turner et al., 1998). Proper wording and contexts for the questions soliciting information on sexual and physical abuse are critically important in the construction of reliable and valid interviews (Stewart, 1996).

An extensive body of literature has developed on trauma, including sexual abuse, and its emotional consequences. Trauma, especially posttraumatic stress disorder (PTSD) may be a risk factor for alcohol and other drug misuse because PTSD appears to share much the same physiological basis as alcoholism. Sexual abuse in women is especially pertinent because of its high rate and the relatively high percentage of such experiences leading to PTSD and/or alcoholism and other drug use.

A study by Miller, Down and Testa (1993) sheds some light on the relationship between sexual abuse and alcohol misuse. It assessed the effect of different kinds and levels of child abuse on the level of adult alcohol consumption and the specificity of the effect. Is sexual abuse a risk factor limited to alcohol misuse or is it a risk factor for a variety of other disorders as well? Miller et al. (1993) studied five different samples totaling 472 lower socioeconomic status women in western New York State. Participants were obtained from: (a) outpatient alcoholism clinics, (b) department of motor vehicles classes for first time drunk driver offenders (DWI), (c) outpatient mental health clinics, (d) shelters for battered women, and (e) a random household sample,

Alcohol problems were evaluated in terms of DSM-III-R criteria as well as additional scales assessing drinking patterns and alcohol related problems. Using these criteria all the women in treatment for alcoholism, 100%, were categorized as having lifetime alcohol-related problems; 62% of the DWI sample, 43% of the battered women sample, 51% of the mental health sample, and 18% of the household sample had an alcohol problem sometime in their lives.

Results indicate that the prevalence of sexual abuse was disproportionately greater among the heaviest drinkers, women in treatment for alcoholism. Prevalence of sexual abuse was significantly greater for women in treatment for alcoholism than for women in treatment for nonalcohol related problems. There is some specificity to the relationship between childhood sexual abuse of females and alcoholism in adulthood.

A relationship between sexual abuse culminating in PTSD and alcoholism is suggested by the results obtained in a national comorbidity survey. Kessler et al. (1995) conducted a national representative face-to-face survey designed to assess PTSD and its comorbidity using the criteria of DSM-III-R defining PTSD as: [a] exposure to a traumatic event that is 'outside the range of usual human experience'; [b] reliving the experience in nightmares, flashbacks, or intrusive thoughts; [c] numbing or avoidant symptoms; and [d] hypersensitivity, either as indicated by general signs and symptoms of autonomic arousal or by hypersensitivity to cues reminiscent of the trauma. These symptoms must persist for at least 1 month' . (Kessler, 1995, p. 1048).

Data were collected from approximately 8000 respondents in a stratified probability sample of the noninstitutionalized civilian population 15 - 54 years old. A structured diagnostic interview was designed to provide diagnoses corresponding to the DSM-III-R classifications of PTSD, affective, anxiety and panic disorders, antisocial personality, alcohol abuse without dependence, alcohol dependence, drug abuse without dependence and drug dependence. Questions were also asked concerning the duration of symptoms of PTSD and their onset in relation to the target trauma. Additonal questions concerned each of 12 different types of traumas that may have been experienced as well as an open ended question about experiences that might qualify as traumas as defined by DSM-III-R.

Results indicated that the overall lifetime prevalence of reported PTSD was 7.8%. There was a significant gender difference. Women were more than twice as likely to have experienced PTSD during their lifetime than men, 10.4% versus 5.0%. The majority of individuals exposed to a traumatic experience, however, did not develop PTSD. Approximately 61% of the men and 51% of the women reported at least one traumatic experience during their lifetimes. The largest proportion of traumas were witnessing someone being injured or killed, and being involved in a life-threatening accident. In each case a higher proportion of men than women experienced these traumas as well as physical attacks, and combat experience. A significantly higher proportion of women than men experienced rape, 9% vs. 0.7% and molestation, 12.3% versus 2.8%. Women exposed to trauma were more than twice as likely to develop PTSD than men, 20.4% versus 8.2%. For men the most upsetting trauma most commonly associated with PTSD was combat exposure, 29%, and witnessing an accident or death, 24%. For women, rape was the experience most commonly associated with PTSD and reported as most upsetting, 30%, followed by sexual molestation, 19%. Almost half the cases of PTSD in women were related to these two traumatic experiences.

A lifetime comorbidity of PTSD with at least one other DSM-III-R disorder was common, occurring in 88% of the men and 79% of the women. The problem is to determine which was primary, had an earlier age of onset and possibly served as a risk factor for the disorder that followed. Results of analyses by Kessler et al. (1995) indicate that PTSD in men and women usually preceded comorbid affective disorders and alcohol and other drug disorders, and in women, comorbid conduct disorder. Alcohol abuse/dependence was comorbid in 52% of the men with PTSD; alcohol abuse/dependence developed in the absence of PTSD in 34% of the men in this sample. For women, alcohol abuse/dependence and PTSD were comorbid in 28% of the respondents. Alcohol abuse/dependence occurred in 14% of the women in the absence of PTSD. For the majority of individuals who had a history of alcohol and other drug abuse or dependence and comorbid PTSD, the PTSD was primary, had an earlier onset than the drug misuse. Posttraumatic stress disorder may therefore serve as a risk factor for alcoholism, but the reverse may also be true, although with a lower frequency. A closer examination of the biobehavioral characteristics of PTSD is necessary to answer the question of how it might serve as a risk factor for alcoholism.

An analysis of the neurobiological research on PTSD has led Yehuda (1997) to formulate a theory of enhanced negative feedback regulation of cortisol that accounts for much of the clinical and neurobiological characteristics of the disorder. It also suggests why PTSD is a risk factor for alcoholism. Yehuda proposes that the neurobiological alterations underlying PTSD are different from the stress reaction observed in most trauma. Only a small percentage of people suffering a traumatic experience develop PTSD as we have seen above. The analogy with the distinction between alcohol consumption and alcoholism is obvious, but there is more than mere analogy involved. Yehuda (1997) suggests PTSD as distinguished from trauma without PTSD is produced by dysregulation of the HPA axis as a consequence of heightened negative feedback from cortisol.

Paradoxically, depression and PTSD manifest different extremes of circulating cortisol levels. Depression is often accompanied by high levels of cortisol whereas

PTSD is accompanied by low levels (Resnick, Yehuda, Pitman, & Foy, 1995; Yehuda et al., 1995). Yehuda (1997) resolves the paradox by observing that two factors are involved in the dynamics of the closed-loop HPA axis. Physiological and behavioral effects of cortisol depend on the level of the steroid and the number and sensitivity of glucocorticoid receptors with which it can bind. The number and sensitivity of such receptors are reduced in clinical depression thereby reducing the physiological and behavioral effects of cortisol. "Down regulation" of receptors occurs in response to excessive levels of cortisol in depression. It brings about a homeostatic adjustment, balancing out the effects of excessive cortisol by decreasing the number of receptors to which it can bind and have a biological and behavioral effect. In PTSD the number and sensitivity of glucocorticoid receptors is greater than in nontraumatized people. It is unclear which came first, the increased number of receptors which lowered the level of cortisol or the low level of cortisol which "upregulated" the number and sensitivity of glucocorticoid receptors. Another interesting question, analogous to one in alcoholism, is whether the unusually low level of cortisol and large number of sensitive glucocorticoid receptors reported in PTSD is a consequence of PTSD or was present prior to the trauma and is a risk factor for PTSD. Regardless of whether the condition was a risk factor for PTSD or occurred as a result, once the HPA axis is characterized by low cortisol levels and high receptor sensitivity, it functions in a characteristic manner, one which produces the kind of behavior seen in PTSD victims. It may also characterize a risk factor for alcoholism.

Evidence of abnormally low cortisol levels accompanying PTSD previously seen in combat veterans was provided in a study of holocaust survivors. The latter trauma victims consisted of one subgroup with PTSD, a second without PTSD, and a matched control group that had not suffered trauma or PTSD. There were no morbid conditions in the three groups other than PTSD in the index group. Results showed that the index group had significantly lower cortisol levels, an effect produced some 50 years earlier, than the holocaust subgroup without PTSD and the control group.

A study of rape victims provides suggestive evidence that low cortisol levels and previous trauma are risk factors for PTSD following later trauma (Resnick et al., 1995). Blood samples for assessing cortisol were drawn from rape victims within two days of their trauma. Approximately three months later they were assessed for PTSD and a history of possible previous assaults. Women who had been raped previously had significantly lower cortisol levels but a higher probability of developing PTSD following the index rape than women who had not been assaulted prior to the index rape. Low cortisol levels are a risk factor for PTSD if trauma is experienced.

As previously suggested, one of the functions of cortisol is to provide feedback to the pituitary gland to reduce its production of ACTH and signal the adrenal cortex to reduce its release of cortisol. This negative feedback results in excessive circulating CRF despite the appearance of normal levels of ACTH. Blocking the synthesis of cortisol, removing its negative feedback inhibition of the pituitary gland, results in more than four times higher ACTH levels in PTSD than control subjects suggesting that there are significantly higher levels of hypothalamic released CRF in PTSD than in control subjects (Yehuda, 1997). Behavioral effects characteristic of anxiety may be produced by CRF (Tershner & Helmstetter, 1996). This is why giving alcohol to alcoholics increases their anxiety. It stimulates the HPA which contributes to already high circulating levels of CRF.

Recall the results of Gianoulakis and her colleagues showing a low basal level of beta-endorphins in FH+ subjects which increases markedly with an alcohol challenge (Gianoulakis et al., 1996). The enhanced endorphin response suggests increased sensitivity due to upregulation of opioidergic receptors. Recall also that Schuckit and his colleagues show low response levels of cortisol and ACTH to alcohol in FH+ subjects (Schuckit et al., 1987; Schuckit et al., 1988), suggesting that there is a heightened negative feedback inhibition in subjects at risk for alcoholism. Low response level individuals at risk for alcoholism appear to have a similar dysregulation of the HPA system as PTSD victims. There is also a reasonable possibility that the dysregulation of the HPA system preceded, is a risk, for PTSD in individuals exposed to trauma (Resnick et al., 1995). High comorbidity of PTSD and alcoholism may be the consequence of the same enhanced negative feedback system of the HPA axis posing a risk factor for alcoholism and PTSD. This interpretation supports in part a compensation theory of alcoholism reinforcement. Low levels of endorphins as a consequence of heredity or PTSD are compensated for by alcohol consumption. This is not the entire story because endorphins are not the sole source of reinforcement for alcohol consumption. It is an important one, but not the only one as we have seen. The complete behavioral sequence of approaching and consuming alcohol includes initially orienting to alcohol and then consuming it with reinforcement of the sequence from dopamine, norepinephrine, serotonin, and other neurotransmitters.

Heavy drinking as a function of the social environment:
Occupational and social variables

For most men and a rapidly increasing percentage of women, half their waking hours at least five days a week are occupied by an income producing activity. One might assume that jobs that are stressful will increase the risk for alcoholism because as we already have seen, certain kinds of stress and trauma are risk factors. If you have a tyrannical boss and for whatever reason you are locked into the position, the job market is poor for someone with your skills, you need the money desperately, the stress experienced may increase the risk for excessive alcohol consumption. A job which is boring, repetitive, uninteresting and over which the worker has little control or social support may also be stressful and lead to increased alcohol consumption (Hemmingson & Lundberg, 1998).

It is not a simple matter to assess characteristics of an occupation that may constitute a risk factor for alcoholism and avoid confounding factors such as self-selection. For example, people with a disposition toward heavy drinking may disproportionately apply for work in certain occupations such as breweries or bar tending. It is possible to address the problem within a longitudinal study: assess people before they enter an occupation and after several years follow up those that remain in the index occupation as compared to those that move into different occupations. A study of this sort has been conducted on brewery workers (Whitehead & Simpkins, 1983). Such an occupation may attract people who are already heavy drinkers, in part because a tradition in many breweries in the past is that they would have "beer breaks" instead of coffee breaks. Nevertheless, it is possible to disentangle self-selection from the occupation per se, and yes, brewery workers are at risk independently of the self-selection factor.

Whitehead and Simpkins (1983) attacked the general problem of occupation as a risk factor by first reviewing the available studies of occupations and work-place drinking and their characteristics considered risk factors for heavy drinking or alcoholism. A bipolar semantic-differential scale (Osgood, Suci, & Tannenbaum, 1957) was then used to assess the relative presence or absence of risk factors by having three sociologists rate on a risk scale each of the 43 structural characteristics of jobs that were isolated in the review of drinking in different occupations. Mean ratings ranged from 1-5 with a 1 meaning the absence of a structural characteristic related to risk and 5 meaning the definite presence of such a characteristic. A correlational analysis was conducted relating characteristics of occupations to the prevalence of alcoholism and the heavy consumption of alcohol. Eight characteristics were retained which correlated at least 0.30 with prevalence of alcoholism and heavy consumption. A mean characteristic rating of 4 or greater was taken to define a high risk profession. These occupations are: "entertainment (4.42); army- based in the United States (4.41); navy- carrier-based (4.41); pipeline construction (4.33); navy- shore-based (4.30); marine corps (4.25); oil rig work (4.17); army- based overseas (4.16); alcohol-beverage work (4.13); sales- on the road (4.09); seafaring (4.09); tavern keeping (4.04); and publicans [innkeeper] (4.00)." (Whitehead & Simpkins, 1983, p. 477). Two characteristics explained 66% of the variance in the rate of alcoholism: social pressure to drink and the ready availability of inexpensive alcoholic beverages. Five characteristics accounted for 68% of the variance in the rate of alcohol consumption in the at-risk occupations: peer approval of heavy drinking, ready availability of inexpensive alcoholic beverages; a preponderance of young workers, official sanction of heavy drinking, and recruitment of heavy drinkers. It is apparent that the three additional risk factors account for a small amount of additional variance.

Risk factors for heavy drinking and alcoholism isolated by Whitehead and Simpkins (1983) are applicable to the analysis of a variety of circumstances and living conditions. Fraternities in particular come to mind. Their members characteristically approve of heavy drinking and there is a ready availability of inexpensive or even free alcoholic beverages courtesy of breweries with policies of two kegs for the price of one, donations of beer kegs to intramural athletic events, etc. Reversal of these risk factors have the opposite effect, a decline in consumption and alcohol related problems. During Desert Storm, fought in Arab countries where the sale and consumption of alcohol by Muslims is forbidden, American soldiers had little opportunity to drink. Rate of disciplinary problems and alcohol abuse was reportedly lower than in any previous overseas army operation.

Changing the culture of an occupation can reduce the rate of alcoholism and heavy drinking. With the cooperation of AA, the union and management, using recovering alcoholics in positions within the heavy drinking culture of sand hogs, the heavy drinking subculture could be changed (Sonnenstuhl, 1996).

An implication of Whitehead and Simpkins' (1983) study is that a particular subculture represented by an occupation may serve as a risk factor for alcoholism in addition to genetic and stress risk factors. When alcoholic beverages are readily available, heavy drinking is approved, and there is social pressure to drink, individuals in such a situation are at increased risk for alcohol misuse problems. Drinking at a consistently relatively high level may escalate into alcoholism in the apparent absence of sources of unusual stress and a family history of alcoholism. Factors of ready availability of inexpensive alcohol and social reinforcement may be all that is needed for an increased risk of alcoholism. Presence of job related chronic stress adds to the risk. Job related stress as a factor based on self-report is difficult to assess (Ames & Janes, 1992). It is correlational in nature and time precedence and directionality are difficult to determine. Which came first, the heavy drinking or the reported stress? Stress may increase drinking but structural characterisics of an occupation will facilitate or prevent drinking on the job and thereby increase or decrease the risk of alcoholism independent of stress. You can't be drinking on the job if you are working in a fast food place all day or are a check-out clerk in a supermarket. You can if you are a jazz musician playing in a bar or night club.

Another approach to the study of alcohol consumption and alcoholism in different occupations was adopted by Parker and Harford (1992). Extensive data have been collected on the prevalence of drinkers and of alcohol dependence in different occupations as a result of a nationwide household survey conducted by the National Center for Health Statistics. Direct interviews of more than 43,000 respondents were obtained. An advantage of such a survey is its size and the number of occupations for which information can be obtained. It also has disadvantages. A household survey does not interview people in the armed services, traditionally characterized as a heavy drinking occupation (Whitehead & Simpkins, 1983), transients, homeless, and many entertainers who are "on the road" playing jobs in different cities, living in hotels, and not having a permanent address. They all would be overlooked and all would tend to be heavy drinkers.

Interpretations of descriptive statistics on the prevalence of alcoholism in different occupations are difficult without further analyses. Many variables may combine to determine the outcome: income, available health care programs, age of workers, gender, etc. Given the above caveats, we can turn to some of Parker and Harford's (1992) results. Descriptively, the prevalence of alcohol consumption seems to be a function of income, a higher percentage of individuals consume alcohol in the managerial, professsional, and technical occupations than in white and blue collar occupations. More than 80% of architects and people in health occupations such as physicians and dentists are current consumers of alcohol. In contrast, 65% of construction workers, coal minors and oil well drillers consume alcohol; less then 65% of truck drivers consume alcohol. Prevalence of alcohol dependence as defined by DSM-III-R is a different matter. Architects show a 9% prevalence of alcohol dependence and physicians and dentists show an alcoholism prevalence rate of only 1%. In contrast, construction workers show an alcoholism prevalence rate of 8% and coal miners and oil well drillers have a 14% prevalence rate of alcohol dependence (Parker & Harford, 1992).

Reasons for the differences between percentage of alcohol consumers and percentage of people suffering from alcohol dependence in various occupations are many. One important factor is the presence of a drinking subculture within the occupation. Development of such a subculture is more likely when there are a group of people working in the same physical location who share similar norms and attitudes towards drinking. A further important condition is that alcohol is available and accepted in the workplace, and social life off the job as well as on the job centers around socializing with co-workers. As I observed, jazz musicians in the '30s and '40s were such a subculture. A similar subculture is unlikely to develop in the operatng room. It is more likely to develop among the workers on a construction site who eat lunch together, interact continuously, have coffee breaks together and ride together to and from work, all occasions when they can drink, once the social norms are established that accept, approve, and pressure individuals to participate in such behavior (Ames & Janes, 1992).

Nationalities, ethnic and religious groups may also vary in rates of alcohol consumption and the prevalence of alcoholism. Studies of these groups have been conducted for many years and the similarities and differences in the prevalence of alcohol consumption as compared to alcohol dependence are intriguing, but difficult to adequately assess. There is no doubt, however, that ethnicity as a subculture is of considerable importance in the consideration of population risk factors (Helzer & Canino, 1992).

Drinking on college campuses

If there is one subculture where alcohol consumption and alcohol problems are primarily determined by the two important environmental variables of ready availability of alcohol and social approval of heavy drinking, it would be on many college campuses, particularly fraternities and sororities. Not every campus, however, is a gin mill. There is variability among campuses as a function of location, historical period, size, academic emphasis, ethnic make-up, and tradition. A large metropolitan university where the majority of students live at home and commute to school will have less drinking on the average than a university located in a small college town where almost all students live in dormitories and fraternity and sorority houses.

Every year we read stories in the newspapers about accidental deaths caused directly or indirectly by excessive drinking, usually in college fraternities. Two young men on my campus died May, 1997 in alcohol related accidents. For some years now fraternities and sororities on the UCLA campus have agreed to conduct "dry rushes" and to control their parties, limit drinks, require IDs and evidence that participants are of drinking age, 21 or older. Ostensibly, the fraternities adher to the rules, otherwise they are in danger of losing recognition from the university and their national organization. Some fraternities follow the spirit as well as the letter of the rule. Others do not. Some circumvent the rule by holding their parties off campus, away from their houses. One fraternity had a weekend party at the Lake Mead Recreational Area where fraternity members and guests had been drinking heavily. Apparently, one of the fraternity members known to be a good swimmer dived into the lake from a cliff. A fraternity brother noticed that he did not surface after the dive and dived in to search for him. Both drowned. Two promising young men died as a result of their disorientation, lack of judgment and motor coordination caused by their excessive alcohol consumption. One of them was underage.

For the past approximately half a century there have been a variety of studies on college campuses investigating correlates of drinking and excessive drinking (Engs & Hanson, 1985; Straus & Bacon, 1953). One of the best and most extensive of these studies has been conducted by Wechsler, Dowdall, Davenport, and Castillo, (1995). They analyzed episodic heavy drinking, or binge drinking as they called it, defined as 5 or more drinks in one sitting for a male and 4 or more for a female, in a representative sample of 17,592 students from 140 four year colleges. Ethnic make-up of the sample was White-Americans, 81%; Asians-Americans, 7%; Latino-Americans, 7%; African-American, 6%; and Native-Americans, 1%. Wechsler et al. observe that college students are at the age of highest binge drinking rates. They drink in this manner at an even higher rate than their noncollege age peers. Very little difference was found in binge drinking below the legal drinking age of 21 and 21 and older among these college students. A much higher probability of drinking for age below 24 than above was found.

Variables that increased the risk for binge drinking were, being White, binging in high school, considering partying an important part of college life and not considering religion very important. Considering athletics very important and community service not very important also were risk factors for heavy drinking. The strongest risk factor was living in a fraternity or a sorority. Living in a sorority was a greater risk factor for women binging then living in a fraternity for men binging. Using marijuana and smoking cigarettes on a typical day were also strong risk factors for binge drinking.

Results obtained by Wechsler et al. (1995) are in accord with results we obtained in a much smaller convenience sample from a single university (Schall et al., 1992) studying a somewhat different set of variables. Our analysis of drinking in a sample of approximately 700 students concentrated on personality and social environment risk factors. We found the usual risk factors of gender and ethnicity, but it must be kept in mind that each of these variables is represented by mean scores that are averaged over a variety of subgroups. There is an apparent gender difference. White men overall drank significantly more than White women. However, the difference is largely due to the fact that more White women were abstinent during the previous month than men. If we examine only those who do drink, there was little difference between White females and males. This suggests, recalling the research on first-pass metabolism, that White college women who do drink are at greater risk for the negative consequences of alcohol than White men.

We found significant ethnic differences. White and Hispanic students were the heaviest drinkers on campus with mean alcohol consumption during the past month of 15.54 oz and 13.02 oz, respectively. Again, means are misleading. Examining results of males and females separately within the ethnic groups showed that male and female Hispanics drank 37.42 oz and 7.17 oz, respectively as compared to White males and females who drank 22.89 oz and 11.50 oz, respectively. These were the only two ethnic groups on campus that showed a significant gender difference but it must be remembered that each of these groups are also aggregates. Hispanics differ depending on country of origin, Cuba, Mexico, Puerto Rico, South and Central American (Office of Applied Statistics, 1998). Our sample was not large enough to examine differences as a function of country of family origin among Hispanics or among Asians where, again, they include students of Japanese,

Chinese, Vietnamese, Samoan, Korean, and Indian origin. There are considerable differences in alcohol consumption among these countries (Helzer & Canino, 1992). Whites can also be subdivided into white ethnic groups differing traditionally in alcohol consumption and problems (McCready, Greeley, & Thiesen, (1983).

Schall et al. 1992 found that mean alcohol consumption for Asians or Pacific Islanders was 4.04 oz, 4.82 oz for African-Americans, and 11.64 oz for Native Americans or Alaskan Natives. None of these groups showed significant gender differences.

Risk factors may also be considered in the light of the area of study selected by the students, remembering that 79% of the students were freshman and data were collected during the fall quarter, before they could be fully acculturated into their major. Lowest levels of alcohol consumption were by women in engineering and physical science 3.24 oz, and 3.12 oz, respectively. Lowest levels of consumption by males were in life science, 10.83 oz, engineering, 16.35 oz, and physical science, 16.97 oz. Heaviest drinking women were in fine arts, 15.73 oz as was true of men, 36.39 oz. Students in the "soft" areas drank significantly more than students in the "hard" areas.

There may well be differences in personality among males and females concentrating in the "soft" areas of fine arts, humanities, and social sciences as compared to engineering, physical and life sciences. I would predict that the former students would score higher on the sensation seeking scales, and lower on socialization than the students in the "hard" areas. Both personality characteristics are significantly correlated with alcohol use. We had the data, unfortunately, we did not analyze these relationships. We should have. Another possible confound which we did not study because of the small numbers of students involved is that Asian-American students tend to major more frequently in the "hard" subject areas, engineering, mathematics and physics, and their levels of alcohol consumption are low. We need, therefore, to analyze Whites, Asians, etc., within each of the major study areas to control for confounds. In other words, compare White students who major in soft versus "hard" areas, Asian-Americans who take soft and hard majors, African-Americans in the two areas of concentration. Unfortunately, we did not have a large enough sample to conduct such analyses. It would not be difficult for large representative surveys of drinking on college campuses to add questions on areas of concentration, ethnicity, and personality and tease apart their relations to alcohol consumption and problems.

We did examine alcohol consumption by residence. Again, relatively small numbers of students in some living arrangements required our combining groups. The two largest groups lived at home with their families or in dormitories. Men and women who lived at home consumed significantly less alcohol than dormitory residents. We also compared consumption of students affiliated with sororities and fraternities, pledges for fraternities and sororoities, those who reported that they might join, and those who reported that they would never join. Heaviest drinkers by far were the male pledges to fraternities. Our study was conducted during the fall quarter and the pledges were being entertained by visits to the fraternity houses. Male pledges drank 48.83 oz of alcohol during the previous 30 days as compared to 29.29 oz for members of the fraternities, 21.20 oz by students who might join and 11.32 oz by those students reporting they would never join a fraternity or sorority. These results suggest that there is some self-selection. Students planning to join a fraternity drink more than those who would never join. Women showed similar trends but with significantly lower levels of consumption then the men.

A statistical model of our results showed that major risk factors for heavy drinking were sensation seeking, particularly the Disinhibition subscale of the Sensation Seeking Scale (Zuckerman, 1979), Availability of Alcohol Drinking Contexts, and drinking to cope with personal problems. These results suggest that personality traits are important risk factors interacting with the ready availability of alcohol and social reinforcement for its heavy use. Paramount among these personality risk factors appear to be impulsive sensation seeking. This is a confirmation of some of the results obtained in an important early "natural experiment."

Students entering the University of Minnesota between 1945 and 1963 received the Minnesota Multiphasic Personality Inventory (MMPI) as part of a project standardizing this widely used personality inventory. Hoffmann, Loper, and Kammier (1974), searched the records of the two largest alcoholism treatment facilities in the state of Minnesota for patients who had been students at the University during the period some 13 years earlier when the MMPI testing had occurred. A group of such men was found. Their MMPI scores were compared to classmates receiving the MMPI who did not go on to receive alcoholism treatment in a Minnesota facility.

Results showed that college students who subsequently developed alcoholism as defined by treatment in a hospital were not distinguishable from their classmates on the basis of anxiety or depression. Students at risk were more extraverted, adventuresome, and defiant of authority. Their MMPI profiles were significantly higher than their cohorts on scales 4 and 9, psychopathic deviate, Pd, and hypomania, Ma. They were not at risk because of anxiety and depression and they were not significantly more maladjusted. These results are contrary to the implication of the tension reduction and stress dampening hypotheses that the anxiolytic effect of alcohol, its ability to reduce anxiety, serves as a reinforcer for greater alcohol consumption. All scores were within the normal range. The MMPI was readministered to the index group of former students as part of an assessment battery following admission to an alcoholism treatment facility. While hospitalized for alcoholism treatment they reported very different personality characteristics than when they were students. They now showed high levels of anxiety, depression, and feelings of inadequacy (Hoffmann, Loper, & Kammeier, 1974; Kammeier, Hoffmann, & Loper, 1973; Loper, Kammeier, & Hoffmann, 1973).

Our hypothesis is that the personality change from extraverted, outgoing sensation seeker to depressed dysphoric alcoholic is due to their chronic alcohol consumption. It resulted in activation of the HPA axis and enhancement of the negative feedback inhibition resulting in excessive release of CRF. The latter produces symptoms of anxiety and sensitizes the individual to such reactions in situations that previously would not induce dysphoric behavior (Tershner & Helmstetter, 1996).

Results of the Minnesota group, Wechsler, our own research, Engs, Hanson, and many others, show that a personality trait of high sensation or novelty seeking and extraversion combined with the availability of alcohol and reinforcement for heavy drinking, the situation found on many college campuses, especially in many fraternities and sororities, is a risk for alcoholism.

DEVELOPMENT OF ALCOHOL DEPENDENCE:

ANIMAL MODELS

Animal models of alcohol dependence have been developed by selectively breeding strains of preferring and nonpreferring rodents or heavy and light drinking animals (Begleiter & Kissin, 1995). Stress as a risk factor has also been illuminated by animal models as indicated in the experiments on the effects of separation and isolation stress. Chronic alcohol consumption as a risk factor for alcoholism independently of inherited vulnerability, prenatal alcohol exposure, and environmental stress, has also been studied via an animal model. It examines sociobiological factors influencing alcohol consumption over the long term and captures variables generating a risk for alcohol dependence by merely having available a free choice between water and different alcohol-water solutions (Wolffgramm & Heyne, 1995). An unusual feature of the core experiment by Wolffgramm and his collaborators is its longevity. It covered the lifetime of a rat, nine months with a choice of water or an alcohol and water cocktail, nine months of alcohol deprivation, and a final nine months of choice of water or alcohol-water solutions with experimental variations including choice of water or an alcohol cocktail spiked with quinine.

Effects of housing

A feature of the studies by Wolffgramm and his colleagues is the investigation of several social variables during the "social drinking" phase of the rats' lives, before they developed alcohol dependence as well as after. For example, Wolffgramm (1991) studied the effects on alcohol consumption of living under different housing conditions. Rats were randomly assigned to group, individual, or housing in contact cages. The latter consisted of individual cages separated by bars from other cages, permitting visual and auditory cues of other animals each in its individual cage. Group-housed rats were maintained in groups of four/cage. To study the effects of separation, each of the group-housed animals was placed in an isolated individual cage one day a week. Once a week social behavior was observed by placing the rats living in group cages in an open field for 15 min and videotaping their behavior for later analysis. Standard chow and water were available ad lib for all animals.

There were four major phases to the study, (a) 4-week base period when only water was available followed by, (b) 9-month period in which water and 5%, 10% and 20% alcohol solutions were available, the free choice situation followed by, (c) as long as nine months abstinence, only water available in the four drinking tubes and, (d) a final phase in which water and the 5%, 10%, and 20% alcohol solutions were again available. A number of subexperiments were conducted during the final phase varying housing conditions and introducing additional choices among other drugs, primarily diazepam. A final six-week period involved a choice between water and the alcohol-water solutions laced with noxious tasting quinine.

Results showed that average alcohol consumption during the first week of the experimental phase did not vary significantly as a function of housing condition.

Differences developed as a function of housing after one week. Animals normally living in group cages and then isolated for one day a week consumed significantly more alcohol during isolation then any other group. Animals housed individually on a continual basis were the second heaviest alcohol consumers. Animals in group housing and in individual contact cages consumed the smallest amounts of alcohol. Differences between the latter two groups were not significant. Variability within each of the groups was high despite the significant differences in consumption between isolated and non-isolated animals. Effects of short-term isolation habituated. After 3-4 months animals temporarily isolated did not differ from the group housed animals. Long-term isolated animals continued to maintain higher levels of alcohol consumption than group-housed animals.

During the first week of the experimental period almost all the animals preferred the 5% solution to the higher concentrations. Preferences shifted after this initial period as a function of social separation. Rats in group housing maintained their 5% solution preference with very little consumption of the 10% and 20% solutions except when they were in temporary isolation where a preference for the 20% concentration appeared. Most animals housed in permanent isolation shifted to the 20% concentration within two weeks. Animals in the contact cages showed a similar decline in preference for the 5% concentration and an increase in consumption of the 20% concentration although their total alcohol consumption was less than the permanent isolation group. Least preferred in all groups was the 10% concentration. Individual differences in drinking patterns were apparent. Animals preferring the 20% solution were analogous to binge drinkers, consuming a high dose at one time and drinking tap water at other times. Animals preferring the 5% alcohol concentration drank this solution almost exclusively. Total fluid intake as well as food intake was similar under all housing conditions.

Individual differences and long-term effects

Wolffgram and Heyne (1991) determined whether individual differences in alcohol consumption within housing conditions were related to state or trait variables. Animals were observed in the open field once a week in "tetradic encounters" at the start of the study prior to introduction of alcohol and other drugs, providing measures of social dominance and play.

Individual differences persisted as a function of dominance level with a significant negative correlation between social dominance and alcohol consumption. Regardless of housing conditions animals that were high in social dominance, determined prior to the introduction of alcohol, drank significantly less alcohol than low dominance animals. Low dominance animals living in isolation, therefore not affected by the stress of lack of dominance, drank significantly more than animals living in isolation who were high in dominance. These results indicate that the individual differences in alcohol consumption as a function of dominance is a trait variable not a temporary state variable induced by the stress of low dominance when encountering animals in the open field. Stable housing conditions were essential for the maintenaince of the negative relationship between social dominance and alcohol consumption. Moving the rats once a week from one housing condition to another disrupted the relationship, increasing alcohol consumption in the socially dominant rats. Their alcohol consumption eventually reached the levels of the socially subordinate animals living in unchanged housing conditions.

Neurochemical effects

A related experiment demonstrated that differences in alcohol consumption as a function of housing have a neurochemical basis (Rilke, May, Oehler, & Wolffgramm, 1995). Rats maintained in isolation and drinking only tap water showed a significant reduction in striatal D2 dopaminergic receptor density in comparison to group-housed animals drinking water. Group-housed animals drinking a 6% alcohol solution also showed a significant reduction in the density of their D2 dopaminergic receptors. On the other hand, long term alcohol consumption resulted in a significant increase in receptor density in the individually housed animals so that their D2 receptor density reached the level of control animals drinking water and living in group housing (Rilke et al., 1995; Wolffgramm & Heyne, 1995). An interaction between alcohol consumption and housing provides striking evidence of the biological effects of the social environment, housing conditions, on brain neurochemistry and alcohol consumption. Evidence is also provided of the dialectical interactions taking place in the maintenance of homeostasis of the internal biological and external social environments mediated by behavior.

Physical dependence on alcohol

Wolffgramm and Heynes (1995) found that continued availability of water and the three alcohol dosage levels resulted in relatively stable individual differences in alcohol consumption for approximately 25-40 weeks at which time the level of alcohol consumption spontaneously increased. Growing tolerance does not seem to be the factor responsible for the increase since tolerance should have increased long before 25 weeks of alcohol consumption. When access to alcohol was interrupted for up to 4 weeks and then made available once again there was a significant increase in alcohol consumption following the return to drinking. During the alcohol withdrawal period the threshold for reaction to foot shock was significantly lower than before or after the deprivation period suggesting that long term chronic alcohol consumption resulted in lower levels of circulating endorphins, increasing the sensitivity to pain. The increase in alcohol consumption after 25 weeks could be due to the down regulation in the number of opioidergic receptors. Increased alcohol consumption was necessary to activate the decreased number of receptors for beta-endorphins. Following a period of alcohol deprivation there was an up-regulation of opioidergic receptors compensating for the lowered level of circulating endorphins. When alcohol consumption was made available following the period of deprivation there was much greater reinforcement from alcohol released beta-endorphins due to the larger number of opioidergic receptors. Consumption of alcohol increased. Down-regulation once more occurred providing a homeostatic balance.

A greater alcohol withdrawal effect and clearer evidence of the development of behavioral dependence on alcohol appears when a longer period of free choice of alcohol is permitted before enforced abstinence. Nine months of alcohol consumption followed by withdrawal of alcohol for approximately 9 months followed by a return to a choice of water versus three alcohol dosages showed that the alcohol experienced animals drank significantly more than matched alcohol-naive animals. They also drank more than the level they attained before abstinence was introduced. A preference for alcohol persisted during abstinence equivalent to a third of a lifetime of the average rat. They then quickly "relapsed" and given the choice of water versus "cocktails" drank significantly more than they ever had in the past. Sound familiar?

Alcohol dependence, the development of a qualitatively different state following alcohol withdrawal, was expressed in several ways. It reflected the irreversibility of the effects of chronic alcohol consumption and a new state: loss of control over alcohol consumption. Not only did the preference for alcohol fail to extinguish during abtinence, but changing living conditions and social dominance or subordination no longer affected alcohol consumption. A test of loss of control was administered in the form of alcohol solutions laced with bitter tasting quinine. Alcohol naive rats and "social drinkers" showed a significant reduction in their consumption of alcohol when they had the choice between tap water and the alcohol-quinine cocktails. Chronic drinkers, the animals that had been drinking for 9 months, abstinent for 9 months, and now given the opportunity to resume drinking, showed some reduction in alcohol consumption but still drank significantly more alcohol-quinine cocktails than tap water. They consumed more alcohol-quinine cocktails than the social drinking rats consumed the usual cocktails. Dependent rats were unable to control their consumption of alcohol despite its negative consequences, its noxious taste.

Further differences in the effects of alcohol on social drinkers and dependent rats became apparent. For dependent rats a low dose of alcohol had a tranquilizing effect whereas a high dose stimulated them. Social drinking rats showed the opposite effect. A small dose stimulated whereas a high dose sedated them. These effects call to mind the results Hodgson et al. (1979) obtained with different priming doses of alcohol given to moderate and severely dependent alcoholics. Opposite effects were obtained: a large priming dose in the morning satiated moderately dependent drinkers whereas it primed severely dependent drinkers to consume more alcohol in the afternoon. These are qualitative differences in alcohol related behavior reflecting a "point of no return". A qualitative change occurs distinguishing the ordinary social drinker, even a heavy social drinker, from one who develops dependence. There is no simple continuum from social drinker to alcoholic. It is not a matter of a continuum of learning or amount of alcohol consumed as behavior therapists claim (Heather & Robertson, 1983; Marlatt, 1979). A qualitative difference develops between the social drinker and alcoholic, a point of no return (Coper et al., 1990). Among other changes, a loss of control over alcohol consumption occurs. Brain dysfunction reflecting the Janus effect underlies the qualitative change.

Wolffgramm and his colleagues observe that signs of dependence were seen only in animals that self-administered alcohol, where they had a choice of fluids, water versus different dosages of alcohol. Rats receiving intragastric administration of alcohol did not show the effects of dependence. In analogous fashion, rats given access to alcohol and water only once a week became dependent whereas animals in the same group housing condition having only alcohol solutions available, had no choice of drinking alcohol or tap water, did not show signs of dependence. On test days when a choice of water versus varying doses of alcohol was available, the latter animals drank significantly less alcohol than the intermittent drinkers (Wolffgramm, 1991). Our hypothesis is that greater ORs were evoked in the intermittent and choice than the forced administration conditions. Intermittent drinking probably included binge drinking followed by withdrawal causing brain cell death, sensitization, and disinhibition of the frontal lobes. Alcohol consumption evokes a greater OR in the choice situation because of the contrast, mismatch, produced by two different tasting solutions. Therefore larger ORs, including greater activation of the dopaminergic system reinforces approaching and consuming alcohol as compared to the other two administration methods where novelty evoked ORs would not occur. Corresponding effects have been reported by other investigators for different drugs, including cocaine. A neuroimaging study by Porrino and her colleagues provides evidence supporting the present interpretation. Neuroimaging of a rat's brain following self-administration of alcohol vs. intragastric administration by the experimenter showed that the mesocorticolimbic system is activated in the self-selection case whereas in the experimenter administered condition activation was limited to the hippocampus and sensory systems (Lyons, Whitlow, Smith, & Porrino, 1998).

Alcohol withdrawal effects obtained following a third of a lifetime of chronic alcohol consumption (CAC) followed by a third of a lifetime of abstinence from alcohol are different from the well-established alcohol deprivation effect (McKenzie et al., 1998; Sinclair & Senter, 1968; Senter & Richman, 1969). Alcohol deprivation effects are obtained following weeks of CAC, either operant or free choice, followed by weeks of alcohol deprivation and then a return to alcohol consumption. Increased alcohol consumption following the re-presentation of alcohol-water solutions occurs relatively quickly, within minutes into the first drinking session following deprivation (McKenzie et al., 1998). Consumption will vary depending on operant or choice situations. After a few days the rate will return to the prior level of alcohol consumption. This alcohol deprivation effect, I believe, is interpretable in terms of increased arousal generated by an OR to the mismatch in beverage, the change from drinking water to drinking an alcohol-water solution. With repeated exposure to alcohol solutions the OR habituates. The cocktail is no longer novel. This is in contrast to the relatively permanent rise in alcohol consumption found by Wolffmann and his colleagues following alcohol withdrawal, as well as the changes in other behaviors observed. Loss of control over alcohol consumption is an expression of sensitization exacerbated by neuronal loss in the frontal cortex, cerebellum, and hippocampus due to the neurotoxicity of heavy drinking, its effects, and withdrawal.

A biobehavioral framework is available that accounts for the nonhuman animal model of alcoholism developed by Wolffgramm and his colleagues and by implication characteristics of human alcoholism as well. It provides an explanation for the point of no return, the phase in which qualitative changes occur marking the transition from alcohol misuse to alcohol dependence, the development of loss of control and why a lapse readily turns into a relapse (Chutuape, Mitchell, & de Wit, 1994). None of this is within the ken of behavior therapy with its quiver of knowledge limited to such notions as expectancy, beliefs, self-efficacy, attributions, and a learning continuum from social drinking to alcohol dependence.

Conclusion

This chapter has been a long and somewhat tortuous journey. It was designed that way so that the reader would have little doubt that alcoholism is not merely a bad habit acquired by the usual principles of learning and stigmatized by a "straight" majority. Alcoholism is a consequence of brain dysfunction, damage, disease, which may or may not be reversible depending on the individual case. One of the glaring errors of revisionists is that they present most alcoholics as ordinary people who drink too much, have simply developed a life style of excessive drinking similar to someone developing a life style excessively focused on playing golf (Fingarette, 1988b). Along with the decline in intellectual capacity (Ciesielski, Waldorf, & Jung, 1995) revisionists fail to consider the changes in personality that occur with the development of alcoholism, changes that are also the consequence of damage to the structure and function of the brain (Hoffmann et al., 1974; Kammeier et al., 1973; Küfner & Feuerlein, 1989; Loper et al., 1973; Pettinnati, Sugerman, & Maurer, 1982). Changes in personality reflect the mechanism of disinhibition, CAC produced loss of inhibition by the frontal cortex over the sensitized circuits in the limbic system that control emotion and motivation. Also lost is the capacity to modulate the dorsal areas of the cortex involved in intellectual processes (Starkstein & Robinson, 1997). Although alcoholics suffer from brain dysfunction there is hope. As we shall see in chapter 7 abstinence oriented treatment does work for many alcoholics. With abstinence brain dysfunction can be reversed in many cases and to varying degree. This should not come as a surprise given the research results by Baxter et al. (1992), Schwartz et al. (1996) and their colleagues. They showed that behavioral techniques of cue exposure and response prevention changed the metabolism of the caudate nucleus in those people who recovered from their obsessive compulsive disorder. There is a continuous interaction between the social environment, behavior, and physiology. We suspect that this is the basis in part for the success of AA, especially as an aftercare program. Close interactions among members of the group raises levels of endorphins and serotonin in the brain as do close attachments generally. The fact that alcoholism is the consequence of a brain disease does not mean that "talk therapy", social interactions, and behavioral methods cannot change the neurochemistry of the brain. That they cannot is one more myth created by revisionists that flies in the face of much infrahuman and human research.

In the next chapter we turn to a very different matter: how some psychologists and government administrators have failed to meet their first public responsibility: Do no harm. We shall have a glimpse of how politics, power, and ineptitude intrude upon the processes and integrity of science and the trust upon which they must rest.

4

THE PLACE OF
FACTS IN A WORLD
OF VALUES

Introduction

I was sitting in my office at UCLA one beautiful fall morning in 1976 when there was a knock on my door. I opened it to see a young man in a dark three-piece suit. Dressed like that I knew he wasn't a student or a faculty member. Must be a book salesman, bibles or encylopedias; thought he was in the social sciences building. I was wrong on all counts. He handed me a summons. I was being sued for $3,500,000 by a Richard Roe as part of a class action suit brought by Mark and Linda Sobell in the name of the former patients in their Patton State Hospital study. Additional defendents were Mary Pendery, Jack Fox who was the chief clinical psychologist at Patton, the medical director of Patton, the hospital, and UCLA, etc. When I closed my office door I didn't realize that I was opening the door to a new career. How did I get into such a pickle? Entirely by chance.

I was chairman of the Psychology Department at UCLA in 1972 when, as part of my administrative duties, I received a proposal for a grant request from an assistant professor in my department. A training program was planned which would prepare undergraduates as behavior modifiers who would treat alcoholics using some of the techniques described by Mark and Linda Sobell (1972) in a monograph published by the California Bureau of Mental Hygiene. The Sobells reported striking success for their controlled drinking treatment program after a six month follow-up of patients. Using behavior modification methods based on laboratory derived principles of conditioning they were able to train alcoholics to control their drinking. It was a rather remarkable accomplishment since the traditional wisdom is that abstinence is the only viable treatment goal for alcoholics.

Physically dependent alcoholics receiving the experimental treatment were said to be functioning significantly better than alcoholics receiving traditional treatment with abstinence as the treatment goal. These results reported by the Sobells were revolutionary, not only because they were counter to traditional beliefs and clinical experience, but because they were purportedly obtained in a rigorously conducted experiment with detailed quantitative results. The Sobells purportedly randomly assigned patients to experimental and control groups. Following discharge from the hospital patients were reportedly interviewed in detail every 3-4 weeks. In later follow-ups each patient and 1-15 collaterals were purportedly interviewed at that rate for a full two years. At each interview the patients' daily drinking disposition was reported: (a) the number of days they were abstinent; (b) controlled drinking days, six drinks a day or less, (c) drunk days, more than 6 drinks a day; (d) incarcerated days in jail resulting from an alcohol related incident; and (e) incarcerated days in a hospital for an alcohol related incident.

The proposal aroused my interest for two reasons. First, there was the intriguing possibility of applying the principles of conditioning to a real world problem with important social consequences. Second, I had some concern over permitting relatively young and inexperienced students to conduct behavior modification with alcoholics. I obtained and read the Sobells' (1972) study on which my colleague's proposal was based. He wanted to broaden the applicability of the Sobells' notion by establishing a buddy system between alcoholics under treatment in the nearby Veterans Administration (VA) Hospital and undergraduate majors in psychology who in their junior and senior years may take individual studies and field work courses. These students would take the recovering alcoholics to local bars and train them to control their drinking according to the methods described by the Sobells. Never drink straight whiskey; do not gulp your drinks; do not drink alone; do not drink when angry...

Even though I had no knowledge of the problems of alcoholism at the time, my colleague's "pet vet" proposal seemed far-fetched to me. It seemed unreasonable in large part because I had little trust in the judgment of the typical undergraduate psychology major. I asked Mary Pendery to comment on the proposal. She also had misgivings, but suggested that we find out more about the Sobells' work by visiting them at Patton State Hospital in San Bernardino, about 75 miles east of Los Angeles, where the research had been conducted. I called the chief clinical psychologist at Patton, Jack Fox, who also happened to be a former Ph.D student of mine, and inquired about the Sobells and their research and whether he thought he could arrange a visit with them. Jack informed me that the Sobells had left Patton and were now working at the Orange County Mental Health facility, south of Los Angeles. The alcoholism treatment unit had been closed, but we were welcome to visit Patton, see the simulated bar built in the hospital, and talk to staff who had worked with the Sobells on the project.

Mary and I visited Patton in June, 1972. During the course of our visit we were urged by Jack and several others on the professional staff, all of whom happened to be former Ph.D students of mine, to follow-up the patients. Jack reported that he was receiving telephone calls from alcohol treatment facilities all over the country asking how they could establish an alcoholism treatment program similar to Patton's. Word had spread about the Sobells' success even though it had not yet been published in a professional journal, since it had already received considerable publicity in the media. Jack was concerned because he was seeing former patients in the study relapsing, and because his clinical experience told him that the treatment program could not work. Another staff member expressed the feeling that the participants serving as experimental and control subjects were not randomly assigned. More seriously ill alcoholics were assigned to the control group. He and other members of the professional staff urged us to follow-up the patients and find out what was happening to them. Mary and I however were busy with our daily responsibilities and we procrastinated, but at least I convinced my colleague to withdraw his grant proposal.

A major factor goading us into action was a public lecture given by the Sobells in San Diego in March, 1973. Linda Sobell's claims concerning the remarkable success of their controlled drinking treatment was on the front page of the Metro section of the daily newspaper. Men in the outpatient clinic came to Mary with copies of the newspaper demanding to know why they were not receiving this remarkable new treatment program that behavioral psychologists had developed.

This event and the urging of colleagues motivated us to initiate a follow-up of the patients who had participated in the Sobells' Patton study: Individualized Behavior Therapy for Alcoholics (IBTA).

I formally applied to Patton's Research Committee and the Medical Director for approval of our research protocol designed to follow-up the patients in the original Patton IBTA study. We thought that tracking the patients should not be too difficult despite the lapse of time since the original treatment study, because San Bernardino and San Diego were in the same catchment area. Patients who were veterans and who lived in the area would be likely to go to the San Diego VA Hospital where Mary was Director of the Alcoholism Treatment Unit. An unforseen event intervened, however, which made it impossible for us to begin the follow-up study.

Following approval of our research protocol on May 5, 1973, it was discovered that the Hospital's research records were incomplete. There was no record of who served in the Sobells' study, much less who served in specific groups. Without the list of names of the subjects in the experiment it was impossible to follow them up and to retrieve their medical records containing the participants' medical history.

Approximately two weeks before the Research Committee meeting which reviewed our protocol, a hospital clerk who had assisted in the IBTA study was known to have had a list of the subjects in her possesion. When asked for a copy of the list of participants' names by a member of the professional staff, the clerk replied that she could not find it. The list was lost. Jack telephoned Linda Sobell on May 15 and asked for a copy of the list of subjects' names. Before hanging up on him, she voiced objections to having Mary on the research team because of her bias. I received a telephone call from Mark Sobell the next day. He was rather upset initially by what he considered to be our unprofessional behavior in not informing him that we planned to conduct a follow-up study of his patients. I replied that I had planned to contact him and was also instructed to do so by the Patton Research Committee. It was obviously essential that I do so in the light of the missing list of subjects' names. We saw no point in contacting the Sobells prior to the meeting of the Research Committee, until we knew that the follow-up study was approved. Following a cordial interchange we arranged to meet at the San Diego VA Hospital to discuss our follow-up study and possible collaboration in its conduct. Before concluding our conversation Mark suggested that Mike Digan, an alcoholism counselor who worked with Mary, and who was listed as one of the investigators on the research protocol submitted to Patton, not be present at the meeting. Mark claimed to have evidence showing that Digan was not a trustworthy counselor. We ignored the suggestion.

Mary, Mike Digan, and I met with Linda and Mark Sobell on May 24, 1973. The Sobells expressed concerns about our proposed follow-up. Patients may be upset by our invasion of their privacy and the Sobells felt they may be sued as a consequence. They suggested that if we collaborate with them we would be covered by their clearance. However, if we were to collaborate, they insisted that we could not use Digan as the interviewer. They showed us Digan's confidential Employee Performance Report from his previous place of employment, the San Diego Detoxification Unit. Digan's overall rating was standard, but improvement was needed in three categories: cooperation, quality of judgment, and public and/or employee relations. Written comments indicated that he was a good alcoholism counselor but had difficulty in following established administrative procedures.

The Sobells made it clear to us that we could collaborate with them if Digan was not a member of the team. We refused this condition because Mary had been working with Digan in the Alcoholism Treatment Unit of the San Diego VA Hospital and considered him to be a person of good character and an excellent alcoholism counselor, one who was known and trusted by a large segment of the chronic alcoholic population in the San Diege area.

We had, the Sobells declared, two alternatives: collaborate with them using a mutually agreed upon interviewer or proceed independently. The latter course involved gaining clearance from the Bureau of Legal Affairs of the State Department of Mental Hygiene. The Sobells would not provide Patton with a copy of the list of subjects because it was their personal list. They insisted that the Hospital's list must have been destroyed or lost during the course of a move or change of quarters in the Hospital. Uppermost in their minds was a concern for their patients' right to privacy, which they suggested would not be respected by Digan. Their continued credibility in the eyes of the patients was also essential because the Sobells were to be interviewing patients again for their two-year follow-up. A concern was expressed that the patients might well sue them if we invaded the patients' privacy. The Sobells insisted that Digan could not be trusted to maintain confidentiality and respect patients' privacy, and we must prove otherwise if we wished to use Digan in a collaborative study. They implied, however, that we would be provided with a list of the subjects' names if we took the independent route of gaining clearance from the State Bureau of Legal Affairs. If this latter course were taken, the Sobells would not be legally liable. It was our immediate feeling that we would have to adopt the latter route in order to conduct a truly independent follow-up study in the manner in which we thought would be most appropriate. Otherwise, we would be placed in a position where we would find it necessary to compromise our beliefs concerning the proper way in which to conduct the follow-up, beginning with the use of Digan as the interviewer.

Following the meeting we felt that there must be something wrong with the study. Why the Sobells' reluctance to provide us with the list of names enabling us to undertake an independent study and their opposition to our use of an experienced alcoholism counselor such as Digan? Their arguments about confidentiality and the invasion of privacy did not impress us. Besides, they must have engaged in a search of our backgrounds within a very short period of time to uncover where Digan had worked and to obtain his confidential employee file without his authorization. It suggested fear of an independent follow-up of the participants in the Patton study. At the time we felt that they may be concerned over a biased assignment of patients to the different treatment groups. The least severely dependent in terms of their status at intake might have been placed in the controlled drinking experimental group. During our meeting with the Sobells they showed us an interview data sheet for one subject filled out in great detail. We did not realize at the time that this was an interview form for the time-line follow-back method. The thought never occurred to us that interview results might be fabricated.

We followed the second course and obtained official clearance from the Bureau of Legal Affairs to conduct the follow-up study. However, the Sobells refused to provide the Medical Director of Patton with a list of participants' names enabling him to complete the hospital records. Requests from the legal staff of UCLA and the State Department of Mental Hygiene were to no avail. During the time between approval of our study by Patton and recovery of a list of names of the participants which would permit us to conduct the follow-up, Glenn Caddy and David Perkins were approved by the Research Advisory Committee of Orange County to conduct a follow-up study of the patients from Patton State Hospital. They were planning to use 15 undergraduate and graduate students from Fullerton State College as interviewers. Caddy and Perkins did not submit their proposal to Patton State Hospital for approval and neither the principal investigators nor the students signed oaths of confidentiality at Patton meeting requirements of California statutes. Their study was undertaken with the full support and cooperation of the Sobells.

A major breakthrough in our attempt to obtain the list of subjects' names occurred when Mary reasoned that some of the alcoholism facilities in the area might have a list of the names because they helped the Sobells track the subjects. One such place would be the San Diego Detoxification Center. She was right. A list was in the possession of the Director of the Center, Walter Kimsey, the same person who had written the critical evaluation in Digan's confidential personnel file acquired by the Sobells. Kimsey assured us that if an official requested a copy of the list, for example the Medical Director of Patton State Hospital, he would give the list to the Hospital permitting it to complete its records. Such a request was made by the Medical Director, but then Kimsey refused to relinquish a copy of the list. For some reason he had a change of heart. He eventually provided a list to the Health Care Agency Administrator of San Diego County. Further legal avenues were pursued and there was an extended series of interchanges among representatives of county, state agencies, and counsel for UCLA.

In the meantime Jack reasoned that there should be a way of retrieving the names of the patients participating in the study through the hospital's admission records, because in their publications the Sobells presented results of individual subjects by their actual initials rather than code. Although it was a slow and cumbersome method, it could work. It did, and we began to reconstruct the list of participants in the Patton study.

Knowing that in one way or another, either as result of the list of names returned to Patton by San Diego County or by means of reconstructing the list through the admissions records, we would be able to conduct the follow-up study, Mary and I submitted a grant proposal early in 1974 to the National Institute of Alcohol and Alcohol Abuse (NIAAA) to fund our follow-up. Our site visit by a team assigned by NIAAA was chaired by Peter Nathan of Rutgers and included Albert Powlowski, Chief of Extramural Research. A charitable description of the site visiting team is that they were unfriendly. They thought that we were hostile and responded in kind. They resented the implication that the Sobells might be guilty of wrong-doing and argued that it would be more profitable to conduct an independent replication of the Sobell study.

Team members suggested that we obtain a new sample of patients and conduct an entirely new experiment and follow-up of these new patients. It was our contention that such an argument reflects an insensitivity to the problems posed by a replication study of new patients. Since individualized behavior therapy is by its nature individualized and the detailed step-by-step procedures were not specified in a manual, it is impossible to replicate precisely the procedures employed by another therapist. If nothing else, the therapists differ in appearance, manner of speaking, etc. Failure to obtain the same results as the Sobells could be interpreted to mean only that Mary or whoever did the therapy was not as effective a therapist as the Sobells or did not conduct the treatment in a satisfactory manner. A failure to replicate can always be explained away without impuning the honesty or effectiveness of the original investigators. Only many replication attempts and repeated failures to obtain comparable results could lead to the conclusion that the Sobells' Patton study was of limited generality. Such a procedure would take years and would be enormously expensive monetarily and in human suffering. In the mean-time the widely publicized Patton study would serve as a model for future treatment programs. Most importantly, replication studies could inflict serious harm upon patients, since controlled drinking, despite the evidence provided by the Sobells, is contrary to the extensive experience of clinicians in the field that it is not a feasible treatment goal for the great majority of alcoholics. It was a nonbeneficent treatment until shown otherwise, and unethical because of the increased risk of irreversible biomedical consequences including brain dysfunction. This judgment has been born out by subsequent research. Even the Sobells now agree that controlled drinking is not an effective treatment for alcoholics (Sobell & Sobell, 1995).

Our project was disapproved. A number of grounds were offered for the decision: (a) subject availability was not assured, (b) the retrospective reconstruction of data three years old was judged to be technically difficult and, (c) there was a lack of confidence that the study could be done in an objective manner. The Committee suggested that evidence of bias on our part was our persistence in attempting to conduct the follow-up. Since we were obviously biased against the controlled drinking procedure, the follow-up could not be completely objective.

This argument is paradoxical. It assumes that the Sobells were not biased, did not wish to see the controlled drinking procedure prove successful. It implies that scientists do not have hypotheses which after all are biases, that they hope will be confirmed, and if they do have such biases, this must affect their results. Conditions of "objectivity" demanded by the site visiting team would make science impossible. Lack of feasibility and lack of benefit to the subjects were additional reasons given for disapproval of the project.

Years later through the Freedom of Information Act we obtained copies of the correspondence between the Sobells and officials in the NIAAA. In September 1973, not long after our application to Patton's Research Advisory Committee, Mark Sobell wrote to Albert Powlowski expressing concern over our planned attempt to conduct a follow-up of their subjects. Sobell indicated that they were in consultation with Peter Nathan about possible courses of action that they might take. Two years later Peter Nathan was chair of the site visiting team, which included Powlowski. Nathan, who later became Head of the Alcoholism Research Center at Rutgers University and Executive Editor of the *Journal of Studies on Alcohol,* played a pivotal role in the Sobell saga including the attempted suppression of my paper approved by peer review for publication in the *Journal of Studies on Alcohol.*

After considerable legal maneuvering, through the efforts of Allan Charles, the attorney for UCLA, San Diego County released a copy of the list of names to the Medical Director of Patton who in turn forwarded a copy to me. We received the list in July, 1975. From the outset it was Charles' legal opinion that there were no grounds for concern over liability on the part of the Sobells. Participants of their own volition entered Patton for treatment. They were known to be alcoholics and we had signed an oath of confidentiality. The Sobells could not be held legally responsible for errors we might make in maintaining confidentiality.

Then came the knock on my office door. An injunction had been obtained by the Sobells preventing us from interviewing patients in addition to the class action law suit:

The plaintiffs claimed that unless the defendants were restrained from contacting the subjects or performing further research they would suffer injury to their character, reputation, and to their social, business, and economic standing in their communities. The plaintiffs also contended that their right of privacy had been violated by the disclosure [of their names to us by the Medical Director] and that it constituted a negligent infliction of emotional distress. (Dorinson to Essaye, March 24, 1982)[1].

Mark Sobell also claimed in his affidavit that our research was nonbeneficial since Caddy and his co-workers had already conducted an independent follow-up of the participants in the Patton study. The brief in our defense was written by David Dorinson, Esq., a counsel for the Regents of the University of California.

In my affidavit accompanying our brief (Maltzman, 1976) I state:

Over the years I have been asked at various times by other investigators to provide them with the original data from my experiments. They wished to analyze it in different ways, test hypotheses of their own, etc. I have always freely provided them with the data. In like fashion I have requested the original data obtained by other investigators so that I might analyze the data to test hypotheses that I held which differed from those of the original investigator. I have had no difficulty in obtaining the necessary information. In the case of these kinds of data the identity of the individual subject is not determined and is unnecessary to the analysis or interpretation of the results. In no case, therefore, is the identity of subjects transferred along with the original data. Such information is unnecessary. In the case of data obtained from patients in a hospital setting, as well as in many other situations, the data must be identified by subject or code and the greatest care is needed to safeguard the right to privacy and confidentiality of the subject. In all such cases the responsibility for safeguarding the rights and welfare of the subjects belongs with the institution. It was for this reason that we obtained approval for the conduct of our follow-up study from Patton State Hospital, the University of California, San Diego, and clearance from the Bureau of Legal Affairs.

Science is a cooperative public enterprise. This is the way it ought to be among a community of scholars seeking an understanding of phenomena and concerned with the implications of the phenomena for science and the common good. My experience, therefore, with the Sobells who have persistently hindered the efforts of Patton State Hospital, the responsible institution, to obtain a copy of the list of research subjects who were patients in Patton at the time of the Sobells' study, is unheard of in my experience (sic).

On the basis of the information I now have I believe I know why Mark and Linda Sobell have persistently attempted to thwart our efforts at conducting a follow-up investigation of their study conducted at Patton State Hospital. I believe they have deliberately misrepresented the results that they have obtained and deliberately misrepresented their follow-up procedures....

I shall not attempt to recount the long and difficult course Patton State Hospital has traveled in attempting to obtain a list of the research subjects needed to complete their files. The latter list of course was essential if we were to conduct our own follow-up study. Nor will I comment upon the distortions present in the Declarations of Mark Sobell in his account... I will only note that while the Sobells repeatedly emphasize that they are concerned about the confidentiality and right to privacy of the patients in the Patton Study they themselves have no compunction to abridge the right to privacy of someone else, namely, Mr. Michael Digan, our collaborator in the proposed follow-up study. When we met with the Sobells in May 1973 we were astonished to be confronted with the confidential personnel report on Mr. Digan. The Sobells used this report in an attempt to exclude Mr. Digan from the project and to justify their refusal to return the list of the subjects' names to Patton State Hospital. Since Dr. Pendery was thoroughly familiar with Mr. Digan's outstanding qualifications as an alcoholism counselor, we were not about to accede to the Sobells' demand that Mr. Digan be dropped from our follow-up study because he could not be trusted to maintain confidentiality or conduct himself in a professional manner.

Dr. Pendery and I subsequently visited Mr. W. Walter Kimsey, Superintendent, Detoxification Center, County of San Diego, Mr. Digan's former supervisor, the person responsible for the personnel report. We requested his objective evaluation of Mr. Digan as an alcoholism counselor and whether or not he believed Mr. Digan was responsible, concerned with the welfare of his patients, and capable of maintaining their confidentiality and respecting their rights in our proposed follow-up study. Mr. Kimsey replied in the affirmative and stated in essence that Mr. Digan had been a fine employee.

Following the receipt of the list of subjects' names by Patton State Hospital a copy was forwarded to me. Between that time and the injunction against Patton State Hospital, Dr. Pendery made initial contact with several patients in order to determine the feasibility of conducting the follow-up study. After her initial one or two contacts Dr. Pendery informed me that she was puzzled and startled by the information she had obtained. The patients had spontaneously commented that they had been interviewed from 1 - 4 times, not the minimum of 24 times required by the Sobells' description of their follow-up procedure. One patient reported that he had been interviewed frequently. But his attorney had complained to the Hospital about the treatment that he had received. I therefore accompanied Dr. Pendery on an initial contact meeting with another subject. This subject stated that he had been called from 2 - 4 times by Linda Sobell during the two year follow-up period to determine how he was functioning. [In recent months he had been called several times by Linda Sobell informing him that a follow-up study by other investigators was planned and that these investigators could reveal his identity as a recovered alcoholic. He was disturbed by this information. He did not want it known publicly that he was a recovered alcoholic for fear that his employer might fire him as a consequence. He had considered bringing a lawsuit against us to prevent the follow-up. He showed us a letter sent to him by the Sobells' attorney informing him that time was of the essence to bring suit and to prevent the follow-up and his exposure as a recovered alcoholic] He was a member of the controlled drinking-experimental group (CD-E). He is now functioning well, and has been for sometime. But he does not engage in controlled social drinking and stated that he believes that this is impossible for an alcoholic to do. He is now functioning well, he claimed, not because of the treatment received from the Sobells at Patton Hospital, he was drunk for six months following release from the Hospital, but because of treatment he subsequently received, and is still receiving, at a different facility which uses an abstinence treatment goal.

I believe it is of fundamental importance to interview as many of the patients in the original Patton study as possible in order to confirm that evidence we already have that the Sobells misrepresented the procedure they employed and the nature of the data that they have obtained. While the patients contacted prior to the court injunction all expressed a willingness to cooperate and to be interviewed, it is entirely possible that other patients may refuse to be interviewed. Their rights in this regard would be respected. We believe that a discrete and thorough effort to respect the rights of the patients is essential, and that we are capable of performing in such a manner. Nevertheless, it is always possible that the right to privacy of some patients may be abridged during the course of even the most carefully conducted study. On the other hand, if the single most important experimental treatment and evaluation study of controlled drinking is not what it has been represented to be, and our preliminary findings indicate that it is not, then untold thousands of alcoholics may be doomed to death or a life of pain and misery, as well as thousands of innocent highway victims of alcoholics. All this because *gamma* alcoholics have been led to believe that they can be trained to practice controlled drinking as the result of the purported findings of the Sobells' study. It must also be noted that many of the patients in the control groups of the Patton Study are still suffering from severe alcoholism. Making contact with them as part of our follow-up would provide an opportunity for the investigators to obtain treatment for these unfortunate men.

If called as a witness, I could and would competently testify to the facts stated herein.

I declare under penalty of perjury that the foregoing is true and correct.

Executed at Los Angeles, Californa on December 22, l976. (pp. 8-11).

Judge Hauk decided in our favor and dismissed the case with prejudice in Federal Court on April 4, l977. "Dismissal with prejudice meant that the court determined that the action that was filed was legally unmeritorious in its entirety" (Dorinson to Essaye, March 24, l982)[1]. Judge Hauk concluded that on balance it was more important to determine how the patients were faring following treatment than any possible breach of confidentiality and invasion of privacy which were protected by their right to refuse to participate in the study.

An obvious criticism may be voiced of the evidence presented in my affidavit suggesting that the Sobells committed fraud. Perhaps the patients were vindictive. The Sobells gained fame and fortune at their expense and they are still suffering from alcoholism. The patients may have been helped at one time, at the time of the Sobells' follow-ups, but now they have relapsed and they blame the Sobells for their inability to continue to successfully control their drinking or abstain, as the case may be.

The above arguments suffer from a number of erroneous assumptions. First, the patients when initially interviewed did not know that the Sobells published papers describing the Patton study and eventually in 1978, a book, and that the study of them made the Sobells famous. Second, they did not know that the Sobells stated that each patient was interviewed at least once a month for two full years. The remark by the first patient interviewed by Mary that he spoke to Linda only two or three times in two years was spontaneous. The thought had never occurred to us before this first interview that the interview procedures could have been intentionally misrepresented and results describing daily drinking dispositions fabricated.

Two books that I read during the '70s helped me realize what I was up against in trying to expose the alleged fraud perpetrated by the Sobells. At the outset there was no way to understand the magnitude and nature of the support afforded the Sobells by their fellow behavior therapists. These two books helped me understand the nature of their support, its pervasive influence and the tactics used to extend that influence. One of the books was a mystery that is on most lists of the 10 best mystery novels of all time, *A Daughter of Time* by Josephine Tey (1951). It taught me about the profound influence of politics and ideology in human affairs using as a background the true story of Richard III, not the theatrical version popularized by Shakespeare, the version driven by politics.

The second book was one I reread after reading it when it was first published, *1984,* by George Orwell (1949), one of my favorite authors in my "youth" and a brilliant social commentator. He delineates in chilling fashion the power an authoritarian regime has in controlling the thinking of its citizens. However, he apparently failed to recognize that the tactics for controlling the thinking of a citizenry can be employed to control the thinking of a delimited group within a democratic society. It can control the thinking of what one might consider a most unlikely group, behavior therapists. This possibility is not surprising once one recognizes that behavior therapists are no different than anyone else when it comes to the powerful motives of greed and the lust for power and the rewards and punishments that shape these acquired dispositions. The Sobells and their supporters are primarily successful academic clinical psychologists relying on the Orwellian principle: IGNORANCE IS STRENGTH. They are revisionists because they rewrite history. A basis for their influence is expressed by another Orwellian principle: WHOEVER CONTROLS THE PRESENT CONTROLS THE PAST AS WELL AS THE FUTURE. Evidence supporting these allegations may be found in almost every chapter of this book.

Ethics Complaints

During the period of the temporary injunction the Sobells informed us that they were bringing a complaint against Mary and me to the Ethics Committee of the American Psychological Association, the Committee on Scientific and Professional Ethics and Conduct (CSPEC). Their complaint was that we were contemplating nonbeneficial research. Our follow-up would have no benefit because an independent follow-up had already been conducted by Caddy et al. and we were planning to use Digan who could not be trusted to maintain confidentiality.

Brenda Gurel, secretary for the CSPEC wrote:

At the Committee's direction, I am writing to let you know that as a result of the Committee's discussion of the Sobells' charges against you, the Committee members agreed that the questions raised by the Sobells were, indeed, legitimate, although CSPEC would not wish to prejudge the matter in terms of possible ethics violation... Therefore, we must respectfully ask for your view of this question, whether or not you believe the human participants' rights to privacy should be considered and any other issues you think it would be constructive for CSPEC to address. (B. Gurel to Maltzman, October 3, 1976).

I replied that these issues and more were under review in federal court as part of the law suit initiated by the Sobells. I would reply when the case was judged. The Sobells also wrote to Jack Fox threatening him with an ethics complaint to the APA. He replied that he welcomed the opportunity to address the issues involved and wrote to the CSPEC saying that he welcomed a discussion of the issues and submitted a copy of the legal brief written in our defense by Dorinson, including our affidavits. Later that summer, following settlement of the lawsuit in our favor and lifting of the injunction, Mary and I received a letter from the Sobells informing us that they prepared a letter which they will mail to subjects on July 11, 1977 and "has been reviewed by the American Psychological Association and by legal counsel (M. Sobell and L. Sobell, to Pendery and to Maltzman, June 13, 1977).

Their letter informs the patients that people who have no connection with the Patton State Hospital research project may try to interview them, that the Sobells sponsored a legal action against these people in an attempt to protect the patients' identity, but due to their lack of personal funds the Sobells were unable to pursue the court action and the case was dismissed. The address of CSPEC was given if they wished to bring a complaint.

The former IBTA patients had no way of knowing that a judge in federal court ruled that we might be able to help them if help was needed, and that the judge decided that the good that might come from our follow-up outweighed its possible harm. Judge Hauk's ruling also determined that the medical director of the hospital is responsible for safeguarding the rights of patients not the Sobells who were employees of the Hospital at the time of the study. The case was not dismissed because of the Sobells' lack of funds. One may also wonder in what sense was this issue reviewed by the APA? And the CSPEC? Did the latter take a vote on this issue?

Mary telephoned Gurel concerning this rather unusual action by the Sobells. She was informed that two members of the Committee assisted the Sobells in the wording of their letter. Without informing us of these proceedings and in the possession of a brief with a signed affidavit alleging that the Sobells committed fraud, the APA Ethics Committee assisted the Sobells in their attempt to prevent or hinder our follow-up study. I wrote to Gurel requesting a rationale for their actions, and included a copy of our brief and my affidavit in case they had not read it. Gurel replied:

"Since I cannot answer for the Committee members, your question concerning their rationale for assisting the Sobells must remain unanswered until the Committee has seen your letter. This will occur at the July 15-16 meeting, and I will write as soon as possible after that time." (B. Gurel to Maltzman, July 13, 1977).

Following dismissal of the law suit against us I asked CSPEC to investigate the Sobells' alleged scientific misconduct. Bases for my allegations were derived from the contacts with patients that were made prior to issuance of the injunction as indicated in my affidavit. Gurel replied:

At its July 15-16 meeting and by mail prior to that time, the Committee spent a considerable amount of time reviewing the materials available to it. As a result of this and after extensive discussion, the members concluded that it would be difficult, if not impossible in the long run, to verify the various claims and counter-claims that have emerged in the situation. The only conviction that emerged from the discussion was an opinion that all parties involved appeared to have formed such strong feelings in the matter that these then came to influence their perceptions of others' motivations and intentions.

The Committee directed me to communicate this to you, Dr. Pendery, and Drs. Sobell, and to also tell you that the Committee declines taking any further action in this matter. CSPEC also wished me to indicate to you all that the members found CSPEC's involvement in the dispute to have been a most valuable educational experience. (B. Gurel to Maltzman, August 22, 1977).

It is apparent that Gurel did not answer my question concerning the justification for Committee members assisting the Sobells in the name of the APA. It is the Committee's job to sift through the clouds of purported feeling on both sides and discern the truth. Their argument implies that murder, bank robbery, etc., cannot be judged when the perpetrator and victim are emotionally involved. I learned then, and subsequently, that the CSPEC, as is true probably of ethics committees in other professional associations, do not exercise much power, even if they have it, for a variety of reasons. The severest sanction at the disposal of CSPEC is that they can expel you from the association. If that happened, as a nonmember I would have to pay more for my psychology association journal subscriptions. The CSPEC cannot fire me from my job as a professor. Their sanctions have some power over psychologists in private practice, but their power is limited by the American Psychological Association's fear of litigation. The CSPEC will recommend expulsion of a member of the Association if a felony has been committed. It is a paper tiger, especially for academic psychologists, because it has no judicial power, no subpoena power, and cannot provide witnesses with immunity. Its primary role is to educate members. The CSPEC permitted itself to be used by the Sobells in their attempt to frighten off patients with a letter having the appearance of approval from the American Psychological Association. The CSPEC, like any other committee is made up of people, and people can be influenced, some more than others. The Sobells apparently found two that could be influenced and the Secretary must protect them. It's politics as usual.

Manuscript submitted to *Science*

With the ethics complaint and the lawsuit behind us, Mary slowly began to interview patients. It was a gargantuan task because the VA refused to consider the follow-up research part of her VA duties. She had to track subjects not only in San Diego County, but everywhere else on her own time and expense. Our failure to obtain extramural funding added years to the impossible task Mary had taken upon herself, to interview every living subject in the experimental and control groups.

In 1979 Mary told Jolly West, an old friend and the head of the UCLA Department of Psychiatry and the Neuropsychiatric Institute about the "Sobell affair". He was sympathetic and was instrumental in raising funds from private donors to cover some of Mary's expenses. It also enabled Mary to take some time off to search for patients who had moved from Southern California. Mary interviewed all the possible patients she could find, an incredible task only she could relate in detail. A manuscript describing our results was finally submitted to *Science* July 9, 1981.

Science eventually published a report of our follow-up study (Pendery, Maltzman, & West, 1982) emphasizing only the past and current condition of the patients in the experimental group showing that the majority were not functioning well and at best one was drinking moderately. *Science* declined to consider material in an earlier draft of the manuscript implying fraud on the part of the Sobells. *Science* was in the midst of litigation with powerful industrial firms for alleged libel concerning the firms' responsibility in the pollution of the Love Canal in upstate New York, the topic of a news article that had appeared in *Science* (Carey, 1982). Three expensive law suits were enough. Lawyers advised the editor, Dr. Philip Abelson, that our initial manuscript may be libelous, this despite Dorinson's objections that the assertions in our manuscript were true, the ultimate defense against libel in the United States. Dorinson also pointed out that eliminating all direct reference to fraud does not eliminate the possibility of legal action. All the plaintiff need do is to find one expert to testify that a reading of the manuscript suggests fraud.

No matter that if the Sobells brought a legal action that came to court they would have to testify and be cross-examined under oath and penalty of perjury and their records would be subpoened. The mere threat of the possibility of legal action was enough to make the journal published by the largest science organization in the United States, the American Assocation for the Advancement of Science (AAAS), become faint hearted. When it becomes a balance of money versus principle, the former usually wins.

Abelson asked us to revise the manuscript and stick to the facts. Our revision was sent to new reviewers and was recommended for publication. By this time the Sobells had learned that a manuscript describing our followup was under review by *Science*. They obtained the services of the prestigious Washington law firm of Arnold and Porter to represent them, and *Science* began to receive threats of legal action. Before publishing our paper Abelson asked us to provide objective independent evidence for each of the assertions in it. Mary and I spent two full days in the editorial offices of *Science* in Washington, D.C. reviewing all of our evidence with members of the editorial staff and Anthony Essaye, Esq., a member of the staff of the law firm of Rogers and Wells hired by *Science* to represent them in discussions with the Sobells and their law firm.

Although I believed that the revisions asked by *Science* represented a failure of nerve and the original version would have had considerably more impact, I felt only admiration and respect for Abelson and his highly skilled and thoughtful editorial staff. This is the real world, where even a powerful and important science association and journal can be forced to bend principles when faced with threats of costly litigation.

I had sent a copy of the original version of the manuscript to Ray Hodgson, a well-known British behavior therapist who I knew, for his comments. He had conducted some interesting experimental studies with alcoholics and I thought he was a cut or two above his typical American counterpart. A copy of this earlier draft was obtained by Marlatt and the Sobells and widely circulated among their colleagues. Marlatt constructed a lengthy critique of our paper and wrote on May 27, 1982 to Hodgson as follows:

> Their goal [Pendery and Maltzman] is to destroy the reputation of two psychologists and to kill the notion of controlled drinking as a viable treatment option once and for all. And that seems wrong to me.
>
> I await your response to all this. In the meantime, I am taking the liberty of sending copies of this letter to Terry Wilson, Peter Nathan and Barbara McCrady, since I have spoken to each of them recently about this matter. I am willing to serve as a clearinghouse for all of us who wish to respond to the issues involved in one way or another. We should all keep in touch regarding developments in what could become the big 'gunfight at the O.K. Corral' in the alcoholism field.

Marlatt (1983) authored the leading article in defense of the Sobells and controlled drinking in the *American Psychologist*, the journal distributed to all members of the *American Psychological* Association. At that time Nathan was Associate Editor of the American Psychologist responsible for reviewing and accepting articles on clinical issues including alcoholism. I was not invited to reply to the article.

Mark and Linda Sobell were invited to provide the standard brief reply to our article in *Science*. It was our understanding that if they were to reply in *Science*, their data would be subject to the same kind of detailed analysis ours had been. Instead, they replied in a lengthy article in *Behaviour Research and Therapy* (*BRAT*) (Sobell & Sobell, 1984a), the leading journal in the behavior therapy field. Their excuse for replying in *BRAT* was that they were not permitted to write a full-length article in *Science*. Ten editors of clinical psychology journals wrote a letter of protest to *Science* (Barlow et al., 1983). Abelson replied, but before publishing his letter and the protest letter, he circulated his reply to each of the signatures of the protest letter. Abelson's description of the events that occurred is worth noting:

> In absence of criticism of experiments and replication of results, the integrity of science would be destroyed. The overwhelming majority of scientists understand this, and most cooperate with those who challenge the validity of their work. The behavior of the Sobells with respect to the research report by Pendery et al., was unprecedented in my experience of more than 20 years as editor.

The Sobells, in writing, threatened us with legal action while we were in the initial phase of considering the paper. Shortly after, we received a letter from their attorney. Under such circumstances, prudence dictates that contact between the principals cease and that one deal with the matter through attorneys.

The report that we published in our 9 July issue [Pendery et al., 1982] was very carefully edited. It was extensively reviewed, including evaluation by an expert statistician. Painstaking efforts were made to ensure an absence of comment about the integrity of the Sobells. We required that assertions made about patients' histories be documented by court records, police records, hospital records, or affidavits. The final draft was checked repeatedly, sentence by sentence, to ensure that supporting evidence was available. In crucial instances, two or more independent documents corroborated statements made... The avenue of a technical comment has been and remains open to the Sobells. They have not so far availed themselves of it. (Abelson, 1982, pp. 555-556).

Apparently two of the original authors of the protest letter withdrew after reading Abelson's letter; 10 did not. Whoever those two are, I congratulate them for their courage in acting independently and refusing to bow to the pressure to conform.

Censorship

I was invited to reply to the Sobells' article in *BRAT* which I did (Maltzman, unpublished a), but the editor, S. J. Rachman, one of those who signed the protest letter to *Science*, informed me that my manuscript was libelous and was rejected without being submitted for independent peer review.

Dorinson reviewed the manuscript and judged it to be free of potentially libelous material. I asked the attorney for Pergamon Press, publisher of *BRAT* to specify which passages were libelous and the legal precedents forming the basis for his judgment. He replied that his judgment stands.

Much of the material in the paper has been cannibalized and distributed throughout various parts of this book. In the paper submitted to *BRAT* I presented the analyses of the time-line follow-back method demonstrating that logically the Sobells had to know they were interviewing patients less than every 3-4 weeks because using the time-line follow-back method necessarily requires that you know the date of the previous interview. The manuscript containing such analyses was sent to the Trachtenberg Committee established by the Alcohol, Drugs, and Mental Health Administration (ADAMHA) to investigate the Sobells' alleged fraud. It was acknowledged by Michelle Applegate, author of the Trachtenberg Report, as an unsolicited manuscript without further comment. They did not follow my advice in what to look for to evaluate my allegation of fraud (see chapter 5).

One part of the manuscript that has not been cannibalized and redistributed in various chapters in the present book will be presented in the following section with the addition of two more current references. It describes a basic strategy employed by the Sobells beginning in the 1970's.

On Paradigms

The Sobells engage in puffery posing as martyrs in the forefront of a scientific revolution battling the unwashed hordes of antiscientists of which Dr. Pendery and I are part. This has been a familiar refrain played by them and their supporters for more than a decade. Appealing to Kuhn (1962) is a common occurrence today on the part of many groups of psychologists, e.g., cognitivists in their attacks on behaviorists, behaviorists, in their attacks on dynamic psychologists, humanists in attacking all the others, etc. A brief comment is, perhaps, in order. More detailed analyses of this situation in the field of alcoholism must await another time and place.

One difficulty with the Sobells' stance as molders of a new scientific paradigm is that Kuhn's analysis of the growth of science has been under attack for years by philosophers and historians of science (Lakatos, 1970; Laudan, 1977; Shapere, 1964; Toulmin, 1970). Masterman (1970) has noted some 21 different usages of the term "paradigm" in Kuhn's work. In which of these senses are the Sobells part of a new paradigm? Furthermore, Kuhn's analysis of the growth of scientific knowledge in terms of scientific revolutions and normal science pertains to physical science, and even here philosophers and historians of science dispute the adequacy of his analyses. It is not generally accepted as an accurate picture of how scientific knowledge grows. Kuhn himself does not believe that his analysis of paradigms applies to behavioral science which he considers to be in a preparadigmatic stage. Critics claim that behavioral science is in a multiple-paradigm phase however these paradigms may be defined (Masterman, 1970).

More to the point, a few poorly designed or conceived studies, some minor laboratory experiments, establishment of a straw man, the disease model as the opposition, may seem impressive and flattering to their architects, but this does not represent a substantial advance in science, much less a revolution, however conceived. This sort of self-satisfying ideologically motivated portrait does an injustice to -- and ignores -- the mainstream of research that has made substantial advances dealing with alcoholism as a biopsychosocial disease (Begleiter & Kissen, 1995, 1996; Kissen & Begleiter, 1983a, 1983b). Claims of a paradigm shift are pointedly vapid when it is remembered that the bulwark of this so-called revolution is the tainted research under discussion and its authors are its standard bearers.

More Ethics Complaints

Considerable media interest was aroused by our *Science* article. There is a cozy and mutually advantageous relationship between major science journals, the science establishment, and the media. It is standard practice for major science journals such as *Science, The New England Journal of Medicine* (*NEJM*) and *Journal of the American Medical Association, (JAMA)* to distribute prepublication proofs of their articles to science writers associated with major newspapers a week or two before publication of the journal. If an article catches the fancy of a science writer he or she would have the time to interview the authors and other experts in the field, gather some additional information, and write an article for their paper before receipt of the journal article in the mail following publication. In order to avoid one writer scooping the others, which is tantamount to having the story appear in only one newspaper, since there is nothing worse than a warmed over, cold, story, the science journal places an embargo on the media story. Science newswriters cannot publish their story until a specified date, which is the day that the journal begins distribution - mailing the journal to its subscribers. In this way, all the writers can publish on the same day without scooping anyone - except the subscribers to the journal who learn about the existence of an article before they receive the journal. For example, my *Los Angeles Times* of September 6, 1996 carried a story titled, "separate human memory systems found" (Hotz, 1996) related to a journal article appearing in my September 6, 1996 issue of *Science* (Knowlton, Mangels, & Squire, 1996) which I received approximately September 16th. As a consequence of this procedure, the story about our article and the implied criticism of the Sobells appeared in newspapers several days before it appeared in *Science*. Mary and I as a consequence were criticized for fighting this controversy in the media rather than in peer reviewed journals. The fact is I contacted no member of the media. Most were contacted in the normal manner by *Science* through its prepublication proofs of the forthcoming issue. Mary had spoken to reporters for the *Los Angeles Time* and the *San Diego Union*. All followed the embargo rule.

The most controversial article, in large part because of where it appeared, in the *New York Times* written by Philip Boffey (1982) states: "in a telephone interview yesterday, Dr. Maltzman said: 'Beyond any reasonable doubt, it's fraud.' " Boffey went on to report that Mark Sobell described the, "new criticism as part of 'an ideological controversy' in which those who favor traditional treatment for alcoholism have made 'lots of vicious attacks' on controlled drinking..." (p. A12). To make clear that a serious issue was at stake and not mere politics, I put my belief in as strong a manner as possible. It is noteworthy that the Sobells did not attempt to sue me for libel as a result of the *NY Times* story - or any other story or article.

The Sobells informed Mary and me that they were bringing an ethics complaint against each of us. We subsequently received letters from the CSPEC to that effect and not long afterwards Caddy brought complaints against us. The two complaints were combined by CSPEC because of their similar nature. I replied for both of us and an exchange of letters followed. The original complaint against Mary brought by the Sobells was dismissed by the Committee because she never made public allegations of fraud. As the result of a miscommunication the Committee however reprimanded her for failing to reply in time to the complaint. My letters were to have been taken as a reply from both of us. Eventually, the misunderstanding was clarified and the reprimand of Mary was rescinded by the Committee. I received a more serious sanction, censure, because of my comments to the media.

During the course of my exchange of letters, and, finally, quite explicitly in the hearing I requested to rebut their censure, a more serious sanction then a reprimand, the real basis for the Committee's concern became apparent. By mutual agreement, the hearing was tape recorded by the Committee. A summary of the Committee hearing follows.

APA Ethics Committee Hearing

When I appeared before the full Committee, I was first asked to briefly describe how I became involved in the affair. The Committee emphasized that they were not attempting to determine the truth or falsity of my allegations but the process I used. It appeared to be sensationalistic. I argued that the truth is not sensationalistic. The Committee was obviously concerned with the excessive use of the media to plead my case. I pointed out that I never solicited an interview from the media. Such reports appeared prior to the full appearance of an article in *Science* by only a few days. It is standard practice for major journals to give prior notice of forthcoming articles to science writers so that they can prepare a story if they wish. This normal procedure was in place, etc.

I was confronted with the results of the Dickens Committee Report (Dickens, 1982) and asked how I could make allegations of fraud in the face of such an extended Report exonerating the Sobells of misconduct. I proceeded to point out the serious flaws in the Dickens Committee Report including the most important one. They never took the essential first step in any such investigation of fraud in science: Obtain all of the raw data and determine whether these data can reproduce the published results. Telephone contacts are not the raw data producing the dependent variables used by the Sobells, daily drinking dispositions. Six-months averaged summary sheets, likewise, are not the raw data. Numbers recorded in each category for each day on the time-line follow-back interview forms are the raw data. If an investigating committee does not know what the basic dependent variable is in a study, the variable that allegedly is fabricated, how can they conduct an investigation that can be taken seriously? Not one of the "investigations" of the Sobells' work took this essential first step of examining all the raw data and from these attempt to reproduce the published daily drinking disposition results given for each subject.

After approximately two hours of questioning a member of the Committee got to the heart of the matter. She was a distinguished clinical psychologist with a private practice on Park Avenue, NYC. I looked her up in the Association Membership Directory as I did the other members of the CSPEC before I went to Washington. She was vice-chair and several years later became chair of the Committee. She said essentially, "this is all very interesting, but it is beside the point. The point is you gave psychology a bad name."[2] I replied to the effect that she does not know this for a fact. She did not survey a national representative probability sample to determine what the public thought about the affair. On the contrary, I added, it is possible that the status of psychology has been enhanced in the public eye because the public sees that members of the Association are concerned about their well-being.

I was being tried for a charge that the Sobells had never brought against me. I realized, finally, why members of the Committee and some fellow psychologists were angry. My damaging the reputation of the American Psychological Association and psychologists generally was the real complaint against me.

I went home and not long afterwards received a letter rescinding my censure. I learned that the view expressed during my hearing was not unique. The wife of an old friend of mine berated me on similar grounds. My allegation that the Sobells committed fraud is giving psychology a black eye. Why don't I investigate fraud and misconduct in psychiatry? I replied that I am a psychologist not a psychiatrist and I found by accident what I believed to be fraud by psychologists not psychiatrists. Furthermore, it is the Sobells who are giving psychology a black eye for committing the alleged fraud in the first place.

How can fraud be proven? It has been argued by some that all that the Pendery et al. (1982) study did was show that years later the men who were no longer drinking moderately had relapsed. One cannot assume that a brief treatment of a few weeks would necessarily last a life time. What the Sobells reported about their patients for two years following treatment and what Caddy et al. reported for a third year are true and what Pendery et al. reported some 10 years later is also true. Why am I making a mountain out of a mole hill? "What's wrong with this guy, anyway?" "What's bugging him?" "Let well enough alone!" "Why am I dragging up stinking dead fish!" "Why the vendetta against these hard working creative young people?" "What do I have against them?" "What's my motivation?" "How can you believe what an alcoholic said he remembers from 10 years ago?" These were some of the complaints conveyed to me. On the other hand, I also received support from colleagues. Two professors in my department collected a petition submitted to the American Psychological Association in my behalf signed by more than 40 departmental colleagues. Questions raised by CSPEC at the hearing concerning the Dickens Committee Report and the purported congressional investigation summarized by James Jensen are treated in detail in chapter 5.

Censorship

Brown, Jackson, and Galizio (1983) published a note that posed a common criticism of Pendery et al. (1982). It is a poor study because we did not compare the experimental and control groups. This criticism is a common diversionary tactic. Whether our study is good or poor does not address the more important question of whether or not the Sobells fabricated much of their interview data and misrepresented their procedures. I wrote in reply (Maltzman, 1984) that we did compare the groups and found a significant order effect which prohibits further comparisons, as well as several additional observations. The Sobells replied to my note in the same issue. Having authors provide a brief reply to a criticism in the same issue of a journal is the usual procedure. What was unusual is that I was not afforded a similar opportunity to reply to the article by Brown, et al. (1983). If I had not subscribed to the *Bulletin of Psychologists in Addictive Behaviors* (*Bulletin*), I probably would never have known about the article, because it was not a widely known and circulated journal. No matter. I wrote a brief reply to the Sobells' brief reply to my paper replying to Brown et al. (Maltzman, unpublished b). At the same time I submitted a letter to the editor in response to an open letter by Marlatt (1984) that appeared in the *Bulletin* in his office as president of the Society of Psychologists in Addictive Behaviors, the society publishing the *Bulletin*.

Miles Cox, the editor, declined to publish my comment and letter stating that they were libelous. I asked him to provide the grounds for such a judgment. He replied that it was the judgment of the Executive Committee which included Marlatt who was President of the Society at the time. Cox also stated that they had decided

124

not to publish further material on the Sobell controversy and controlled drinking since it was settled and the Sobells had been exonerated of wrong doing. A lengthy article on controlled drinking appeared in the next issue (Marlatt et al., 1985). Similar articles favorable to some form of controlled drinking and the Sobells' work have continued to appear in the *Bulletin* (Graber & Miller, 1988; Peele, 1986).

The Society of Psychologists in Addictive Behaviors is now Division 50 of the American Psychological Association and has an important voice in establishing criteria for specialization in the area of substance abuse.

More Ethics Complaints, Some Mine

I brought an ethics complaint against Cox to the CSPEC. They declined to consider the case. A similar reaction was elicited by my ethics complaint against Marlatt. I also brought an ethics complaint against the Sobells for failing to adequately inform the public concerning their research errors as reported by the Dickens Report. The CSPEC judged that the Sobells had adequately informed the public about their careless errors. The CSPEC did not investigate the raw data of the Sobells' study, only their current published statements and leaned heavily upon the Dickens Committee Report for guidance. The CSPEC concluded that the Sobells were careless but did not intentionally misrepresent the frequency of their follow-ups.

Events that led to my ethics complaints against Marlatt and Cox were not the last of my experiences with the *Bulletin*. In my reply to Brown et al. (1983) I stated:

Cases of alleged fraud are not resolved by opposing authors in conference. Nevertheless, we are willing at any time to sit down with the Sobells and Caddy and his colleagues and review all of their data and they ours, in the presence of an impartial third party such as a government investigating body or a congressional committee. The Canadian Dickens Committee was not a disinterested third party. The inadequate nature of their report, for example accepting telephone contacts as basic data rather than the detailed interviews generating daily drinking dispositions, the Sobells' basic dependent variable, reveals as much. (p.72).

Bernard Dickens a professor of law and Committee chair, and Anthony Doob, the psychologist on the Committee also from the University of Toronto, brought an ethics complaint against me as well as veiled legal threats. The CSPEC took the complaint under consideration and requested a statement defending my actions. A 22-page single-spaced statement accompanied my letter submitted in reply (Maltzman to Mills, June 6, 1985). These materials resulted in the dismissal of the complaint against me. My letter formed the basis for a manuscript that I submitted to the *British Journal of Addiction*.

In the meantime Caddy brought an ethics complaint against me because of statements I made concerning his character during my talk at the University of Washington. Grounds for my statements were not accepted by CSPEC and I was reprimanded.

And More Censorship

I sent a manuscript to the *British Journal of Addiction (BJA)* , (Maltzman, unpublished c) replying to an article by Doob (1984). My paper examined some of the inadequacies that I believed were evident in the report by the Dickens Committee (Dickens et al., 1982), the Trachtenberg Committee (Trachtenberg, 1984), and Doob's article.

Griffith Edwards, the editor of the *BJA,* wrote that my paper ought to be published, but in all fairness he wished to obtain replies from all parties concerned, including the Sobells, Dickens and Doob, and Trachtenberg. The latter was chair of an investigating committee convened by the Alcoholism Drug and Mental Health Administration (ADAMHA). I suggested that if he did, the Sobells and others would threaten a libel suit and inquired what he would do then. He replied that he would cross that bridge when he came to it. Three years later he came to it and on advice of attorney rejected my manuscript because of the threat of legal action on the part of the Sobells, Dickens and Doob. Excerpts from Edwards' initial letter follow:

On the basis of advice which I have received from a senior colleague, and my own view of your paper, I would now like to come back to you with the following suggestions. Let me say that the background to the approach which I am proposing is my belief that the B.J.A. ought to be absolutely open to all views and non-partisan. It should attempt to be fair and humane towards all parties. We should support honest and open debate without fudging contention, but I believe that the cause of good debate is best served by aiming at a tone which does not unnecessarily inflame matters.

1. I believe that this paper ought to be published. Every now and then there is a phrase or two which might sound all right in the ding-dong of live verbal debate, but, which set down in cold print, seems perhaps unnecessarily stinging-let's forget about what the other side may have said in the past, and simply concern ourselves with the tone of the present text. I am returning to you a copy of your paper on which I have done some minor editing with these issues in mind...

2. When we have got the paper to that stage, I would like your permission to show it to the Sobells, to Dr. Doob, to Professor Dickens, and perhaps also to Dr. Trachtenberg... I would need to ask the parties concerned whether they considered the text in any way libelous or whether they would agree to its publication. My previous experience is that such open dealing leads to an open and generous response. (G. Edwards to Maltzman, December 20, 1985).

When I submitted my manuscript to the *BJA* I did not realize that the libel laws in Great Britain differed from those in the United States. Here, the truth is the ultimate defense against libel. It is not in Great Britain where the test is whether or not assertions damage the reputation of an individual. Three years after my submission Edwards rejected my manuscript because of the threat of legal action by the Sobells, Dickens, and Doob.

My fourth experience of attempted censorship and also the influence of ideology on a scholarly journal involved a manuscript I sent to, at the time, the most prestigious journal in the field, the *Journal of Studies on Alcohol (JSA*) in

January 1986. It was a reply to Cook's (1985) article on the "controlled drinking controversy". My cover letter accompanying the manuscript requested that it not be reviewed by the field editor for psychology, Marlatt, or by Nathan who at the time was Executive Editor of the *JSA*, head of the Rutgers Center of Alcohol Studies, and president of the corporation that was publisher of the *JSA*. My request was honored. It was reviewed by the editor for the field of sociology and two ad hoc reviewers and was accepted with a request for a minor revision. I received a letter from Geraldine Howell, Managing Editor, of the *JSA*, June 12, 1986, formally accepting the paper and asking me to sign and return a copyright assignment form. It was scheduled for publication in the November, 1986 issue and was listed among the articles accepted for publication in the July, 1986 issue.

After an unduly long delay in receiving the galley proofs, the managing editor called to say that Nathan found that my manuscript may be libelous. I wrote to Nathan explaining that the manuscript had been reviewed by counsel for the University of California and found free of libelous material. I asked him to indicate which material was considered libelous. He never responded to the query. On November 21, 1986 Nathan wrote:

The decision to refer your critique of Cook's ... paper to our University Counsel derived from two factors: 1) Two of those who read the critique raised the possibility of a libel suit ... 2) My own reading of the critique caused me to wonder about the same matter... As a consequence, I did decide to refer the critique to our University counsel in order to protect the University... Parenthetically, I found the critique surprisingly moderate, given the nature of your previous public pronouncements on the Sobells and their work.

Mendelson, editor of the *JSA*, on December 28, 1986, wrote:

Following your notification of acceptance of this article we invited Dr. Cook and Drs. Sobell to prepare a response which could be published along with your contribution. The Sobells responded to our invitation by stating they felt many of the comments you made in your article were libelous and they further stated that if your material were published, a suit against you and the Journal, its editors and publishers could ensue ... [We] requested an evaluation of the potential threat of a libel suit... by the University.... Counsel... [who] stated: 'After review [sic] the manuscript and the letter ... from the Sobells threatening such a suit, I have concluded there is a significant possibility of a libel suit over this article.

My reply to Mendelson is in the Notes to this chapter[4]. Examination of the letters by Nathan and by Mendelson raises some questions. Why did they wait so long before informing me of the threat of a potential law suit by the Sobells? Why wait until November, the publication date for my article, to contact me? Why the different descriptions of events by Mendelson and Nathan? Nathan makes it appear as though two independent reviewers suggested that my paper may be libelous whereas Mendelson states it was sent to the Sobells and Cook. I subsequently discovered that Marlatt (Marlatt & Forseth, 1991) tells a very different story; one that is more plausible than the above vignettes of what purportedly transpired.

Suing the Journal of Studies on Alcohol

I was fortunate to obtain the services of a large and prestigious Los Angeles law firm which accepted my case pro bono, in the public interest, and brought a law suit against the *JSA* and others. How did I obtain the services of the most prestigious law firm in Los Angeles, O'Melveny and Myers, Secretary of State Warren Christopher's old law firm, to represent me, pro bono ? I was lucky. Years before, I let Ken O'Rourke, an undergraduate friend of one of my graduate students, Rick Anderson, hang out in my lab. He lived in an animal house of a fraternity and needed a quiet place to study. In due time he graduated from UCLA and went to law school. Following graduation from law school Ken was hired by O'Melveny and Myers. He happened to be visiting Rick one afternoon while I was engrossed in the *JSA* dispute. I described the problem to Ken. He asked for a brief written description of the affair which he would present to a committee of the senior partners of O'Melveny and Myers for consideration. A few days later he told me that O'Melveny and Meyers would take the case pro bono. What luck!! It meant that I would not have to pay lawyers' fees. He thought, however, that I might have to pay some peripheral expenses such as xeroxing and his travel costs to New Jersey to discuss legal issues with the Rutgers attorney. I asked how much these minor supplies and expenses might be. Ken thought that they could be in the neighborhood of $30,000. I guess the stunned look on my face, the disbelief upon hearing that "free legal help" would cost only $30,000, suggested to him that I was unfamiliar with real legal costs. A few days later he called to tell me that upon further discussion the senior partners decided to waive the "minor" expenses involved.

A complaint was brought against the *JSA* and others for breach of contract and torts. This legal action followed repeated attempts by my attorneys, Ken O'Rourke, and Bob Vanderet to amicably resolve possible differences. Ken's request for information concerning which specific passages in my paper were libelous was never honored by the attorney for Rutgers. At considerable expense, I assume, to Rutgers, the State University of New Jersey, and the taxpayers of New Jersey, a large and prestigious Los Angeles law firm, Latham and Watkins, was hired to represent them. Faced with going to court they finally capitulated. After a delay of more than $3^1/_2$ years during which time there were numerous interchanges among attorneys and the court including a trip by a Latham and Watkins attorney to Toronto, my paper was published in the September 1989 issue of the *JSA* (Maltzman, 1989). It was preceded by a Prefatory Comment from Nathan (1989) and followed by replies to my paper by the Sobells (1989), Cook (1989), and Baker (1989).

We hear a great deal about how sleazy attorneys run up costs due to frivolous law suits, defraud senior citizens, are ruining the country, etc. There probably is some truth to that. There are sleazy untrustworthy lawyers, just as there are sleazy psychiatrists, clinical psychologists, physicians, auto mechanics, bankers, stock brokers, government officials, etc. No matter what occupation, there are some good ones, some bad ones, and a lot in between. One never knows until they are tested. I must say that my experience suing *JSA* left me impressed with the intelligence, integrity, knowledge, and drive of O'Rourke and Vanderet, and also with Van

128

Arsdale, the attorney from Latham and Watkins who was hired to represent *JSA* and Rutgers. Van Arsdale was not responsible for the kind of people he represented. Despite that happenstance he impressed me with his intelligence and fairness. After the case was concluded I thought about writing to congratulate and tell him that I admired his intelligence and integrity. I never got around to it. A few months later I learned that he had died of cancer.

Now let's return to sleaze. An interesting article was brought to my attention. It contained a revealing interview with Marlatt by Roger Forseth, editor of *Dionysos:* "the literature and intoxication triquarterly" published at the University of Wisconsin-Superior. It gives a different and more plausible account of how the *JSA* purportedly came to face the possibility of a libel suit from the Sobells and was forced to reject my manuscript. In the course of the interview, Marlatt (Marlatt & Forseth, 1991) states:

> Maltzman, who has apparently experienced some frustration with the acceptance of his views about the alleged scientific misconduct of the Sobells, has continued to try to have an article published that he believes will substantiate his claims that somehow the data in the original Sobells report were faked.... So he sent this article first to the *Behavioral Research and Therapy* (sic) where the Sobells published their original work. The editor, Jack Rachman... looked at it, judged it to be libelous, sent it to lawyers who said it was indeed libelous, and on those grounds rejected the article. Next Maltzman sent it to the *British Journal of Addiction*. The editor, Griffith Edwards, read it, also judged it to be libelous and rejected it. Finally, Maltzman sent it to *Journal of Studies on Alcohol (JSA)*, along with a note to the editor asking that I not be involved in the review process!... I first learned about the plan to publish it when I read in *JSA* the list of forthcoming articles. I saw it on the list, and the Sobells and Peter Nathan (the executive editor of *JSA*) saw it, and we all said, 'What's this?' 'What's this article?' We asked Mendelson and he said, 'Well I haven't really read it that carefully because we allow the field editors to make their own decisions.' We pointed out that the manuscript had been judged libelous by a couple of other journals, and that he might want to have the lawyers (at the Rutgers Center for Alcohol Studies, the publishing home of *JSA*) take a look at it, because the Sobells might sue if this gets in. Nathan and Mendelson consulted the lawyers, and the lawyers agreed that the article was libelous, so on further review would not be published. That, we thought, was the end of it. Maltzman then hired a law firm in Los Angeles and said, in effect, the field editor told me this has been accepted and now you're telling me it has been rejected. Breech (sic) of contract. We are going to sue Rutgers. (pp. 19-21).

I shall comment only briefly concerning some of the more obvious misrepresentations and distortions in Marlatt's interview. Contrary to Marlatt and Nathan's published comments my article was accepted on the basis of its scientific merit as the result of peer review. Efforts to reject it after its acceptance were the consequence of the intrusion of ideology and politics into the process. Ordinarily, the intrusion would have succeeded as it had in the past. Circumstances this time permitted me to obtain the pro bono services of a prestigious law firm. The manuscript published in the *JSA* was not the same manuscript "judged libelous by a couple of other journals". They were different manuscripts (Maltzman, 1992). Griffith Edwards, editor of the *BJA* did not judge my manuscript libelous out of hand as I have already indicated. He wanted to publish my paper until threatened by litigation.

Once my paper was published the Sobells did not turn around and sue the *JSA* and me for libel. In an interview reported in the *Chronicle of Higher Education*, the Sobells admitted that they never planned to sue the *JSA* (McDonald, 1989). Their little game of chicken in collaboration with Nathan and Marlatt cost Rutgers University and the taxpayers of New Jersey hundreds of thousands if not millions of dollars in legal fees. By the nature of his control over the *JSA*, Nathan was able to write an editorial comment making it appear that the *JSA* was forced to publish my unmeritorious paper and Cook, the Sobells, and Baker, could safely rationalize their defense. My reply (Maltzman, unpublished d), again, was censored and never published.

Nathan, the Executive Editor and chief officer of the corporation that owns the *JSA* wrote a Prefatory Comment (Nathan, 1989) that precedes the series of articles. In it he likens my relentless attacks on the Sobells to the Ayatollah Khomeini's ruthless pursuit of Salman Rushdie. He states in his Comment that I was requested to withdraw my paper, which is false. He states that the *JSA* was publishing my article because they are honoring a commitment, which is false. They were forced to honor their commitment by my legal action. Nathan's comment is falsified by the objective record, including legal documents on file in the Superior Court of the County of Los Angeles (Maltzman v Alcohol Research Documentation,1988).

In an interview in the Chronicle of Higher Education:

Mr. Sobell acknowledged that he and his wife, Linda, had threatened lawsuits against the British journal and the journal at Rutgers after reading advance copies of Mr. Maltzman's papers, but maintained that it was 'utter nonsense' to suggest that they had sought to intimidate the editors of the journals to prevent their publication... Mr. Sobell, who called the whole matter 'unfortunate,' said he had no plans to sue the journal or Mr. Maltzman over publication of Mr. Maltzman's paper. (McDonald, 1989, pp. A5, A19).

Why is it that when I read the Sobells, Marlatt, Nathan, W. Miller, etc., I am reminded of Orwellian "doublethink"[3] , and "Newspeak"? In his letter Nathan complimented me on my moderation. Now to the *Chronicle of Higher Education* Nathan says:

he objected to the paper because of "Mr. Maltzman's '*ad hominem* ' attacks on the Sobells", which, he added, "repeated charges that he made in print before" and, "Mr. Maltzman's article 'raises no new issues and provides no new insights. Instead, it repeats a series of allegations that have been considered and rejected by five separate and competent investigative groups" (McDonald, 1989, p. A13)

The Sobells threatened a lawsuit but did not plan to sue and think that threatened law suits are not intimidating? Doublethink. I brought an ethics complaint against Nathan. My letter to Mills, Director of the Office of Ethics stated: "His 'Prefatory Comment' published in the *Journal of Studies on Alcohol*, ... copy enclosed, makes intentionally false and misleading statements and therefore violates... Ethical principles... Some of the evidence confirming these violations is indicated in my reply to the Prefatory Comment,...a copy... enclosed." (Maltzman, to Mills, December 26, 1989). Six months later I received a reply from Betsy Ranslow, Administrative Director of the Office of Ethics:

Your complaint has been evaluated independently by the Chair of the APA Ethics Committee and by me. On the basis of those independent evaluations, we have unanimously decided that the evidence simply does not support a charge of an ethics violation and we are, therefore, closing this matter and will take no further action.

While I am sure this comes as a disappointment to you, Dr. Maltzman, I hope you can understand that well meaning individuals can read the same materials and come to somewhat different conclusions. Nonetheless, in this case, we feel that there was no ethics violation involved. (B. Ranslow to Maltzman, June 27, 1990). More doublethink.

Censorship by failure of nerve

In 1989 I submitted a manuscript for a chapter in an edited book on values and human development. Part of the chapter was a case history of my experiences in attempting to expose the alleged scientific misconduct by the Sobells. It was used to illustrate the inherent role of values in science. I titled my chapter, "The place of facts in a world of values", which was a play on the title of a classic book by Wolfgang Köhler, one of the founders of Gestalt psychology, *The place of values in a world of facts* (Köhler, 1938). My chapter was accepted by the book editors and forwarded to the series editor for the publisher, John Wiley. I had told one of the book editors who was an old friend of mine that I thought it best that the manuscript be reviewed by attorneys for Wiley, because I did not wish to mislead them with respect to the controversial nature of some of its contents. After a delay of approximately a year I found myself engaged in conference calls with an editor and an attorney for Wiley concerning the specific wording of various parts of the manuscript. After further long delays I was informed that I would have to remove the entire case history, a critical part of the paper, and all references to it. I refused. The Wiley editor on advice of counsel said that they wanted to publish the chapter but I must remove the material in question because of the possibility of legal action and the attendant costs of the defense against such action. They admitted such legal action was remote given the history of my experience and the interview published in the *Chronicle of Higher Education* (McDonald, 1989) in which Mark Sobell stated that they never intended to sue the *JSA* over publication of my paper. Nevertheless, legal action remained a logical possibility.

After further delay, I had an idea. I proposed that the law firm that had represented me in legal action against the *JSA*, O'Melveny and Myers might represent Wiley in case of legal action against them. I was told that it was an interesting idea, but it would be costly if they should lose the case. Attorneys for Wiley recognized that legal action against them was a very remote possibility given the legal as well the financial burden involved in bringing a libel complaint against a publisher represented by a major law firm, but it still was a logical possibility. Wiley therefore could not accept the offer. I must remove the case history and all references to it in the manuscript.

I had another idea several days later. I inquired and discovered that it was possible to obtain an insurance policy from Lloyds of London covering a single event, e.g., a single ship voyage - or publication of a single book. I informed the

Wiley editor that I personally would obtain insurance indemnifying them as well as providing legal representation. The editor thought that was a creative idea. He would get back to me. Wiley legal advisors thought it was an interesting idea. Nevertheless they rejected the proposal because it could give them a "bad image". I withdrew my manuscript. An editor said I was being self-righteous. I said I refused to submit to censorship. The book has now been published without my chapter, entitled, ironically, *The role of values in psychology and human development* (Kurtines, Azmitia, & Gewirtz, 1992).

One more failure of nerve

A relatively new journal appeared, *Ethics and Behavior*, that I thought would be an ideal vehicle for the chapter I withdrew from Wiley. I sent the manuscript to the editor. It came back with mixed reviews. It was much too long and rambling but very interesting and relevant. The editor, Gerald Koocher, asked me to shorten the paper. It was originally written as a chapter in a book which is much too long for an article in a journal. I shortened it a bit, but cutting it felt like cutting flesh from my body. It hurt. Again, it got positive reviews for interest and relevance, but was too long. This time one of the reviewers who Koocher said was a lawyer as well as a psychologist suggested that the next revision be first sent to the Sobells. They should have the right to review it and decide whether or not they object to its publication. I thought this was entirely unreasonable, a decision driven by fear of litigation, not the norms of professional journal review and I could foretell the outcome. I withdrew my manuscript.

One has courage

A magazine for alcoholism and drug counselors edited at the time by Cliff Creager had the courage to publish a paper of mine in which the "F" word was allowed to appear. After review by an attorney for the publisher a brief article called, "The winter of scholarly journals" was published in the *Professional Counselor* (Maltzman, 1989). Neither the publisher nor I have been sued for libel.

Ideology and the withering of scholarship in professional journals

Chapter 1 was originally written as a paper submitted to the *JSA*. After my legal dispute with the *JSA* quieted down there was a reorganization of its editorial board. Mendelson was replaced by an acting editor who eventually was replaced by a permanent new editor, Marc Schuckit. Marlatt was no longer on the editorial board. He claims (Marlatt & Forseth, 1991) that he resigned because he did not wish his colleagues to believe that he was responsible for the publication of my article. Nathan was no longer Executive Editor of the *JSA* since he left Rutgers University to go, the irony of it, to the University of Iowa, my alma mater. He was appointed Provost and given a chaired professorship in the Department of Psychology. Whether or not the fiasco that cost *JSA* and Rutgers a fortune in legal fees was responsible for these changes, I do not know.

Ideologically driven editors can practice censorship by following the form but not the substance of using impartial experts as reviewers of papers submitted for publication. All that is necessary is to choose a reviewer whose ideological biases agree with yours, one who would be a willing apologist for the Sobells, Marlatt, etc., and their revisionist distortion of past and present research and theory.

Since Marlatt and Nathan were gone and there was a new acting editor and an associate editor for psychology, I assumed that I might receive an impartial review from the *JSA* of a paper that I had written on why alcoholism is a disease. In its early form the paper was a critique of Fingarette's (1988b) popular book, *Heavy Drinking*, which was a succinctly written book summarizing the revisionist misconceptions and distortions of Marlatt, Miller, Peele, and the Sobells, with the addition of several whoppers of his own. One of the great things about teaching a college course is that it forces you to keep up with the literature in a field and it forces you to understand in detail the nature of the relevant research literature and theory under study. If you have to explain a particular research project or theory to a class of undergraduate students you have to make it interesting to keep them awake and intelligible to avoid a sea of blank faces. In a way, teaching the substance of a subject is a matter of self-preservation. Few things are so humbling and frustrating as to receive a term paper or exam filled with gibberish - which at least in part is your fault.

Furthermore, if you are going to do intellectual battle, you better be sure that you know more about the field and your adversary's position than they do. Teaching in the area helps. After several years of teaching about why I thought alcoholism is a disease in my undergraduate course on alcoholism, I started writing a critique of Fingarette's book (1988b). It could not be entirely negative, so I shifted the main point to a presentation of the bare bones essential characteristics of a disease, what it has meant over the course of history to call a condition a disease and why alcoholism meets these conditions. After quite a long delay following submission of my manuscript I received a letter from Howard Blane, the associate editor for Psychology, with three reviews and a cover letter explaining the process and the reason for rejecting my manuscript.

The initial two reviews were divided in their opinion. One was very brief, a few paragraphs and was relatively negative, obviously missing the main points of my paper. The second review was very positive and considered my paper an important contribution. Blane then asked for a third review, the tie breaker. It was a three page review that gave detailed criticisms. They were the kind of remarks that Marlatt would make. Blane rejected my paper on the basis of the third review. I wrote a 46 page reply, covering the third review literally line-by-line, disarming the arguments, pointing out its errors of fact, misinterpretations, and omissions. I also took heed of reasonable criticisms and made the paper less abrasive, including a change in title. I sent my detailed criticisms of the reviews to Blane asking him to reconsider his evaluation of my paper in the light of my rebuttal of the negative reviews. A copy was also sent to John Carpenter, acting editor. Blane wrote back that his judgment stands. He does not reconsider decisions. I submitted the paper to the *Journal of Psychoactive Drugs* where it was accepted after minor revisions. Chapter 1 is a slightly updated version of that paper (Maltzman, 1992) combined with a reply to a critic (Maltzman, 1998).

Follow the party line

An indication of the widespread acceptance of behavior therapy and the productivity of its practitioners is that for more than a decade an annual review was published each year with chapters written by different specialists summarizing behavior therapy publications in major areas of clinical psychology including a chapter on addictive behaviors. Volumes regularly reported controlled drinking studies and theory. When the Pendery et al. (1982) article was published, the "Sobell affair" received prominent coverage. Regardless of the author of the chapter on addictive disorders, Brownell or Foreyt, both specialists in eating disorders, a biased presentation supporting the Sobells was provided, often taking their cue from Nathan. In the final volume of the series, Foreyt (1990) wrote:

I know that I promised in the previous volume of this series that final comments on the Sobell and Sobell... controlled drinking controversy had been written and that the story had been laid to rest. Unfortunately, another article, along with several rejoinders has been published; thus, some comment needs to be made for those readers still following the saga. Readers unfamiliar with the history are referred to the original articles... and reviews of the controversy in Volumes 9, 10, and 11 of this series (Brownell, 1984, 1985; Foreyt, 1987b).

The latest article is one by Maltzman (1989) in which he states the same allegations he has made over the past seveal years. Reading his article, I could not find anything new in it that I had not read previously. The article appears to me to simply repeat what he has already written (e.g., Pendery et al., 1982).

In the same issue of the *Journal of Studies on Alcohol* is a strong editorial statement by Nathan (1989). He comments that the Maltzman article was accepted by a field editor and that the journal later requested that it be withdrawn because parts were thought to be inappropriate. The request was refused and the article was published to honor the journal's commitment. Nathan also writes that, in his reading, Maltzman raises no new issues....

I was again impressed with how thoughtfully and impressively the Sobells handled each of the attacks on them and their work. Although minor errors in the reporting of their data were found, none of these errors appeared to have affected the study's outcome. Only because the Sobells kept such detailed records of their study, including original tapes and notes, were the inquiries able to arrive at their conclusions. The outcomes of the inquiries indicate that the results of their study are correct. This latest article by Maltzman does not add any new information as far as I can determine... Their study has been essentially vindicated by five separate inquiries. It has been drawn out long enough, and it has diverted attention away from the growing number of reports investigating the role of controlled drinking with individuals who have difficulty handling alcohol. The Sobells write that they anticipate that their calling a halt will be welcomed by most who have followed the controversy. I for one agree with them. Let's call it quits and turn our priorities to other issues in this field. (pp. 215-217).

I wrote to Foreyt with copies to editors of the volume stating my intention of bringing a complaint to CSPEC. I received conciliatory letters from Foreyt and from editors of the volume denying that he was unethical or biased. I submitted a complaint to the APA Ethics committee and replied to Foreyt.

My complaint was that Foreyt violated principal 4g of the Ethical Principles and that his misrepresentations may directly affect the well-being of the public by misleading clinical practice. Ranslow, Director of Investigations for the Office of Ethics, replied several months later:

I have now had the opportunity to carefully evaluate your complaint against Dr. John P. Foreyt of Houston, Texas. Your complaint has been evaluated independently by the Chair of the APA Ethics Committee and by me. On the basis of the review of all of the information related to this matter, we have decided not to open this matter up as a formal ethics case and to close it under the provisions of Part V, Section 5.4 of the 1992 *Rules and Procedures* .

While I am sure this comes as a disappointment to you, I hope that you can understand that we took your complaint seriously and made the decision that seemed most fair in light of all the materials received. (B. Ranslow to Maltzman, May 17, 1993).

The rule in question, Part V, Section 5.4 states:

If the Director and chair do not agree that there is cause for action by the Committee, the matter shall be closed. The matter shall also be closed if the Director and Chair agree that, although cause for action otherwise exists, the allegations even if substantiated would constitute a trivial violation or one likely to be corrected. In the event of closure, the Director shall so inform the complainant in writing. A case closed pursuant to this subsection may be reopened only if the complainant presents significant new evidence, as defined in Part II, Section 6.

Apparently the Ethics Committee considers misrepresenting the truth, exaggerating, distorting, and failing to present relevant information concerning the treatment of individuals with a disorder that may cause serious harm to themselves and to others of no real importance. If this is the attitude expressed by the APA Ethics Committee which purports to educate the membership in values basic to the science and profession, then it is no wonder that the norms of appropriate professional behavior have sunk to the level they have.

I will give a final example of the biasing effect of ideology on the conduct of gatekeepers, the professional journals. I wrote a reply to the paper published by Marlatt, Larimer, Baer and Quigley (1993) appearing in the journal *Behavior Therapy* a publication of the Association for the Advancement of Behavior (AABT). It was an expansion of Marlatt's presidential address to the Association. With a few additions and deletions to avoid redundancy with material in other chapters of this book my manuscript which was rejected is now chapter 8.

Following rejection by *Behavior Therapy* I thought I would try my luck with the *Journal of Psychoactive Drugs*, since they published my paper "Why alcoholism is a disease" after its rejection by *JSA*. Although I felt that publication in *Psychoactive Drugs* is a bit like preaching to the choir because it is a journal directed towards practitioners in the field. It is not oriented towards behavior therapy or any other specific "school". I felt that at least the objections I raise to Marlatt's evident lack of scholarship and the Sobells' alleged misconduct would receive an airing. It was somewhat of a surprise to receive a prompt rejection from the Managing Editor, Jeffrey Novey, without benefit of input from reviewers. He wrote that the paper should be published in the journal in which the original article I am criticizing had been published. I replied that I agreed, but that the journal in question had rejected my paper. I included with my letter the reviewers' comments and my reply to the reviews. Novey replied that his original position is unchanged. The argument is between the editor of *Behavior Therapy* and me and that's where the paper should be submitted.

I made one final attempt to publish the paper in a journal, submitting it to *Psychological Reports,* a general psychology journal that publishes articles covering the entire range of psychology. Quality of its articles varies considerably. It ranges from brief articles and preliminary investigations to long, detailed, and thoughtful conceptual articles by such giants in the field as Paul Meehl. Accompanying my manuscript was a cover letter and the reviews and my reply to the editor of *Behavior Therapy.* The Editor of *Psychological Reports,* Carol Ammons, obtained extensive reviews which she forwarded to me. She did not provide her reviewers with the reviews from *Behavior Therapy* or my reply. Reviews obtained by Ammons were generally favorable, with a variety of suggestions for modifying the manuscript, including the elimination of quotations from Bronowski's work and pejorative terms such as "revisionist", and "pettifogging". Ammons agreed with these suggestions. I thanked her for the thoughtful reviews and withdrew my manuscript from consideration explaining that I could not accede to the proposed revisions. Ammons wished me luck and requested that if I obtain publication elsewhere I should kindly send her six reprints for the reviewers some of whom would like to cite my paper. I thought that any further submissions to journals would be a waste of time. It is time to write a book.

NOTES

1. This and the later quotation of Dorinson to Essaye are from a letter David Dorison, Esq., an attorney on the staff of the Regents of the University of California wrote to Anthony Essaye, Esq., an attorney representing *Science* in its response to threats of litigation from the Sobells. The letter was written in response to Essaye's request for some background to the dispute with the Sobells.
2. Due to the poor quality of the tape and transcript in addition to my chronologically disadvantaged memory, these are not the exact words she used, but the statement captures her essential point.
3. Orwell (1949) describes doublethink as follows:
   To know and not to know, to be conscious of complete truthfulness while telling carefully constructed lies, to hold simultaneously two opinions which cancelled out, knowing them to be contradictory and believing in both of them; to use logic against logic, to repudiate morality while laying claim to it, to believe that democracy was impossible and that the Party was the guardian of democracy; to forget whatever it was necessary to forget, then to draw it back into memory again at the moment when it was needed, and then promptly to forget it again: and above all, to apply the same process to the process itself. That was the ultimate subtlety: consciously to induce unconsciousness, and then, to become unconscious of the act of hypnosis you had just performed. Even to understand the word 'doublethink' involved the use of doublethink." (pp.29-30).
4. Letter to Mendelson, editor of the *Journal of Studies on Alcohol.*

UNIVERSITY OF CALIFORNIA, LOS ANGELES UCLA

BERKELEY · DAVIS · IRVINE · LOS ANGELES · RIVERSIDE · SAN DIEGO · SAN FRANCISCO   SANTA BARBARA · SANTA CRUZ

DEPARTMENT OF PSYCHOLOGY
LOS ANGELES, CALIFORNIA 90024

2/9/87

Jack H. Mendelson, M. D.
Alcohol and Drug Abuse Research Center
Harvard Medical School
McLean Hospital
115 Mill Street
Belmont, MA 02178

Dear Dr. Mendelson:

Re: A REPLY TO COOK, "CRAFTSMAN VERSUS PROFESSIONAL: ANALYSIS
OF THE CONTROLLED DRINKING CONTROVERSY"

I have received your letter of December 28 in which you state, "Since
the university counsel has determined that the contents of your article
engender a significant possibility of a libel suit, we have decided that we
will be unable to publish your article. I regret that this situation has
arisen, but I'm sure you understand I cannot permit publication of
libelous material in the Journal based upon recommendation of the Office
of University Counsel from the State University of New Jersey, owners
and publishers of the Journal."

No, I really do not understand how the most prestigious journal in its
field and an established university and its press can be so easily
intimidated by the mere threat of a libel suit and be so insensitive to the
implications of their actions for the alcoholism field and for society as a
whole.

Your statement, "I cannot permit publication of libelous material in
the Journal.." is inaccurate and misleading. My paper is not libelous
merely because the Sobells or their attorney say it is. It is libelous if it
is so established in a court of law.

I have been on record since 1976 stating my belief that the Sobells
committed fraud. My allegation was accurately quoted in the NY Times in
1982. The Sobells have never brought suit against me. They never have,
because the best defense against libel is the truth, and I believe they
know I am telling the truth. For them to win a law suit against the
JOURNAL for publishing my paper the Sobells must prove in court that I
demonstrated a willful disregard for the truth and a malicious intent to
do them harm. Do you seriously believe that my paper approved by peer

Figure 4.1 Letter to Mendelson. Page 1 of 3.

2

reviewers as worthy of publication in the JOURNAL lends itself to such proof? Do you really think the Sobells are prepared to be cross-examined under oath, have all of their records subpoened, permit the patients to testify, etc.?

In 1982 the Sobells brought an ethics complaint against me before the American Psychological Association Ethics Committee because of my allegations of fraud publication by the NY Times. The Ethics Committee censured me; I appealed, and in an appearance before the Committee presented the bases for my belief that the Sobells committed fraud and that the Dickens Committee Report exonerating them was fundamentally flawed. The Ethics Committee rescinded their censure of me and stated that I had a reasonable basis for my beliefs. A few years ago I wrote a brief note pointing out that our critics, including the Dickens Committee Report, inappropriately criticized our Science article for failing to compare the Sobells' experimental and control group. We did compare the two groups and found a significant difference in the order of appearance between the experimental and control subjects. Any further comparison between the two groups would violate the fundamental assumption of any statistical analysis we might conduct, the assumption of random assignment. In passing I mentioned that the Dickens Committee Report was not disinterested. Professors Dickens and Doob threatened a libel suit and brought an ethics complaint against me. The American Psychological Association Ethics Committee dismissed the complaint against me following the presentation of my case against the Dickens Report. Professors Dickens and Doob have never sued me.

I have affidavits from 10 of the 13 living patients in the Sobells' experimental group that Caddy states he interviewed for his follow-up study. They and their collaterals swear that they never received his 80 minute tape recorded interview. Do you think that Caddy is willing to go to court and testify under oath and the penalty of perjury that he conducted these interviews when he cannot produce records of the interviews, which certainly would be subpoened, and the patients and their collaterals would testify to the contrary?

I submit that these threats of a libel suit from the Sobells and their suggestion that Dickens and Caddy would also sue is an empty threat.

Before I submitted my manuscript to the JOURNAL it was reviewed by counsel for the University of California and found free of potentially libelous material. This university counsel is familiar with the case since 1976 when the Sobells, in the name of a fictitious patient, brought a law suit against me, the University of California, and others, in an effort to prevent us from interviewing the patients. The judge in federal court ruled in our favor on the basis of the brief written by this same university counsel.

It is to the Sobells' advantage to prevent my manuscript from being

Figure 4.1 Letter to Mendelson. Page 2 of 3.

3

published, because I believe that any reasonably impartial reader will conclude from it that the Sobells in fact committed fraud. It costs the Sobells nothing to threaten a law suit. To actually mount one is an entirely different matter. It seems to me that a science journal and a university must be willing to take some risk in the defense of the pursuit of the truth, in the defense of the values science and our society deem to be important. What is a university, a university press, a science journal, science, for? What are they worth, if they are so easily intimidated? I do not believe that science as a serious enterprise worthy of public trust and support can survive when as a consequence of the mere threat of litigation it is willing to suppress the expression of criticism and the exposure of scientific misconduct.

I do not believe that I have been dealt with fairly. My manuscript was accepted following peer review and I transferred my copyright to the JOURNAL. Your subsequent rejection of my manuscript I feel is a breach of contract and of trust. I was not afforded the privilege of reviewing and commenting upon Cook's paper prior to its publication in the JOURNAL. Nevertheless, after the entire review process of my paper had been completed it was sent to the Sobells for comment and the opportunity of a reply. I believe that anyone at all familiar with the Sobells' history of litigious threats could have predicted the outcome.

Sincerely yours,

Irving Maltzman
Professor

cc: David Dorinson Esq.
   Associate Counsel of the Regents
   Office of the General Counsel
   590 University Hall
   2199 Addison St
   Berkeley, CA 94720

Figure 4.1 Letter to Mendelson. Page 3 of 3.

5 HOW NOT TO CONDUCT AN INVESTIGATION

DICKENS REPORT EXONERATES SOBELLS

The first and most extensive investigation of the Sobells' alleged fraud was conducted by the Dickens Committee appointed by the Sobells' employer at the time allegations of misconduct appeared (Boffey, 1982), the Addiction Research Foundation, a state supported research and treatment foundation in Toronto, Canada. Chairman of the Committee, Bernard M. Dickens was a professor of law at the University of Toronto, as well as a professor in the Department of Preventive Medicine and Biostatistics, and a member of the Graduate Faculty in Law, Criminology, and Community. A second member was Anthony N. Doob, Professor of Psychology at the University of Toronto and Director of its Center of Criminology. He was also a member of the Professional Advisory Board of the Addiction Research Foundation. O. Harold Warwick, M.D. was the third member of the Committee, a professor emeritus of the University of Western Ontario. William Charles Winegard, a physicist and former President and Vice-Chancellor of the University of Guelph was the final member of the Committee. It was a distinguished group, in the sense that all had illustrious careers within their professions. None, however, had any apparent experience in the investigation of fraud in science or in the conduct of treatment outcome studies.

I had previously described their Report as not being disinterested (Maltzman,1984). The Dickens Committee Report (1982) and subsequent comments by Doob (1984) are not uninvolved, neutral, free from bias. Most importantly, I believe, the Dickens Report is seriously flawed. It cannot be taken as a vindication of the Sobells. It is not a document demonstrating that the Sobells are innocent of scientific misconduct. Three basic allegations are made against the Sobells: (a) they knowingly did not interview the patients as frequently as they stated in their publications, every 3-4 weeks; (b) detailed drinking dispositions of the kind the Sobells described in their publications were not obtained from the majority of patients when they were interviewed; (c) subjects were not randomly assigned to experimental and control groups; some were intentionally reassigned. I believe that the Dickens Committee failed to investigate these allegations in a disinterested and thorough manner as befits the seriousness of the issues involved. Instead, they diverted attention from these issues by attacking the methodology of Pendery et al. (1982).

From the outset, an investigating committee appointed by a foundation whose employees are alleged to have committed scientific fraud is suspect (Kilbourne & Kilbourne, 1983). The Addiction Research Foundation administration, finding itself in a situation where two of its employees are accused of fraud, perceives itself as having much to lose in credibility and nothing to gain by finding evidence of fraud. There is a loss of credibility because their judgment would be questioned: they hired two young people against whom allegations of fraud had already been made (Maltzman, 1976) and apparently had not acted upon that information when it was initially received. Under these circumstances the Dickens Committee had a significant obligation to avoid any appearance of a conflict of interest by conducting an exhaustive and comprehensive investigation. I believe that the Report demonstrates that the Committee failed to overcome the presumption of partiality. I will now turn to the grounds for my belief that the Dickens Committee Report is not disinterested and is fundamentally flawed.

Requirements for an effective investigation of fraud in science

By fraud I mean any one or more of the following: (a) the fabrication of data, the intentional creation of fake results, (b) the intentional misrepresentation of procedures, (c) the intentional misrepresentation of the significance or import of results.

The self-evident first step in an examination of alleged fraud in science by an investigating body is to demand the basic evidence, the raw data: Do these raw data reproduce the results found in the allegedly fraudulent publications? The most important raw data in the Sobells' study include the interviews with the subjects. These provided the data for the basic dependent measure employed by the Sobells, daily drinking disposition. The latter has five components, days drinking moderately, days abstaining, days drunk, days hospitalized, and days in jail for alcohol related reasons. The latter two measures are public, readily verifiable, and have never been questioned by me. The first three are the critical measures dependent upon interviews with the patients. In all of their published reports of the study the Sobells asserted that they interviewed their patients and as many collaterals as possible every 3-4 weeks for two full years. An exception was a handful of difficult to find participants:

subjects were told that the follow-up was to be conducted with both themselves and their CIS [collaterals] approximately every month. They were told that the mode of contact (phone, letter, or personal) would be the method deemed easiest to obtain the necessary information. While subjects were not aware of the specific kinds of questions to be asked, nor the particular criteria used to evaluate their functioning, they were aware that questions would be asked about the specific amounts of alcohol they consumed each day and about other areas of life health functioning. (Sobell & Sobell, 1978, p. 108).

During each interview the Sobells obtained the days drunk, days abstinent, and days drinking in a controlled manner for the previous month purportedly using the time-line follow-back method. Their basic dependent variable, daily drinking disposition, is derived from these measures. Their measure of days functioning well is derived from the first two, days abstinent and days drinking in moderation. The first three measures constituting the daily drinking disposition are the critical measures dependent upon interviews with the patients.

One of the most effective techniques for filling in the time-line is to identify anchor points, generally defined as distinctive time-bound events (e.g., holidays, weekends, birthdays). Other more idiosyncratic anchor points include days marked by arrests, hospitalizations, illnesses, and entry into treatment. As anchor point events are identified and recorded on the calendar, subjects are asked to recall their drinking on the day of those events, as well as the days preceding and following those occasions. (Sobell et al., 1979, p. 158).

A first step in a reasonable investigation of fraud is the examination of the raw data and the reconstruction from them of the dependent variable(s) reported in publications. This obvious first step was never taken by the Dickens Committee. The Dickens Report lists the data base it used, the data provided to them by the Sobells (Dickens et al., 1982, pp. 35-40). This extensive list of data does not include the most essential raw data of all, the interview sheets that yield the daily drinking disposition. Listed in the data base employed are previously published tables and graphs of individual drinking profiles, but not the interview forms containing the original raw data from which the tables and graphs are purportedly derived.

The Committee appears to lack an understanding of what constitutes the critical raw data out of which the Sobells constructed their basic dependent variable, daily drinking dispositions and from that, days functioning well. Daily drinking dispositions are purportedly obtained by the time-line follow-back method and reported on a form for each interview. The Committee's apparent lack of understanding of the nature of the essential raw data is reflected in their comment following the listing of their database:

> No amount of data, notes , letters and attestations would convince an atheist that God exists, or a believer that He does not. Similarly, it is possible that no amount of data would convince someone who believed that the Sobells had fabricated their results that they had not. (p.40).

I submit that the above is an example of the biased comments that pervade the Dickens Report. No amount of the sort of data that they describe would convince me because the contents of their database are largely irrelevant and the critical data are absent. It is obvious that the kind of data available and used are critical, not the amount. This gratuitous remark is one of many expressions of a lack of disinterestedness in the Report.

Instead of examining the raw data on the interview sheets purportedly obtained by the time-line follow-back method, the Report discusses at length the number of hospitalizations reported by the Sobells as compared to the number reported by Pendery et al. However, the number of hospitalizations of the patients are a matter of public record, relatively easy to confirm, and were never in dispute. In dispute was the cause of the hospitalizations and their interpretation, not the number. Our evidence supported by personal and institutional collateral information and examined in the editorial offices of *Science* showed that the hospitalizations were caused by excessive drinking. The Sobells claimed that many of the hospitalizations were the consequence of the subjects' desire to avoid excessive drinking.

Further evidence of the Committees' lack of understanding of the relevant data is reflected in the following statement:

> In the setting we faced, much of the Sobells' data had been made available to Pendery et al. through the Sobells' publications. Pendery et al. had been able to examine these, and had either challenged them or had decided not to contest them in their independent research. (Dickens et al., 1982, p.32).

Summary statistics, means and totals of the days drunk, etc. in a six-month period are not the raw data. These are the published summaries of the raw data and are easy to invent. Information on the interview sheets or the scraps of paper containing the information to be recorded on interview sheets are the raw data. They are summarized by the totals presented by the Sobells, 282 days abstinent, 57 days controlled drinking, 27 days drunk, etc. Subjects' individual data for the second year presented in their book (Sobell & Sobell, 1978, pp. 34-36), sums of raw data purportedly taken from the subjects' interview sheets, are the material which must be examined by an investigation of fraud in science. Means of 6 months or a year are not the raw data. They are summaries. The summary totals reported for the individual subjects are the data that must be reconstructed from the interview sheets or papers the Sobells ought to have given the Committee. Instead, we are told that the Committee's database, provided by the Sobells, contained summary sheets by subject for each six months period for the two years of follow-up.

There is another glaring omission in the relevant data base. The Report states: "We did not consider it right for us to attempt to approach the original subjects of the Sobells' 1972 investigation and the follow-up studies who were traceable, or their study 'collaterals'... and to seek their evidence." (p. 33f). Why not? Ostensibly to protect the confidentiality of subjects. However, this hurdle could easily have been overcome. The medical director of Patton State Hospital could have been asked to request the patients' permission to be interviewed and their identity could have remained confidential by coding. Other avenues were available; none were pursued. On the other hand, affidavits and communications from the staff were obtained by the Committee to support the Sobells' claim that patients were randomly assigned to their treatments. Neither interviews nor affidavits were requested from even a randomly selected group of patients to report on their memory of the frequency and kind of interview they experienced. There was no hesitancy on the part of the Committee to rely on the memory of staff when it came to recall coin tosses for assignment to treatment. It is important to note that staff members were not asked to recall which persons were randomly assigned to which group as a result of the coin toss. In contrast, no subjects were interviewed or asked to submit written answers to relevant questions.

A disinterested Commttee had within their reach the means of refuting my allegation of fraud: Interview Subject #14 and compare his description of the interview March 23, 1972 with the procedures and raw data found on the interview sheets for that specific interview which had to cover the 5.5 months back to October 9, 1971. Although the Committee had the means of refuting my allegation of fraud, putting the entire case to rest, it also ran the risk of proving that my allegation of fraud was true: Detailed interview sheets containing raw data reproducing the published results for Subject #14 and others did not exist. Interviewing patients put the Committee on the slippery slope that could prove fraud. The overwhelming majority of the patients would have reported that they were only occasionally interviewed and that the interview was not a detailed day-by-day reconstruction of their daily drinking disposition as required by the time-line follow-back method. A thorough investigation of fraud in science would have responded to the allegations in my affidavit accompanying the brief in the 1977 legal action brought by the Sobells.

The Committee list Pendery's and my affidavit in their database and comment upon the affidavits in their Report:

> Dr. Pendery appears not to have made use of the word 'fraud' in her published or reported language. Her Declaration prepared in 1976 for the Sobells' 1977 litigation, for instance, is notably lacking in any of the express charges of

deliberate misrepresentations which figure for instance in Dr. Maltzman's public statements. (p. 28).

The Report also states:

Dr. Maltzman's allegations in his sworn statements prepared for the 1977 litigation and, for instance, in the New York Times' unrepudiated quotations, also provided a clear guide to the nature of the allegations against the Sobells, and allowed the Committee to identify the major and minor issues upon which we required the Sobells to defend their scientific and personal integrity in their conduct and presentation of their challenged work. (Dickens et al., 1982, p. 31).

Frequency of patient interviews and patient contacts

The Dickens Report confirms (p.75ff) and the Sobells now admit that the majority of subjects were not contacted every 3-4 weeks as stated in the published reports of their research. Evidence that the Sobells did not do what they said they did is presented in the Dickens Committee Report. This evidence consists of the purported number of patient contacts. Nowhere does the Dickens Report present evidence that the dependent variable, the daily drinking disposition derived from the interview obtained from each patient, was collected using the time-line follow-back method in each purported contact.

Patients and other collateral sources who have seen the Dickens Report assert that even the reduced numbers of contacts reported therein are inflated. They insist that they did not have as many contacts as listed by the Dickens Report (Table 1, p. 78). These contacts are shown in Table 5.1.

The Dickens Report (1982) states:

The records showed that in a number of cases subjects were not contacted for periods of three to six months. This break in contact with subjects was not stated or otherwise disclosed in the Sobells' published papers directed to follow-up results of their original study. The technique that was developed to track back over the time lapse in order to fill in details of subjects' drinking history with a degree of reliability, is called "time-line follow-back" interviewing. It is dependent upon such methods as identifying anchor points consisting of distinctive, time-bound events around which other events can be constructed, and has been described in independent literature by the Sobells... No mention of the need or the means to develop this technique appears, however, in published reports of the Patton State Hospital study follow-up research. The Sobells did not do what they said they did; and, until the committee actually counted the number of recorded contacts, they have never apparently questioned whether their goal of monthly contacts had been achieved. (p.80).

Table 5.1 Frequency of Follow-up Contacts for Experimental Subjects and Randomly Selected Control Subjects (Dickens et al., l982, p.78)

All Experimental Subjects	Year 1	Year 2
1	11	17
2	17	8
*3	6	5
4	12	3
5	10	2
6	15	5
7	10	5
8	5	6
*9	9	7
10	7	5
11A	5	8
12	2	1
13	7	5
*14	10	6
15	9	7
16	9	7
17	7	6
18	8	7
*19	8	11
20	7	3

Random Control Subjects

2	This subject was never found	
1	9	5
9	5	2
14	8	5
17C	11	1
19D	4	5

A - Jailed for 4 months
B - Noted difficult to find
C - In hospital for 9 months
D - Lost for several months
* - Randomly selected by Dickens Commission for more detailed study

A striking lack of disinterestedness is evident, I believe, in the above passage. The Dickens Committee states as fact, not something to be investigated, the Sobells' use of the previously undisclosed procedure for interviewing the Patton patients, the time-line follow-back method. The Committee made no effort to determine whether or not in fact the Sobells had employed the method in the Patton study. It simply accepted the Sobells' word for it. Whether or not the Sobells actually used the time-line follow-back method is of critical importance. Otherwise, they could hardly claim to have obtained reliable daily drinking dispositions, for example, from Subject #5 who was interviewed only twice in the entire second year (Dickens et al., 1982, p. 78). One would assume that a disinterested investigation would explore the possibility that people under investigation for alleged scientific fraud might not be entirely trustworthy. Instead, the Dickens Committee accepts as fact the assertions of the Sobells. The Dickens Report does not state that it believes the time-line follow-back method was used, or that the Sobells state that the time-line follow-back method was used. They never examined the interview sheets to determine that such was the case, or that interview sheets exist, or the data necessary to complete interview sheets exist. They simply state as a fact that the method was used with no supporting evidence. I do not believe that this is the way in which a competent investigation proceeds.

Another kind of evidence supports the assertion that the Dickens investigation was not disinterested, was ineffectual, or both. Item #26 in their data base (p.40) lists my (Maltzman, 1976) affidavit prepared in the 1977 litigation. This affidavit read by the Sobells when it was submitted and in the possession of the Dickens Committee and also read by them, as previously noted here and in chapter 4, states:

On the basis of the information I now have I believe I know why Mark and Linda Sobell have persistently attempted to thwart our efforts at conducting a follow-up investigation of their study conducted at Patton State Hospital. I believe that they have deliberately misrepresented their follow-up procedures.... patients had spontaneously commented that they had been interviewed from 1-4 times, not the minimum of 24 times required by the Sobells' description of their follow-up procedure. (pp.3, 9).

The Dickens Committee Report found that the Sobells did not interview the patients as frequently as alleged. However, the Dickens Report states as fact that there was no intention on the part of the Sobells to deceive. The Sobells discovered their careless error, overestimating the frequency of contacts, as a consequence of the Dickens investigation. This apparent rationalization on the part of the Dickens Committee stretches one's credulity, since evidence in their possession shows that the Sobells knew of my allegation since 1976. Intent to deceive is critically important. It is the difference between a careless error and fraud. One would think that a disinterested investigation would study this issue with the greatest care. Such apparently was not the case with the Dickens Committee investigation.

The Report states:

The Committee found that the Sobells had never counted contacts since their manner of data collection (reconstruction of drinking behaviour of the subjects from reports of the subject and others using a technique they subsequently refer to as "time-line follow-back" interviewing) did not demand it. Thus, when the Committee's count indicated that the Sobells had not been as successful in contacting subjects and CISs as they had reported, the Sobells were *visibly surprised*. The Committee concludes that in this matter the Sobells did not do what they said they did. They were careless in reporting their procedures and in writing their report. They did not go back to their original data (as the Committee did) to see exactly how successful they had been in contacting subjects and CISs. The Committee notes, however, that the Sobells made frequent contact with the subjects where it was possible for them to do so. (Dickens et al., 1982, p. 9f). (italics added).

I believe that the above passage is not the observation of a disinterested committee. It is the biased statement of a Committee attempting to rationalize the discrepancy between what the Sobells said they did and what the Committee found they did: a glaring discrepancy in their stated procedures and the facts. Note that the Committee states as fact that the Sobells were surprised at the discovery of the Committee. As previously indicated, the Sobells could not have been surprised by the discrepancy between their stated procedures and the actual frequency of their interviews. They knew of my allegations since 1976. If it is true as the Dickens Report states that the Sobells used the time-line follow-back interview method, then the Sobells had to have known the frequency of their interviews. The procedure necessarily demands that knowledge.

The Sobells concede that they were careless in stating the number of contacts (Sobell & Sobell, 1989). An important point made by the Dickens Report is that the Sobells were visibly surprised when the deficient number of contacts was revealed to them. The implication is that if they had not been surprised, then they would have had prior knowledge that the number contacts was less than stated. If this were true, they would be guilty of intentionally misrepresenting the frequency of interviews. Furthermore, if the interviews were less frequent than stated, the data obtained from these interviews, the daily drinking dispositons, might also be missing, therefore summary results based upon them fabricated.

Contrary to the assertion of the Dickens Report and the Sobells' current position, there is evidence that the Sobells knew from the outset that the frequency of interviews was less than every 3-4 weeks. Furthermore, the Dickens Committee had to know the Sobells possessed this knowledge. These conclusions follow from (a) the nature of the time-line follow-back method, which the Sobells insist they used, and (b) mine and Pendery's affidavits that are listed in the data base of the Dickens Report (p.40). Comments on these affidavits indicate that the Committee had read my allegations.

Table 5.2 shows the results for one of the four experimental patients randomly selected by the Dickens Committee (p.81) to illustrate frequency of patient interviews. He is experimental Subject #14, HC. Note the gap of approximately 5.5 months between the last contact in October 9 of the first year, 1971, and March 23, 1972, the first contact in the second year. There were only 10 days between the second and third contacts, January 15 and January 25, 1971. Contacts were not evenly distributed. In the case of the 5.5-month interval, as in every other time interval, the daily drinking disposition is reported as days abstinent, controlled drinking, drunk days, days incarcerated in hospital or jail. The first three are reconstructed from the interview, dependent entirely upon the daily drinking

---

Table 5.2   Contact Dates for Experimental Subject #14. Discharged from
Patton State Hospital, October 9, 1970 (Dickens et al., 1982, p.81

Year 1 subject contacts	Year 2 subject contacts
November 8, 1970	March 23, 1972
January 15, 1971	May 24, 1972
January 25, 1971	July 3, 1972
February 24, 1971	August 3, 1972
March 15, 1971	August 31, 1972
April 13, 1971	September 27, 1972
June 2, 1971	
June 17, 1971	
September 10, 1971	
October 9, 1971	

---

disposition for every day of the previous 5.5 months. Since such data are reported for this subject, how did the Sobells know that they had to reconstruct the drinking dispositions for 5.5 months? Since they reported data for two years for this subject, they had to know that they were not interviewing him on a monthly basis, otherwise they could not know when to stop their time-line follow-back procedure - how far back to reconstruct to have complete information for every day of the previous 5.5 months.

Daily drinking dispositions for every day of the year obtained by the time-line follow-back method necessarily requires knowing when a subject was last interviewed, and therefore how frequently he was interviewed. If the Sobells did not fabricate their results for experimental Subject #14, and in fact used the time-line follow-back method to reconstruct his daily drinking disposition, they had to reconstruct 5.5 months of daily drinking dispositions; to do so, they had to know they did not interview him every 3-4 weeks. This could be true of all their subjects. As Table 5.1 indicates, the majority did not receive a minimum of 26-34 contacts, but they have published summaries of purported daily drinking dispositions for every day of these two years. One cannot have the latter drinking dispositions using the time-line follow-back method, and *not know* that interviews are not occurring every 3-4 weeks.

Figure 5.1 shows a time-line follow-back interview form (Sobell et al., 1985) of the kind purportedly used by the Sobells (1978) for all of the interviews. It is designed for a one month target interval, the interval purportedly used. Note the space for the date of the previous interview in the upper right corner. How could Linda Sobell fill out such forms for 5.5 months for Subject #14, requiring six forms rather than the one needed for the stated monthly interview and not know she is interviewing less frequently than every 3-4 weeks? I believe the above argument suggests that if the Sobells used the time-line follow-back method as they insist they did (Sobell & Sobell, 1989), then they intentionally misrepresented the frequency of their interviews. As I noted elsewhere (Maltzman, 1992), Timothy Baker who was an undergraduate research assistant on the

148

Sobells' project, now a professor at the University of Wisconsin, Madison, has written in their defense. In the course of his comments I believe he confirms the above allegation that the Sobells intentionally misrepresented their procedures.

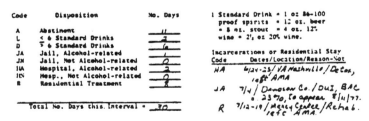

MONTHLY FOLLOW-BACK TIME-LINE

Subject I.D. Code: *044*
Interviewer I.D. Code: *J.H.*
Study Code: *TO-III*

Date of Interview: *7/24/77*
Follow back Interval Dates:
6/24/77 thru *7/23/77*

Monday	Tuesday	Wednesday	Thursday	Friday	Saturday	Sunday
☒	☒	☒	☒	24 June / HA	25 / HA	26 / A
27 / A	28 / A	29 / A	30 / A	1 July / L	2 / D	3 / D
4 Holiday / JA	5 / A	6 / A	7 / D	8 / L	9 / D	10 / D
11 / D	12 Birthday / R	13 / R	14 / R	15 / R	16 / R	17 / R
18 / R	19 / R	20 / A	21 / A	22 / A	23 / A	☒

Code	Disposition	No. Days
A	Abstinent	_11_
L	< 6 Standard Drinks	_2_
D	> 6 Standard Drinks	_6_
JA	Jail, Alcohol-related	_1_
JN	Jail, Not Alcohol-related	_0_
HA	Hospital, Alcohol-related	_2_
HN	Hosp., Not Alcohol-related	_0_
R	Residential Treatment	_8_

Total No. Days this Interval = _30_

1 Standard Drink = 1 oz 86-100 proof spirits = 12 oz. beer = 8 oz. stout = 4 oz. 12% wine = 2½ oz 20% wine.

Incarcerations or Residential Stay
Code — Dates/Location/Reason-Not
HA — 6/24-25/ VA Nashville / Detox, left AMA
JA — 7/4 / Dawson Co. / DUI, BAC .23%, to appear 8/11/77.
R — 7/12-19/ Mercy Center / Rehab. left AMA.

Figure 5.1 Example of a completed time-line follow-back data sheet for a one-month target interval of the kind purportedly used by the Sobells in their IBTA study (Sobell et al., 1985).

Baker (1989) states: "We knew the previous contact date so that we knew exactly how many days had to be accounted for." (p.482). The Sobells therefore had to know that, for example, for Subject #14 there was a gap of 5.5 months between interviews. They therefore necessarily knew that subjects were interviewed less frequently than every 3-4 weeks as reported in their publications.

Furthermore, we are expected to believe that, for example, Linda Sobell conversed with a recovering alcoholic on the telephone, and in the absence of a calendar gradually reconstructed for every day of the previous 5.5 months, whether he abstained; drank in a controlled fashion, not more than 6 oz or 7-9 oz on an isolated sequence of days; was drunk, drank more than 10 oz, or was incarcerated in a hospital or jail for alcohol-related incidents.

How could the Sobells (1978) report that Subject #5, JPr had 282 days abstinent, 27 drunk, 57 controlled drinking days from only two telephone interviews and not know only two interviews were conducted if they used the time-line follow-back method as they insist they did? How would Marlatt et al. (1993) explain how that is possible? Neither the Sobells (1989), commentators, nor investigations have explained how such is possible.

How is it possible that an almost universally accepted investigation by the Dickens Committee never asked this obvious question and never demanded the interview sheets purportedly used on the stated interview days, examined the raw data recorded on them and from these raw data attempt to reconstruct the published results? How could a credible investigation neglect to take this obvious step? How could so many commentators on the Sobell controversy have failed to raise this issue?

The Dickens Report (1982) concluded its discussion of the issue of frequency of contacts obtained by the Sobells by stating:

> The Committee finds that the Sobells did not achieve the frequency of follow-up contacts which they claimed. The Committee also finds the report by Pendery et al. in the Draft to be wrong: contact with subjects and collateral information sources was considerably more frequent than reported by Pendery et al. but less than that reported by the Sobells. The Committee does not know whether the frequency of the follow-up contacts affected the results of the study. The Committee concludes that in this matter the Sobells did not do what they said they did. They were carelesss in reporting their procedures and in the writing of their report. They estimated a statistic they never calculated. There is no evidence of fraud. (pp. 85-86).

Again, the Dickens Committee states as fact, not a matter of hypothesis, that the Sobells were careless in their statements concerning the frequency of contacts. The Committee Report further attempts to explain away the lack of interviews, especially in the second year, as the result of underfunding. Although the lack of funding may explain the absence of interviews, lack of funding does not explain the lack of candor in reporting the frequency of interviews.

Finally, the Dickens Report concludes that there is no evidence of fraud. The Report never states what it would take as evidence of fraud. The latter is usually distinguished from error on the basis of evidence that permits a reasonable inference that the conduct in question was intentional, i.e., it was motivated by the intent to

150

deceive. Such an inference is often difficult to make. It requires "triangulation" from a variety of kinds of evidence. As in the case of fraud, careless conduct may also have misleading consequences, but the latter is characterized by the absence of an intent to deceive. The assertion that certain conduct was careless therefore also requires an inference, the absence of an intent to deceive. Certainly it is as difficult, if not more so, to infer an absence of intent as it is to infer its presence. It is therefore astonishing, I believe, that the Dickens Commission concludes that there was an absence of intent to deceive on the part of the Sobells. Evidence provided for such an inference purportedly is the assertion that the Sobells were "visibly surprised" by the Committee's discovery of the discrepancy between the number of telephone contacts and their published experimental procedures. This "evidence" cannot be taken seriously. At another place (p. 84) the Dickens Report states that the Sobells appeared "demoralized" by the Committee's revelation, a very different emotional state than surprise, one suggesting guilt rather than innocence. Hypothetical inferred emotional states are not evidence.

Bias in background of Sobell affair

Additional evidence of bias may be found in the presentation of background information provided by the Dickens Report. Much of the bias and misinformation present there could be attributed to the fact that the Sobells were their sole source of information. However, one important form of background information is presented in a biased manner for which there is no such excuse as a limited source of information. In question is the inaccurate presentation of the litigation against Dr. Pendery, me, Dr. Jack Fox, and the Medical Director of Patton State Hospital. There can be no excuse for the biased exposition of this issue because Dickens is a professor of law and holds a degree in law.

The Report states:

The Sobells' decision not to collaborate with Drs. Maltzman and Pendery by giving them access to subjects' names, and their unsuccessful litigation which obstructed the latter in pursuing interviews with subjects until some months into 1977, have been considered by some as evidence supporting the allegation of the Sobells' fabrication, fraud and wish to conceal wrongdoing.

The reason the Sobells gave for deciding not to collaborate with the Pendery team was that one proposed team member had a reputation with respect to maintenance of research subjects' confidentiality which the Sobells found unsatisfactory. Assurances were sought on the issue as the Sobells' condition for their collaboration, which were not forthcoming... No negative inference may be drawn, however, from an investigator declining to share confidential data with others who in the investigator's judgment do not warrant trust. Indeed, Dr. Pendery declined to participate in our Committee's proceedings on a comparable basis... but we drew no inference adverse to Dr. Pendery from this. (p.105).

The statement, "one proposed team member had a reputation with respect to maintenance of research subjects' confidentiality which the Sobells found unsatisfactory" I believe is a malicious invention. The person in question, Mike Digan, an alcoholism counselor never had taken part in a research project. What had been questioned by his supervisor in Digan's confidential personnel file was Digan's determination to make independent judgments concerning aftercare which he thought were in the best interests of patients rather than blindly follow the wishes of his supervisor. This is one more example of misinformation probably floated by the Sobells and uncritically repeated by the Dickens Committee. Why did not the Committee investigate and independently determine the truth status of such a defamatory attribution?

An aside is worth quoting and commenting upon, because I believe it is another gratuitous attempt to interpret the Sobells' behavior in the most benign light possible, a process incompatible with the ostensibly disinterested posture of an investigating committee. Thus, the Report states:

> When Pendery et al. acquired the list of subjects' names, however, they had immediate access through the Sobells' publications to what the Sobells claimed to have done and to have found regarding each of them. This presented the individualized data which, some years later, the subjects contacted by Pendery et al. denied were true. Had the Sobells presented data only by code, fraud and fabrication would have been easier to conceal. This is not to suggest, of course, that subject anonymity is indicative of intent to deceive, but to observe that fabrication of data is scarcely suggested by revelation of personal identities, with its potential for traceability, especially when untraceable coding is a reputable and even recommended alternative. (p. 107).

By this logic, the Sobells' carelessness in using the subjects' initials suggests their innocence of fraud. By the same logic, Nixon's failure to destroy his tapes indicates his innocence of any attempt to obstruct justice. No such inference can be drawn in either case. Why then does the Committee raise this possibility?

To continue with the implications of the Sobells' litigation, the Report states:

> The terms upon which the Sobells' unsuccessful litigation was concluded in April 1977, namely, *"with prejudice"*, have been taken by some to be more significant than is warranted in law. The litigation which was launched for the purpose of defending confidentiality of subjects was influenced by the principle that subjects were entitled to protection against having strangers approach them with information of their alcoholic addiction and history. This was the principle which required the Sobells themselves to introduce their subjects to the intended study by Caddy et al.
>
> The Sobells funded from their own private resources their action in the California State Court, but, because Dr. Pendery was in federal employment and the Sobells owed obligations of subject confidentiality to the federal agency which contributed to their research, the litigation became a federal case. This exhausted the Sobells' financial means before evidence and argument could be presented in court. Accordingly, the defendants became entitled to judgment in default of the plaintiff presenting a case, and to protection against becoming involved in further litigation by or on behalf of the same plaintiff, regarding the same issues.
>
> The judgment was therefore not based upon the legal or other inadequacy of the plaintiff's application to the court, nor upon a determination of the respondent's case. Neither side presented a case. Defendants who endure the inconvenience and expense of resisting a claim the plaintiff does not continue

are entitled to be protected against having to suffer that experience again. Accordingly, they recover judgment in terms preventing repetition of the experience. The legal language expressing this is judgment "with prejudice", which bars a subsequent proceeding in the same court on the same issue. The Federal Court in question adopted the strict form in the judgment of stating that if the matter could be reformulated so as to state a permissible cause of action under state law, the judgment did not bar the commencement of an appropriate action in the State Court of California. The language of legal procedure has no bearing upon the merits of the issue, therefore, and justifies no conclusions of irregularity against the Sobells. (pp.107-108).

The Dickens Report thus presents the Sobells' argument, which has been widely circulated, that they initiated litigation against us to safeguard the confidentiality of the patients and they discontinued their legal efforts towards that end because they exhausted their personal funds. It must be noted that almost from the beginning of my efforts in the "Sobell affair" I have had the support of the Administration of UCLA and when necessary, of the statewide University of California system. My efforts to ascertain the truth in this matter would have been impossible without such support. At times, that support has been quite concrete. When the litigation was brought against me the University provided me with an attorney on the staff of the Office of the General Counsel of the Regents of the University of California who is an expert on the protection of human subject rights and questions of confidentiality. He prepared the motion to dismiss the Sobells' complaint. He was asked to comment upon the passages concerning our litigation when the Dickens Report appeared in 1982 because they were at such odds with my layman's knowledge of the relevant law. The following passages are quoted from a 1982 letter received from David Dorinson, Esq. in response to my request to comment upon the above and related passages in the Dickens Report that discussed the litigation brought by the Sobells:

I agree with the statement in the report that no negative inference may be drawn from an investigator declining to share his or her confidential data with others. And I concur that the Sobells had the right to seek to persuade San Diego County not to give the records back to Patton and Patton not to provide you and Mary with the names of the subjects. However, all records identifying the names of participants in the study were not the sole property of the Sobells, and in my opinion, the report should have made this clear.

I do not know why the Sobells initiated litigation. If it was launched for the purpose of defending confidentiality of subjects and was influenced by the principle that subjects are entitled to protection against strangers approaching them with knowledge of their alcoholic addiction and history, the lawsuit could only have been brought to *establish* that principle as a legal requirement, i.e., as a matter of law only the researcher who has conducted a study on human subjects may permit another person to contact the subject for a follow-up study, even if the researcher conducted the study under the auspices of his or her employer and the research records are the property of the employer...

The litigation was removed to federal court. No inference can be drawn because the case was removed to federal court that the nature of the case changed. The statement on page 107 that the case was removed to federal court...'because... the Sobells owed obligations of subject confidentiality to the federal agency which contributed to their research' is inaccurate. It was removed for the sole reason that Mary was employed by the Veterans Administration and the U. S. Attorney elected to have the case removed. The removal had no effect on the nature of the litigation and did not result in any increased cost to the Sobells. The arguments that I made to the federal court would have been made to the state court, had the case remained in Orange County Superior Court...

The judgment was in fact based upon the legal inadequacy of the plaintiff's 'application to the court', i.e., complaint... The statement that neither side presented a case is inaccurate. The defendants presented (oral and written) arguments why the complaint stated no legally cognizable claim and those arguments were sustained. The language of legal procedure has a significant bearing upon the merits of the issue, and I take exception with the report in this regard. The case and the legal theory upon which it was based, i.e., the principle the Sobells sought to establish by the litigation, was deemed legally unmeritorious by the court. The Sobells were of course free to attempt to reformulate a claim in state court but it would have had to be a different claim than the one originally brought....

The Sobells neither appealed Judge Hauk's decision nor did they commence any other action in state court as permitted by Judge Hauk... I cannot understand how the committee could have concluded that the judgment of dismissal with prejudice was not a determination of the legal inadequacy of the complaint. (D. A. Dorinson, Esq., personal communication, November 19, 1982).

Random assignment and related issues

Our *Science* (Pendery et al., 1982) article demonstrated that there was a statistically significant difference in the order of assignment of patients in the experimental and control groups. We agree with the Dickens committee that by itself a significant deviation from randomness does not indicate fraud. However, the Dickens Report devotes more space to this specific allegation than any other, and I believe the Committee did so in an effort to demonstrate that the nonrandomness was not intentional. The Sobells apparently provided to the Dickens Committee reports of Patton State Hospital staff who signed statements indicating that they observed a coin toss ceremony that served as the basis for assignment of the patients to either the experimental or control groups. Subjects for this assignment volunteered and were approved to participate in the experiment with controlled drinking as its treatment goal. A purported random assignment then determined whether they would be in the experimental group that received controlled drinking treatment or in the control group that would receive behavioral treatment emphasizing abstinence as the treatment goal.

It must be noted, obviously, that if a staff person observes a coin flip ceremony for one or more patients, there is no guarantee that: other patients were not assigned to a group in the absence of a coin flip; or that after the coin flip and assignment, the subjects were not reassigned; after the coin flip and assignment, the subject was not dropped from the experiment entirely. None of the statements or arguments presented by the Dickens Report preclude any of the above. Furthermore, as far as can be determined, the Dickens Report never even considers the above possibilities. The Report is concerned with only one issue: demonstrate that the Sobells did not intentionally bias their assignment of patients. This is not the manner in which an unbiased investigation proceeds. Nor does an unbiased report rationalize ignoring our alleged evidence of reassignment of subjects, as may be found in hospital records, by the claim that hospital records are unreliable.

A glaring example of the bias manifested by the Dickens Report, I believe, may be found in their failure to note that a necessary consequence of the nonrandom assignment of the patients - for whatever reason it may have occurred, intentional or otherwise - is that the two groups cannot be compared, since any statistical test that could be conducted comparing the two groups assumes random assignment of subjects. Experimental and control groups cannot be compared, and we did not compare the two groups in our *Science* paper because of the significant order effect reported there and other reasons indicated in the paper.

Despite this necessary consequence of statistical evidence of nonrandomness, the Dickens Committee, which after all is investigating the Sobells' alleged fraud, not our *Science* article, makes the following statement:

by choosing not to compare the Controlled Drinking Experimental subjects' outcome with data from an appropriate control group, Pendery et al. implied that the long term prognosis of the Controlled Drinking Experimental subjects was worse than would have occurred with routine treatment. No form of treatment of alcoholism known to the Committee is clearly perfect for any group; hence comparisons must be made of treatment groups in order to evaluate any particular treatment. This is, of course, the nature of the design the Sobells used: for each experimental group, there was an appropriate control group... From their investigation, Pendery et al. conclude that the outcomes for the controlled drinking patients were not favourable. Pendery et al. do not, however, compare group outcomes. Without comparisons of any kind, we are left, for example, with tragic stories (played up by the mass media) of four Controlled Drinking Experimental subjects' deaths (relating at least in some cases to alcohol). Deaths are often tragic. As unpleasant as they might be, however, drawing inferences from them with respect to treatment effectiveness DEMANDS a comparison. Science, the activity, would have demanded such a comparison even though *Science*, the magazine, did not. (pp. 15-16).

The above criticism of our *Science* article, unjustified on methodological grounds, and irrelevant to the purpose of their investigation, served as the rallying point for subsequent attempts to discredit our report (e.g., Marlatt, 1983; Marlatt et al., 1993), and thereby divert attention from a critical issue: my allegation of fraud on the part of the Sobells. This insistence that the experimental and control groups should have been compared in our *Science* paper ignores the statistical and methodological impropriety of such a comparison, regardless of the reasons for the nonrandomness, an issue never addressed by the Report (Dickens et al., 1982) or by Doob (1984).

I believe the Report's treatment of the issue of the different lengths of hospitalization for experimental and control groups provides a justification, which is actually an apology, for the Sobells' actions. Thus, the Report states:

It should be noted with respect to the allegation of different times in treatment that the Sobells made no claim in any of their published work that their subjects spent identical times in treatment.. Indeed, *the purpose of their study was to contrast their experimental treatments to standard hospital treatment, however long a subject agreed to participate in either ....* length of hospital stay is not really the relevant figure to look at, since it is 'time in treatment' that is really the issue. Had the *more relevant data shown that there was differential time spent in treatment (or differential treatment completion rates), the difference* might have been more relevant. Pendery et al. do not indicate that this was the case, but it is worthwhile observing that even if there were a difference, *this would be relevant to the meaning of the results, and not to the integrity of the Sobells.* (Dickens et al., 1982, pp. 59, 67).

The latter is a stunning conclusion. Significantly more control than experimental subjects failed to complete their treatment. Because of AWOLs the control subjects spent less time in the hospital than the experimental group. Not reporting the differential AWOL rate is a matter of integrity, regardless of the meaning of the results. Interpretation of the results, especially the manner in which the Sobells have espoused controlled drinking as a treatment for physically dependent alcoholics, is an ethical issue, one of integrity. Fraud may occur with respect to intentionally misleading conclusions as well as the intentional fabrication of results. Differential length of stay in the hospital confounds the particular treatment with length of hospitalization. The experimental group not only received a different behavioral treatment, they were in the hospital and received conventional hospital treatment for a longer period than did the control group. Therefore, one cannot interpret an apparent superior outcome on the part of the experimental group. It just as well could be due to a longer hospital stay and longer conventional treatment as to training in controlled drinking. This confound affects the outcome, the interpretation, and the integrity of the Sobells for failing to note the significant difference in hospital stay, protestations to the contrary.

Noteworthy in each of the above treatment of issues by the Dickens Report is that the interpretations all fall on one side, favoring the Sobells. I believe that this evident lack of impartiality in an investigating body undermines the integrity of the Report.

Doob (1984) asserts, as does the Dickens Report, that Pendery et al. (1982) provided no new information. I believe such information follows, indicating the intentional reassignment of a subject. Figure 5.2 is a copy of the Nursing Notes for control Subject JZ for the treatment period during which he participated in the Sobells' individualized behavior therapy experiment. It indicates that he was drinking as part of the research project and subsequently became belligerent. If he was drinking on the project, he had to be a member of the experimental group at the time. However, JZ is reported in all of the Sobells' papers, chapters, and book, as a member of the control group (Sobell & Sobell, 1978, p. 128). This discrepancy between the Nursing Notes and the Sobells' reports I believe suggests that JZ was reassigned from the experimental to the control group following the incident described in Figure 5.2.

156

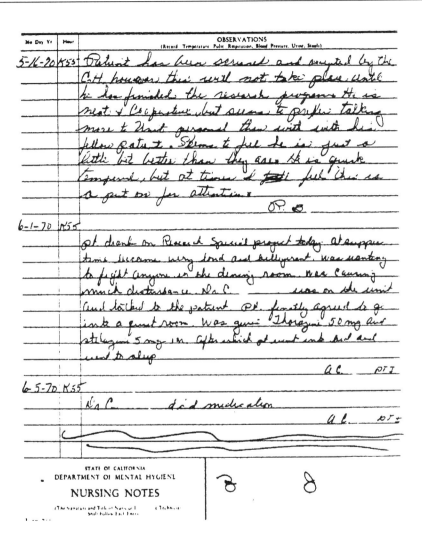

Figure 5.2 Nursing Notes for subject JZ during his participation in the Sobells' IBTA experiment. The full name except for the first letter of the first and last name was oblitered from the photographic copy of the hospital record. Other idiosyncratic personal identifiers were also obliterated as well as names of hospital staff except for initials.

When the allegation that some subjects were reassigned was submitted to the Trachtenberg ADAMHA Committee, the Sobells' reply, presented in the Trachtenberg Report (1984), suggests that the periods of treatment were confused by the patients. Many of the patients in the Patton study were hospitalized several times prior to the hospitalization during which they participated in the Sobells' individualized behavior therapy experiment. Patients consumed alcohol in several basic research, nontreatment, experiments conducted prior to the one in question.

The Trachtenberg Report (1984) states:

The Sobells explained that the simulated bar at PSH (Patton State Hospital) might have been used in pilot studies for basic (nontreatment oriented) research and that some of the control subjects, who claimed they were switched from an experimental to a control group because they remembered drinking at the simulated bar, may actually have drunk at the bar as a participant in some informal pilot study unrelated to the Sobells' research. The Sobells denied that any subjects were 'tried out' or switched from one group to another after assignment. (p. 23).

According to the Sobells (1972), the individualized behavior therapy treatment experiment, "was conducted during the period April 1970 through March 1971." (p.64). Figure 5.2 shows the Nursing Notes describing the experience of JZ drinking during research as occurring 6-1-70, June 1, 1970. The incident in question occurred during the time frame of the Sobells' treatment experiment. There is no mistake in experiments, the possibility the Sobells suggested to the Trachtenberg Committee. There was no random assignment of JZ as claimed by the Sobells, the Dickens Report, and Doob. Drinking in the experiment is not based on a memory error by the control subject JZ.

The only alternative interpretation to the obvious one of intentional switching of JZ from the experimental to control group is that the hospital records are in error. The Sobells and the Dickens Report have resorted to such suggestions because they claim that they have found other errors in the medical records. However, to claim that such detailed statements as shown in Figure 5.2 are in error, refer to someone else, were a mistake on the part of the nurse, etc., stretches credulity beyond reasonable bounds. The burden of proof that the medical record in the case of JZ is incorrect must weigh upon the Sobells and the Dickens Committee. Until such evidence is forthcoming, I believe that the most reasonable conclusion is that the Sobells intentionally switched group assignment in the case of JZ. The arguments presented by the Dickens Commission in defense of random assignment by the Sobells are without merit.

Doob's defense of the Dickens Report

In addition to the Report, Dickens and Doob have expressed themselves in the media and elsewhere, and such expressions further substantiate, I believe, my assertion that the Report is not disinterested. My own experience suggests that quotations and attributions in the public press are not always accurate. I cannot assume bias on the part of the source simply because statements attributed to them are biased. I therefore shall restrict my comments to the one work, by Doob, that has been published in a professional journal (Doob, 1984). This is the article that appeared in reply to Walker and Roach (1984). I believe that the reply by Doob is even more obviously biased as well as flawed than the Committee Report. The following are the grounds for that belief.

Doob, at the outset of his article, purports to describe the difficulties confronting the Committee attempting to conduct the enquiry in question. His use of obloquy, sophistry, and selective presentation of interpretations, all confirm my belief that Doob was not a disinterested party to the Committee investigation. Doob asserts:

> The Committee on which I served had its own set of ambiguities handed to it: we had to determine what the charges were that we were going to investigate. On the one hand, one of the authors of the *Science* article, Irving Maltzman, said quite directly that the issue was fraud.... On the other hand, his senior author, Mary Pendery, appears to take the view publicly that fraud wasn't the issue at all. For example, on CBS television's news-entertainment programme 'Sixty minutes'... she stated that 'people don't understand that the Committee was just addressing whether or not they had committed fraud which wasn't the question that I was interested in at all. I was interested in... did this treatment work or did it fail.' It is difficult for defendant and court alike when nobody is willing to make a consistent set of specific charges. (pp.170-171).

I believe the above statement is a rather striking example of the biased presentation by Doob. To Pendery, the primary issue in the Sobell affair was to determine whether a new treatment goal for physically dependent alcoholics, controlled drinking, really worked, and worked to the remarkable degree claimed by the Sobells: 85% of the subjects were functioning well 85% of the time during the last six months of the follow-up (Sobell & Sobell, 1978, p. 127). For me, the primary issue was the alleged fraud. We agreed both issues are important and both should be addressed by a serious investigation. There is no inconsistency. These issues are not mutually exclusive. Pendery and Maltzman simply prioritized the issues differently. It escapes me why these different comments by different people should cause difficulty for the Dickens Committee. Both issues should have received serious attention by a disinterested investigation. It turns out that neither did.

I believe Doob's sophistry is most apparent in his treatment of the so-called Draft of the article finally published in *Science* (Pendery et al., 1982). He states:

> the status of the Draft itself is rather ambiguous. *Science's* associate editor is quoted as saying that 'We concluded on reading [the original manuscript] that it was libelous, and we asked for another draft... It was an expensive process, but it seemed to be a reasonable thing to do, something we ought to do'... Since 'truth' normally negates libel - that is, a true statement normally cannot be defamatory - I presume that *Science's* associate editor was acknowledging some rather serious problems with the draft manuscript. (p.170).

The presumption by Doob is false. Truth negates libel, but a purported libelous statement has not yet had its truth status determined. I believe *Science* did not wish to risk the expense of going to court to demonstrate the truth of my allegations of fraud or the bases upon which it could reasonably conclude that scientific fraud occurred. The timidity of publishers punished by rising insurance costs in a litigious age is at issue not the falsity of any allegations of fraud in the Draft.

Doob continues his criticism of our Draft by stating:

From a telephone conversation with Dr. Pendery, the committee found that Pendery et al. no longer stand behind [all of their assertions in the Draft] ... This certainly should explain why the Draft was not appended to the Report, as the authors of the Critique suggest ... Little light would be shed on the issue by further circulating a paper, some aspects of which none of the interested parties would defend. (p. 170).

The Dickens Report (p. 31) promotes a similar inappropriate criticism, and by so doing implies that our results were unreliable and our methodology suspect. What happened was that some patients upon reinterviewing, reported somewhat more interviews, rather than a maximum of four, which was the general case. The change in the final version was an effort to be scrupulously accurate and fair. It was, and is, my belief that the evidence of fraud remained unchanged: the Sobells knowingly interviewed the patients far less than they reported, far less than the minimum of 26 required by their stated procedure. To argue, as does the Dickens Report, that the patients were interviewed many times and therefore at worst the Sobells were careless, is a perversion of science and ethics. One cannot be half pregnant. Either the Sobells did what they said they did or they did not. I believe they did not and knowingly maintained the fiction that patients were interviewed 26 times or more. I believe this also suggests they invented much of the data constituting the daily drinking disposition.

Doob, as was also true of the Dickens Report, criticizes and minimizes the importance of affidavits by patients which state that they were not interviewed a minimum of 26 times by the Sobells and that when they were occasionally interviewed, it was usually in a perfunctory manner. He states:

As is pointed out in the Report, affidavits taken years after the events show at best 'only the conscientious beliefs of those who make them, of course, and not that those beliefs are actually true. The gap between belief and truth may grow with the passage of time. (p. 170).

Doob, the Report, Marlatt (1983), and others claim that memories after so many years would be unreliable, and therefore an affidavit from a patient is of no great import. It is noteworthy that they do not use the same argument when the Dickens Report discusses the statements of Patton State Hospital staff obtained by the Sobells for the Committee. These staff statements and memories are accepted as incontrovertible and irrefutable evidence by the Dickens Committee that procedures were employed by the Sobells to ensure randomness. The Report, Doob, and other critics (Marlatt, 1983) fail to note research indicating that the permanence of memories varies enormously depending upon the significance of those events (Neisser, 1982). It is a reasonable assumption that the memory of the pain of withdrawal, waking up in the morning in a cold sweat, sick and vomiting following a period of excessive drinking, is more likely to be recalled several years later by a patient, than the possible observation of a coin tossing ceremony, who the patient was for whom the ceremony was performed, and whether such patients and no others were in the experiment, i.e., a casual and incidental part of a day, if it happened at all.

I believe further evidence of bias on the part of Doob and in this, again, he repeats what is evident in the Dickens Report, is his selective treatment and misrepresentation of the meaning of information contained in hospital records and the meaning of rehospitalizations. He states:

The hospital records could, under certain circumstances, have been more important to the Committee. However, those circumstances did not exist because Pendery et al. quite properly published the most important (and presumably, from their perspective, the most damaging) data - the detailed reports of the readmission to hospital of these subjects. The Committee had no reason to doubt the accuracy of the reporting of these rehospitalizations, especially since *Science* had apparently carefully checked the data in the article against the actual hospital records... Since the Committee could then presume a one-to-one correspondence between the report in the Pendery et al. article and the actual hospital records, what was left to the Committee was the job of checking whether each of the hospitalizations in Table 2 of the Pendery et al. article was in the Sobells' original data and then whether these data noted on data sheets actually match the Sobells' published data. For example, Table 2 of the article noted 'CD-E 1 Readmitted to Patton 1 month 27 days after discharge.' The Committee then went to the Sobells' data to see whether there was a hospitalization noted for this date. The Committee then checked to see whether the number of days matched. We did this for each person and found that the Pendery et al. and the Sobells' data coincided. (Doob, 1984, p. 171).

The above passage was quoted at length because it raises two important points that I believe illustrate the bias and some of the serious inadequacies found in the Dickens Report:

(1) The Report and Doob do not address the real reason for concern over the hospital records and rehospitalizations. They divert attention from the real problem and create a straw man: is the frequency of hospitalizations reported in Pendery et al. and the Sobells' report comparable? It is. It was never alleged that frequency of hospitalizations or arrests are underreported by the Sobells. If one were attempting to fabricate results, these would be the least likely candidates, because they are a matter of public record, could be obtained by any responsible authority, and are therefore the most likely to be discovered in the case of fraud. Pendery et al. (1982) presented the hospitalizations in detail because they demonstrated the devastating effects of alcoholism - despite the controlled drinking treatment the Sobells had hailed as being strikingly effective. Hospitalizations for alcoholism including serious withdrawal effects with medical complications cast doubt upon the "miraculous recovery" within the next year when Linda Sobell became solely responsible for follow-up interviews. Former patients do not voluntarily admit themselves to a hospital for detoxification following a week of social drinking. What is in question is the meaning, the significance, of the rehospitalizations, not their frequency. The Sobells claim that many of these hospitalizations were sought by the patients to avoid excessive drinking. The detailed hospital records including nurses' and physicians' notes indicate that the rehospitalizations were the consequence of excessive drinking. This point is never addressed by the Dickens Report or by Doob, only the straw man of the accuracy of the number of hospitalizations.

(2) The second issue is the nature of the raw data examined by the Dickens Committee. Doob's comments are revealing in that they show that the Dickens

Committee studied the raw data of the Sobells in relation to the non-issue of frequency of hospitalizations. If they had conducted the same investigation of the critical raw data, the interviews of the patients concerning their daily drinking disposition, I would have no quarrel with the Dickens Report. Since they did not, I can only conclude that they were not disinterested or that their investigation was inept, or both. Why did the Dickens Committee not do the obvious: obtain, for example, the raw data for Subject #5 who is LL in the Sobells' reports and is listed in the Dickens Report (p. 78) as having had only two contacts in the second year of the follow-up period? The Dickens Committee could determine whether the time-line follow-back method was actually used to reconstruct daily drinking dispositions which yielded exactly 197 days of controlled drinking and 164 days of abstinence, as reported by the Sobells for this subject.

I question why the Dickens Committee spent time reconstructing noncontroversial information, frequency of hospitalizations, and not the critical controversial data of the frequency and nature of the daily drinking dispositions that are dependent upon interviews. In fact, the Dickens Committee does not even list the raw data for the daily drinking disposition, the raw data from interviews, in their data base. I believe, again, this is not the manner in which a disinterested and effective investigation proceeds. This is the style but not the substance of a disinterested investigation of fraud in science.

Further evidence of Doob's bias is evident in his discussion of the kinds of intentional misrepresentations that may constitute scientific fraud:

My perspective... I do not expect that it differs much from that of most scientists. I would have thought that once one accepted the integrity of the data as presented, the interpretation of results is exactly that: *an* interpretation. Methods and Results sections tell the reader what the authors did and found. Science is based on changing interpretation of (fixed) data. I see nothing embarrassing or wrong in an author saying what he or she *thinks* are the implications of a set of data, even though somebody else may disagree with these inferences. (p.172).

Doob apparently is unfamiliar with Ethics Principle 4.g of the American Psychological Association, of which he is a member. This principle states:

Psychologists present the science of psychology and offer their services, products, and publications fairly and accurately, avoiding misrepresentation through sensationalism, exaggeration, or superficiality. Psychologists are guided by the primary obligation to aid the public in developing informed judgments, opinions, and choices. (Ethical Principles, 1981, p.635).

One of his most striking instances of bias may be found in Doob's discussion of the question of the frequency of contacts. He states:

As anyone who has followed this controversy knows, the Committee discovered that the Sobells did not contact their subjects as often as they had reported. The Committee concluded that this was an error on the part of the Sobells, but that it was not done with an intent to defraud. Errors, unfortunately, are not unheard of in scientific research. (p.173).

Doob then provides an illustration of a personal experience: He found a statistical error in a published article. An author had apparently incorrectly calculated a statistical test. He concludes, "Nobody I know thought that the error involved fraud, perhaps because the study did not challenge a widely held ideology." (p. 173). I submit that the latter gratuituous comment is inappropriate and reveals, again, the bias present in its author. Doob ignores the critical issue that the context of the Sobells alleged fraud and the context of the attempted analogy are fundamentally different, which is why the analogy is inappropriate. It is logically impossible for the Sobells not to have known that the frequency of contacts was less than reported, if they followed the procedures, the time-line follow-back method, that the Dickens Committee and the Sobells claim they used.

Doob is not finished with his gratuituous remarks. He asserts:

One unfortunate aspect of life is that people make mistakes. The Sobells are no exceptions...The important point to keep in mind... is that a mistake does not make a fraud... Alternatively, if the reader agrees with Irving Maltzman, who appears to believe that any error automatically constitutes a scientific fraud, the reader can come to his or her own conclusions without further expenditure of effort. (p. 173).

Doob concludes his paper with a statement that, I believe, more than any other in his paper, manifests his bias: "One might hope that something could be learned from this controversy. Others [28] have written thoughtful and provocative pieces on it." (p. 174). Doob's reference [28] is to the paper by Marlatt in the 1983 *American Psychologist* , "The controlled drinking controversy: A commentary" which elicited letters to the Editor critical of its bias in a subsequent issue of the *American Psychologist* (March, 1985). This is the same Marlatt discussed in chapters 4, 6 and elsewhere in this book, a major supporter of the Sobells and controlled drinking who wrote the widely circulated infamous "shootout at the OK Corral letter" quoted in chapter 4.

Conclusion

The Dickens Report had the form but not the substance of a carefully considered disinterested investigation of the alleged scientific misconduct of Mark and Linda Sobell. It failed to meet the basic desideratum of an adequate investigation of alleged scientific misconduct: It did not examine all of the raw data. In particular, it did not examine all, or even randomly selected, interviews with patients and from these attempt to reconstruct the basic dependent variable employed by the Sobells, the daily drinking disposition. Evidence it did report demonstrates that the Sobells did not interview the patients as frequently as they claimed. The Dickens Report conclusion that the Sobells were surprised by this discovery by the Dickens Committee, and that the Sobells were careless in counting the number of contacts is contradicted by the evidence available to the Dickens Committee itself. The Report's explanation that the Sobells used the time-line follow-back method to obtain interviews is contradicted by the nature of the interviews described in the Trachtenberg Report (1984) discussed below. Assertions in the Trachtenberg Report attributed to the Sobells indicate that they did not consistently use the time-line follow-back method and did not consistently obtain daily drinking dispositions in the manner described in their publications.

I believe that the evidence demonstrates that: (a) the Dickens Committee Report is seriously flawed, (b) the Report was not disinterested, and (c) its conclusion that the Sobells are guilty of nothing more than carelessness in the conduct and reporting of their research cannot withstand scrutiny.

TRACHTENBERG COMMITTEE REPORT EXONERATES SOBELLS

A second investigation that had the form but lacked the substance of an adequate investigation of fraud in science was conducted under the aegis of the Alcohol Drugs and Mental Health Administration (ADAMHA). The Trachtenberg Committee was established consisting of administrators, a steering group, and in-house investigators who reported to them. A description of the nature and extent of the investigation has been lacking in secondary sources commenting on the Report, invariably citing it as a vindication of the Sobells. One needs to read the Report to understand the enforced incompleteness and superficiality of the investigation. Commentators have uniformly ignored the admitted shortcomings of the investigation by the Trachtenberg Committee or are simply unaware of these shortcomings, offering their comments on the basis of secondary sources or knowledge only of the Report's conclusions published in various media. The Report (Trachtenberg, 1984) states:

When the investigative team met with the Sobells on March 3, discussion of procedural issues centered on what information the investigators could take with them. The Sobells made it clear that the investigative team had full and free access to any and all of their records on the PSH (Patton State Hospital) study, but they insisted that no detailed notes of the data in their records should leave their house unless the investigative team could absolutely assure them that these notes would forever be for the eyes and ears of the investigative team only. The Sobells explained that some of the data in their records could be damaging to some of the study subjects and could perhaps be used by those bringing a civil suit against them and the State of California. The team members explained that because of the Freedom of Information Act, subpoenas, and congressional inquiries, they could not give the Sobells this assurance. After further discussion, the investigative team devised a coding system to protect the identities of the study subjects, and the balance of the day was spent reviewing the records and taking notes. The next morning the Sobells expressed dismay that they had allowed the investigators to take notes of detailed data and insisted that the investigators curtail their note-taking. They said that overnight they realized that the investigators were taking such detailed notes that those familiar with the study could easily identify the subjects. After prolonged discussion, the investigators left the Sobells' house, having decided that the limitation on note-taking would preclude them from having sufficient data to write and support a detailed report-- the kind of report they felt was necessary to respond fully to the allegations. The DMSR [Division of Management Survey and Review] investigators pursued the matter further with Brenner, the Sobells' attorney, and arranged a meeting with him on March 20. At that meeting, Brenner told the investigators that he was aware of the 'problem' because he had spoken with the Sobells after the investigators' visit. He said he felt that any detailed notes recorded by the investigators could create problems for his clients in the area of patient confidentiality and with the pending litigation in California. Further, he stated that he had advised the Sobells against meeting with the investigators again and against sharing any information in their records with them and that the Sobells had agreed to follow his advice.

The Steering Group's executive secretary, technical advisor, and investigative team discussed other ways of obtaining access to the records, and it was decided that the technical advisor would explore the possibilities of obtaining a subpoena. Within the DHHS [Department of Health and Human Services], only the Office of the Inspector General has the authority to issue subpoenas in an investigation of this type. In discussion with representatives of that office, the technical advisor was told that, because the Sobells and their records are located in Canada, there would be no means to enforce a subpoena for the records. The Steering Group had determined early on that an investigation of the allegations against the Sobells, including any possible misconduct by the Sobells in relation to the Caddy et al. study, required full and free access to all of their records. After this meeting with Brenner and the discussion regarding a subpoena, it was clear that the investigators could no longer expect to have access to the Sobells records and, as a result, that the investigation could not be completed. Therefore, it was decided that the investigation should be terminated and a report prepared. (pp.19-20).

Specific results of the limited examination of materials were described as follows:

As noted above, four members of the investigative team met with the Sobells on March 3 and 4, 1984, and examined some of their notes, data, and tapes for several subjects selected by the team members. The team members saw notes from follow-up telephone conversations describing the drinking pattern of several subjects for the time period between contacts. These notes were sometimes quite precise about the amounts of alcohol reportedly consumed on specific days. At other times, the notes were more general in describing the amounts of alcohol consumed by the subjects during certain time intervals (for example, 1 to 2 12-ounce cans of beer per day consumed 2 or 3 days a week since the last contact, denied any other drinking). From this information, the Sobells estimated the number of days in each of the various drinking dispositions (e.g., controlled drinking, drunk, abstinent) for each subject for each follow-up interval and reported these data in the form of percentage of days in each disposition for each 6-month follow-up period... Due to constraints described earlier in this report, the team members were unable to determine the accuracy with which the Sobells converted their follow-up notes into the reported results. (p. 21).

The last sentence above is significant. It indicates that the Committee could not take the first essential step in the investigation for even one, much less all of the subjects: Determine whether or not the interview raw data can generate the published results.

As I have previously asserted (Maltzman, 1989), and ignored by all critics, the information obtained above, "1 to 2 12-ounce cans of beer per day consumed 2 or 3 days a week since the last contact..." cannot reproduce the kind of results reported by the Sobells in their book and articles. The Sobells report specific numbers of days in one or the other drinking disposition for the entire second year for each subject (Sobell & Sobell, 1978). For example, as previously noted, Subject #5, JPr, is reported as having 282 abstinent days, 27 drunk, and 57 controlled drinking days based on two interviews in the entire second year. If the above raw data seen by the investigators for the Trachtenberg Committee were prorated for the year, the Sobells would have to report either 180 days of controlled drinking or 120 days of controlled drinking. What did the Sobells report for the above subject described by the investigators? These raw data cannot reproduce the kind of numerical results presented by the Sobells for the second year of the follow-up study (Sobell & Sobell, 1978, pp. 134-136). I explicitly advised the Committee to obtain and examine the interview forms for subjects such as #5, JPr, and #14, HC, (Trachtenberg, 1984, p. 14). There is no indication that they did.

The Sobells were given an opportunity to comment on a preliminary version of the Trachtenberg Report. Pendery and I did not receive this privilege. The Report states:

In responding to a draft of this report, the Sobells objected to the observation that their term 'daily drinking disposition' was 'ambiguous', and they asked that this 'erroneous' observation be deleted from our report. The Sobells pointed out that detailed definitions of the various 'drinking dispositions' have appeared in their publications... They claimed to have questioned subjects as to how much alcohol was consumed during the interval since their last contact with the subjects, rather than how much alcohol the subjects consumed on each calendar day. Further, the Sobells asserted that they obtained enough information to calculate estimates of the number of days that each subject spent in each of the previously defined drinking dispositions. (p. 19).

Does "2 or 3 days a week " enable the Sobells to present numerical data in each drinking disposition for a subject interviewed only twice in the second year, such as JPr? Does the interview sheet purportedly used in the time-line follow-back method permit estimates or does it obtain information as to how much a subject consumed on each calendar day (see Figure 5.1)?

The Trachtenberg Report continues:

After carefully reviewing information provided in the Sobells' response, the Steering Group made certain changes in the report, but decided that the observation regarding ambiguous terminology should remain.. Words such as 'daily' and 'each day' appeared in the Sobells' publications and were used in phrases like 'daily alcohol consumption,' daily drinking disposition,' and 'alcohol consumption on each day'. The Steering Group believes this usage is ambiguous and subject to misinterpretation. The Sobells also have stated that the issue regarding the use of the words 'estimates' and 'ascertained' is a minor one involving semantics. However, we believe that the latter term implies more exactness to the data gathering process, and its use may have contributed to misinterpretation of the type of data the Sobells obtained and reported. The Steering Group is not suggesting that the Sobells had any intent to mislead by using words like 'daily', 'each day', and 'ascertained'. However, we do believe that the Sobells could have selected more precise words to describe what they did. (p. 22).

Above is one more example of Orwellian DOUBLE THINK as the Report attempts to squirm out from under the weight of the apparent conclusion that the sample of raw data they reviewed does not correspond to the Sobells' published descriptions of the kind of results obtained using the time-line follow- back method. The Sobells (1978) state in their book, "prior to the hospital discharge, all subjects...

were told the reason for the follow-up... they were aware that questions *would be asked about the specific amounts of alcohol they consumed each day.*" (p.108) (italics added). They subsequently state, "alcohol consumption for each day of the follow-up interval was then coded into one of five mutually exclusive categories." (p. 110).

There is no ambiguity. Despite the incompleteness of their study, investigators for the Trachtenberg Committee found raw data that do not conform to the kind of results obtained with the time-line follow-back interview procedure the Sobells insist they used. Evidence the investigators uncovered from one of the few subjects' raw data they were permitted to examine cannot reproduce the kind of results published by the Sobells. The Committee never addressed this problem. Why not? Is it nothing more than semantics or is it fraud compounded by a bureaucratic whitewash, incompetence, or both?

Accompanying the Report is a memorandum by Trachtenberg, Deputy Administrator, ADAMHA, to the Administrator of ADAMHA which states:

Based on the investigative team's necessarily limited review, the Steering Group did not find evidence to demonstrate fabrication or falsification of data reported by the Sobells. However, we did note some errors and use of ambiguous terminology in their publications which indicate to us that the Sobells were careless in preparing their manuscripts for publication. (p.1).

The section of the memorandum concerned with recommendations states:

Since this matter has been investigated as far as is practicable, I recommend your acceptance and issuance of the Steering Group's report... Further, the Steering Group recommends that if ADAMHA receives a grant application or contract proposal in the next 2 years from the Sobells, the investigation report should be made available to persons considering the application or proposal. The purpose of this recommendation is to ensure that the agency's official report, rather than personal recollections and public accounts of this case, is considered. This would help to ensure that there is a clear understanding of the results of the investigation and the bases for these. Since we were not able to reach any definitive conclusions regarding alleged scientific misconduct, we are not making any other recommendations. (p.2).

How reasonable is the conclusion reached by the Trachtenberg Report that the Sobells were careless in the use of their ambiguous terminology? How reasonable is the Sobells' insistence, in response to the Trachtenberg report, that they did not obtain drinking dispositions on specific days, but only estimates, this was their intent, and this is what they published?

In Table 8 of their book the Sobells (1978, pp. 134-136) list the drinking profiles of each of the subjects for the second year follow-up. Total number of abstinent days, number of controlled drinking days, type of drink, number of drunk days, days per week in a particular disposition, and social environment are listed for each subject. Total number of drunk days, style of drinking, maximum binge, type of drink, number of drinks, social environment, and where the drinking occurred are also presented. Number of days in an abstinence oriented environment is a final category provided. Numerical results are given in each category. Results are not labelled estimates. Nor is there any information concerning how estimates are determined. As in the example of Subject #5, JPr, would the data for the subject described in the Trachtenberg Report as drinking one or two beers a day two or three days a week be presented as 180 days or 120 days of controlled drinking? How would a decision be reached? There are no discussions of estimates and rules for their use in the Sobells' articles and book. In contrast, the Sobells (1989) insist that they used the time-line follow-back method which requires filling in a specific disposition for each day of the 3-4 weeks since the previous interview (see Fig. 5.1).

The Trachtenberg Committee did not, could not, take the essential first step necessary in an investigation of fraud in science: Obtain all of the raw data and from these attempt to reconstruct the published results. They did not attempt the reconstruction with the data they did observe. Why not? It is significant that not one commentator on the controlled drinking investigations considers the admitted incompleteness of the Trachtenberg (1984) report and its misleading conclusion.

Conclusion

Contradictions between the contents of the Trachtenberg Report and its conclusions and the contents of the Dickens report reflect the influence of political pressure, incompetence, or both. Pressure by whom and for what reason, I do not know. Although lacking specific evidence in its support, the above hypothesis provides the only plausible account for the obvious contradictions within the text of the Trachtenberg Report, between the Dickens and Trachtenberg Reports, and the fact that competent scientist members of the Committee's Steering Group apparently approved the Report. Again, this fundamenally flawed investigation shows the unfortunate consequences of an institution investigating itself. An inherent conflict of interest is present. If the institution finds the defendants guilty, it finds itself guilty, and loses credibility, because of its poor judgment in providing grant support to the defendants. Furthermore, finding the Sobells guilty of scientific misconduct would put ADAMHA and NIH at risk for malpractice lawsuits by patients who had suffered as a consequence of the Sobells' research. Worst of all, it could bring down the wrath of Congress with resultant budget slashes, loss of credibility by individual administrators, and their careers in government potentially damaged or destroyed.

In-house scientists on the Steering Committee are captives of the political context. If they do not "play ball" with the bureaucrats, their careers are in jeopardy; their space and budget needs are hostages of the bureaucrats. They play ball. This scenario demands that institutions, whether police departments investigating alleged police brutality, universities investigating alleged fraud by faculty, or professional societies investigating its membership, should not be solely responsible for the investigation, if at all.

Widely circulated in the media, the conclusion of the Trachtenberg Committee that no evidence of misconduct was found was used to advantage by the Sobells, their supporters and academic "bystanders" who reported the conclusion in textbooks, articles, and handbooks without examining the original Report.

A CONGRESSIONAL INVESTIGATION?

The Sobells have asserted that they have been exonerated by a congressional investigation. I became aware of this claim during the course of an appeal of my censure by the American Psychological Association's Committee on Scientific and Professional Ethics and Conduct (CSPEC) for my statement quoted in the NY Times (Boffey, 1982) that I believe the Sobells had committed fraud.

I rejected the judgment by CSPEC and requested, as was my right, an appearance before the full board. Prior to my visit before the CSPEC meeting scheduled for June 17, 1983, I received a letter outlining the issues that would be covered in my hearing. Included in the list was the following:

The Subcommittee on Investigations and Oversight of the U. S. House of Representatives investigated this matter and its investigator, Mr. James E. Jenson [sic] writes in a letter to the Drs. Sobell (dated March 23, 1983) that he has concluded that 'there is no evidence to support the allegation that your study was based on fallacious, falsified or otherwise invented data.' How do you reconcile this conclusion with your statements that there was fraud involved in this matter? (D. H. Mills, June 1, 1983).

I had received a copy of the letter in question from neither Jensen nor the CSPEC prior to my hearing. Near the end of my hearing a Committee member asked me to respond to Jensen's letter. I said I could not because I was unacquainted with its contents other than its conclusion and could not evaluate the nature of the inquiry purportedly conducted. I was given a copy of the letter. Since I was unfamiliar with its contents until that moment, the Committee felt it was inappropriate to demand a response from me.

Pendery was also to appear before the Committee because she was reprimanded for not responding by letter within 30 days to a query from the Committee. She was represented by an attorney, Thomas Dyson, Esq. Her reprimand was ultimately rescinded. Following our meetings with the CSPEC the three of us went to the House of Representatives office building to talk to Jensen. An administrative assistant informed us that Mr. Jensen was away for the day. She further informed us that there had been no subcommittee hearings on the Sobells and that no subcommittee hearing was planned. We then proceeded to Congressman Gore's office, since he chaired the subcommittee. His staff informed us that he was unavailable at the time. They also informed us that there had been no subcommittee hearings on the Sobells and that none were planned.

Not long after my return home from Washington I received a letter from the administrative officer for CSPEC. He indicated that they rescinded their censure because I had a plausible basis for my belief reported in the NY Times that fraud was involved in the research in question (D. H. Mills, June 17, 1983). Shortly thereafter a colleague sent me a copy of Jensen's letter and the cover letter accompanying it written by the Sobells. He had received it from the Sobells who had apparently circulated it widely. Their cover letter states that a congressional inquiry had taken place based on "a full investigation of the evidence from both sides". The "Congressional inquiry also provides independent and strong confirmation of the "findings and conclusions of the Dickens' Commitee.(Sobell & Sobell, nd).

In their reply to Walker and Roach (1984) the Sobells state:
 Our records were subsequently independently examined and cross-checked in
the course of an inquiry conducted by the Subcommittee on Investigations and
Oversight, Committee on Science and Technology of the United States House of
Representatives. In a letter informing us of the results of the Congressonal
inquiry, the Investigator wrote: 'My review of all available [sic] supports the
findings of the Commission convened by the Addiction Research Foundation
(also known as the 'Dicken's Commission')'. We cooperated fully with both of
these investigations, and the Congressonal Investigator had access to
Congressional subpoena power. Apparently, Pendery et al. did not co-operate
with either investigation. (p.158).

Note that the outcome of a congressional inquiry is claimed in their letter, one
which was based on a "full investigation of the evidence from both sides". There
was no such congressional inquiry and no such "full investigation of the evidence".
I had received one telephone call from Mr. Jensen. He asked me whether or not I
had made the allegation quoted in the NY Times.. I said I did. He also asked if he
could have a copy of the letters I had written to the CSPEC concerning my
allegations of fraud against the Sobells. I sent him copies.

Figure 5.3 is a copy of Jensen's letter to the Sobells. There are several
interesting aspects to its form as well as its content. There are glaring typographical
errors. It obviously is not a report of the conclusions of a congressional committee,
but Jensen's personal observations It is noteworthy that the portions of the letter
describing the nature of Jensen's inquiry purporting to confirm the validity of the
Sobells' data are characteristically omitted from commentaries (Brownell, 1984;
Hunt, 1999; Marlatt, 1983, 1984; Roizen, 1987; Sobell & Sobell, 1984, 1989).

Jensen states that his investigation involved "the correlation between... notes of
contacts with patients, phone logs and tape recordings of those contacts..." These
are not the raw data out of which the dependent variables, daily drinking disposition
and days functioning well, are constructed. Confusion over the nature of the tape
recordings is also apparent. They do not provide the data contained in purported
monthly interviews providing the daily drinking disposition, the basic dependent
variable. Jensen appears unaware of the nature of the pertinent dependent
variables. The statement,"errors in calculating the number of collateral contacts"
makes no sense. What kind of errors? Did they have too many collaterals or too
few? How would Jensen know what the appropriate number of collaterals or
contacts with them ought to be? Was there an interview with drinking dispositions
obtained from each contact with a collateral? Jensen's statement makes little sense
and does not seem to focus on any critical issue. The complete letter describing the
investigation raises serious doubts concerning the adequacy of the inquiry, Jensen's
understanding of the task facing an investigator of fraud in science, Jensen's
motivation in writing the letter, and the Sobells' presentation of the affair.

Given the absence of relevant subcommittee hearings and the unusual nature
and circumstances of Jensen's letter, David Evans, Esq., a colleague of Thomas
Dyson, Esq., wrote to Jensen. Mr. Evans shared his letter and the reply with me.
Figure 5.4 is a copy of Mr. Evan's letter to Jensen.

Congress of the United States
House of Representatives
Washington, D.C. 20515

March 23, 1983

Drs. Mark and Linda Sobell
Addiction Research Foundation
33 Russell St.
Toronto, Ontario
CANADA M59 25 L

Dear Drs. Sobell & Sobell:

This is to formally advice you of the results of the Subcommittee on Investigations and Oversight;s inquiry into the allegations concerning your study of controlled drinking.

Based upon my review of the evidence, I have concluded that there is no evidence to support the allegation that your study was based upon fallacious, falsified or otherwise invented data.

The correlation between your notes of contacts with patients, your phone logs and the tape recordings of those contacts have convinced me that your report of your study was made in good faith. With the exception of errors in calculating the number of collateral contacts, your representation of the study conducted is an accurate one, and there is no evidence of willful manufacturing of data.

My review of all available supports the findings fo the Commission convened by the Addiction Research Foundation (also known as the "Dicken's Commission") and fully supports their conclusions.

Lasly, the Division of Survey and Management Review at the National Institutes of Health, at the request of the Department of Health and Human Services, is in the process of conducting a review of this controversy. Because the Department of HHS is the funding agency involved, I beleive theri review is a necessary one, in that they are ultimately the apprppriate U.S. Government agency to be conducting any review or investigation of this matter.

If anyone should require any confirmation or further dicsussion of the Subcommittee on Investigations and Oversights conclusions, please have them contact me at (202) 226-3639, or by writing me at Rm. 822, House Annex #1, Washington, D.C. 20515

Sincerely,

James F. Jensen

Figure 5.3 Jensen's letter to the Sobells.

ımerican Bar Association

CHAIRPERSON
...
Washington D C 2000?

CHAIRPERSON ELECT
Martha W. Barnet
P O Drawer 810
Tallahassee FL 32302

VICE-CHAIRPERSON
J David Ellwanger
555 Franklin Street
San Francisco CA 94102
SECRETARY
Abner J Mikva
U S Court of Appeals
3rd & Constitution Ave N W.
Room 3108
Washington DC 20001

RECORDING SECRETARY
Sara-Ann Determan
815 Connecticut Ave N W.
Washington DC 20006

SECTION DELEGATE TO TH
HOUSE OF DELEGATES
Peter F Langrock
P O Drawer 351
Middlebury VT 05753

IMMEDIATE
PAST CHAIRPERSON
Cruz Reynoso
350 McAllister Street
San Francisco CA 94102

COUNCIL MEMBERS
The Officers and

E Clinton Bamberger Jr
Baltimore MD
Robert F Drinan
Washington DC
Alexander D Forger
New York NY
Michael Franck
Lansing MI
Deborah M Greenberg
New York NY
Gary C Huckaby
Huntsville AL
Yale Kamisar
Ann Arbor MI
Philip A Lacovara
Washington DC
James H Manahan
Mankato MN
William L Robinson
Washington DC
Clifford C Stromberg
Washington DC
LeRoy W Wilder
Portland OR

LAW STUDENT
REPRESENTATIVE
Susan Mann
Tacoma WA
YOUNG LAWYERS
REPRESENTATIVE
J Elizabeth Gee
Atlanta GA
BOARD OF GOVERNORS
LIAISON
Richard F Donahue
Lowell MA
STAFF DIRECTOR
Steven G Raikin
1800 M Street N W.
Washington DC 20036
ADMINISTRATIVE ASS STA
J Wade Carey
1800 M Street N W.
Washington DC 20036

July 27, 1983

Mr. James E. Jensen
Investigator
Subcommittee on Investigations
  and Oversight
Room 822
House Annex #1
Washington, D.C. 20515

Dear Mr. Jenson:

In the June 1, 1983 issue of The Journal, published by the Addiction Research Foundation, in Canada, there was an article which mentioned an investigation by the Subcommittee on Investigations and Oversight into the work of Drs. Linda and Mark Sobell. The Sobell's have claimed favorable results in teaching alcoholics to be "controlled drinkers". As far as we can determine, the theory that alcoholics can become controlled drinkers is held in disrepute in the alcoholism field. This has been confirmed by every leading organization in the alcoholism field. The academic research in the alcoholism field also confirms this, and, as a result, there is not a single alcoholism research center in the United States that has adopted controlled drinking as a policy. In the face of this, the Sobells rely on research they conducted years ago as graduate students, research which has been effectively refuted on it's merits by Drs. Mary Pendery and Irving Maltzman and others. Why then did your committee in Congress issue a report which supports the Sobell's research?

My Committee is working on a number of projects that touch this issue, therefore, we would be very anxious to have you answer the following questions:

1. On what legal authority did your Committee conduct this investigation?

2. Who specifically authorized the investigation?

3. Why was this investigation authorized?

4. Who initiated the investigation?

5. Who conducted the investigation?

6. Who was interviewed during the investigation and when?

SECTION OF INDIVIDUAL RIGHTS AND RESPONSIBILITIES

1800 M STREET, N W, WASHINGTON, D C 20036 • (202) 331-2279

Figure 5.4 Evans letter to Jensen Page 1 of 2.

Mr. James Jensen
Page 2
July 27, 1983

7. What documentary evidence was considered?

8. Were the parties you were aware of who have evidence contradicting the Sobell's research given ample opportunity to comment and present documentary evidence? When and how were these people contacted?

9. Were there Congressional hearings on this matter? If not, why not?

10. Will Congressional hearings be scheduled? If not, why not?

11. Why didn't you use your subpoena power to compel evidence on this matter to be brought forward?

12. Who authored your final report?

13. Who approved your final report?

14. Were the parties who have evidence contradicting the Sobell's research given an opportunity to comment on your report before it was released? If not, why not?

15. Will the parties who have evidence contradicting the Sobell's research be given an opportunity _now_ to refute the Sobell's research? If not, why not?

16. Are you aware if and how the Sobell's are using the results of your report?

If a report is issued in the name of Congress, it is imperative that it be a fair and well reasoned analysis based on open debate.

We are looking forward to hearing from you as soon as possible.

Sincerely,

David G. Evans, Esq.
Chair, Alcoholism and Drug Law
Reform Committee

DGE/nhd
cc: Members Subcommittee on Investigations and Oversight

Figure 5.4 Evans letter to Jensen Page 2 of 2.

D-)N J UUIA (R4 L Chairman

P. "F A ROE N J
GE-NE L E PRINN JR CALIF
DAVIS H SCHUER N Y
RICHARD L OTTIN/ER N Y
TOM HARKIN IOWA
WLM L.OYD TENN
DOUG WAL GREN PA
DAN C.CEYMAN KANS
A.TINT GORL JR TENN
BOB "A YOUNG MO
MARGOE L VOLKMER MO.
BILL NELSON FLA
STANLEY N LUNOINE N.Y.
RALPH M HALL TEX
DAVE McCURDY, OKLA
MERVYN M PYMALLY CALIF.
PAUL SIMON ILL
NORMAN J MINETA CALIF
RICHARD J DURBIN ILL
MICHAEL A ANDREWS TEX.
BUDDY MAC KAY FLA
TIM VALENTINE N C
HARRY M REID NEV
ROBERT G TORRICELLI N.J.
FREDERICK C BOUCHER VA.

U.S. HOUSE OF REPRESENTATIVES

COMMITTEE ON SCIENCE AND TECHNOLOGY

SUITE 2321 RAYBURN HOUSE OFFICE BUILDING

WASHINGTON, D.C. 20515

(202) 225–8371

August 5, 1983

LARRY WINN, JR RAN*
MAN. EL LUJAN JR N MEX
ROBERT S WALKER PA
WILLIAM CARNEY N Y
F JAMES SENSENBRENNER JR WIS
JUDD GREGG N H
RAYMOND J McGRATH N Y
JOE SKEEN N MEX
CLAUDINE SCHNEIDER R I
BILL LOWERY CALIF
BOB CHANDLER WASH
HERBERT H BATEMAN VA
SHERWOOD L BOEHLERT N Y
ALFRED A McCANDLESS CALIF
TOM LEWIS FLA

J H POORE
Executive Director
ROBERT C KETCHAM
General Counsel
DAVID S JEFFERY
Minority Staff Director

David G. Evans, Esquire
Chair, Alcoholism and
  Drug Law Reform Committee
Section of Individual Rights
  and Responsibilities
American Bar Association
1800 M Street, N. W.
Washington, D. C. 20036

Dear Mr. Evans:

Receipt is acknowledged of your letter of July 27, 1983.

The Subcommittee on Investigations and Oversight conducted a review of allegations of falsification of scientific data in connection with the study by Drs. Mark and Linda Sobell of treatment of alcoholics by controlled drinking undertaken at Patton State Hospital. This inquiry was conducted as part of the Subcommittee's ongoing interest in the issue of fraud in science.

There were no Subcommittee hearings held on the subject, nor did the Subcommittee issue a report.

The Subcommittee is currently monitoring the efforts of a task force convened by the Department of Health and Human Services to resolve the controversy.

If you should have any further questions, or should you desire a meeting to discuss this matter further, please contact Mr. James Jensen of the Subcommittee staff at 226-3639.

Sincerely,

Albert Gore, Jr.
Chairman
Subcommittee on
  Investigations and Oversight

cc: Members, Subcommittee on Investigations and Oversight

Figure 5.5 Letter sent in reply to Evans' queries by Congressman Albert Gore, head of the subcommittee that employed Jensen as an investigator. No reply was received from Jensen.

It is apparent from Congressman Gore's letter that there was no congressional inquiry, no congressional investigation, and no hearings that characteristically accompany a congressional investigation. It is also apparent that Congressman Gore evaded answering the specific questions concerning the circumstances under which Jensen undertook his "investigation" and "report".

Nevertheless, the Sobells (1984a) asserted, "We were able to reconstruct for the ... Congressional inquiry the actual procedure [weighted random-assignment] followed." (p.422). According to a report in the *APA Monitor*, a monthly newspaper published by the American Psychological Association and distributed to all members, Jensen stated:

'Unlike a Canadian committee that investigated the charges last fall, 'I just waded into the data' rather than first identifying specific questions to be answered, he said. In investigating other alleged scientific frauds, he said, he has found that false data 'don't hold up for a minute' when the scientist is asked for original materials. The Sobells had an entire safe full of tapes and records, including 'documents from the patients' own hand'. (Fisher, 1983, p.48).

A more recent assertion by the Sobells (1989) concerning Jensen was more circumspect than earlier published comments and the cover letter accompanying the Jensen letter mailed to various people. By this time the Sobells were undoubtedly aware of Congressman Gore's letter to Mr. Evans. They state, "the conduct of the IBTA study was further scrutinized by an investigator from the United States Congress. The investigator had complete access to our data." (p.474). They go on to cite a news story in the *APA Monitor* which asserts that Jensen was making a preliminary inquiry to determine whether an investigtion by the subcommittee of the House Science and Technology Committee should be undertaken.

Circumstances surrounding this investigation remain clouded in the absence of answers to the questions raised in Evans' original letter to Jensen and Congressman Gore's evasive reply. It is clear, however, that an adequate investigation of an allegation of fraud did not occur, and certainly not one conducted by a congressional committee.

PATIENTS MALPRACTICE LAWSUIT EXONERATES SOBELLS

According to the Sobells (1989) the most recent exoneraton following an investigation, one cited by other commentators as well, (Baumeister et al., 1994; Hunt, 1999; Nathan, 1989) purports to be the result of a medical malpractice suit brought by subjects in the experimental group or their estates. "... beginning in 1983 ... we were named as plaintiffs [sic] in a $96 million lawsuit filed by some former subjects and their collaterals in the Superior Court of California .... more than 4 years after it was filed, the suit was finally dismissed." (Sobell & Sobell, 1989, p. 475). In fact, the suit initiated in July 1983 named only the State of California, University of California, Riverside and Patton State Hospital as defendants. In September 1983 an Amended Claim was filed against the State of California, Patton State Hospital, Mark and Linda Sobell, Orange County, Glen Caddy and David Perkins and additional John Does. A third and final Amended Complaint was filed in December 1987. The Sobells were *not* named as defendants in the latter final form of the complaint.

As the quotation from the Trachtenberg memorandum indicates, it was considered impossible for the Inspector General to subpoena the Sobells' data since they resided in Canada. In similar fashion, it was impossible for the attorneys representing the patients to serve a summons on the Sobells residing in Canada. Although they were named in the second Amended Complaint, they could not be sued by the patients because of their residence in a foreign country. As a result, the Sobells were not named as defendants in the final Amended Complaint. The latter complaint was dismissed by Judge Kayashima of the Superior Court in San Bernardino, California on technical grounds. The statute of limitations had run out for each of the individual plaintiffs, and after such a long lapse of time between the alleged malpractice at Patton State Hospital and their current medical condition, it was impossible to prove that the current state of the patients was due to the events occurring so many years earlier. The latter is the basis for the judgment that the complaint "was uncertain as a whole". There was no investigation of the Sobells or anyone else.

The following is from a letter sent to the plaintiffs by Susan Sweetman, Esq., of the law firm of Scolinos, Slater & Sweetman representing the patients or their estates:

Re: Carroll, et al. v. State of California, et al.
Case Number: 236924
File Number: 63114

It is with a sad note that I inform you that the above-entitled action against defendants, State of California, Patton State Hospital, California State University at Fullerton, Glenn Caddy and David Perkins, has been dismissed in its entirety. " (S. Sweetman, December, 22, 1987).

Recall Nathan's (1989, p. 465) assertion: "Five separate and competent investigative groups" considered and rejected" my allegations. What is the evidence for this categorical statement by the executive editor of one of the most prestigious journals in the field of alcoholism and alcohol studies? As we have seen, there is none.

Conclusions

If we take an account of the investigations exonerating the Sobells we find: one fundamentally flawed investigation by the Dickens committee; an incomplete and ambiguous investigation by the Trachtenberg Committee that finds evidence contradicting the published results and remarks of the Sobells but refuses to face the contradictions obtained in their limited effort to investigate; a mysterious note by Jensen a staff member of a congressional subcommittee claiming in incoherent fashion to have confirmed the findings of the Dickens Committee exonerating the Sobells; the distinguished head of the congressional subcommittee denies holding hearings; the Sobells claim that an investigation as part of a law suit for malpractice exonerated them; the case was dismissed on technical grounds and did not name the Sobells in the final form of the complaint because they were residents in a foreign country. The APA Ethics Committee's actions described in earlier chapters surely cannot be considered an investigation of alleged misconduct exonerating the Sobells.

I believe at least three firm conclusion can be reached concerning the investigations of the Sobells alleged misconduct: (a) There has been no careful disinterested investigation of my allegations of data fabrication and misrepresentation by the Sobells. (b) The Sobells do not flinch from massaging events to fit their purposes. (c) A science that provides the opportunity for the practices described in this chapter and others to follow suffers the consequences: a loss of trust, misspent funds, resources and time, inadequately educating a generation of students, and most important of all: causing harm to people in need of help, their significant others, and the public at large.

6 THE RISE AND FALL OF CONTROLLED DRINKING

Introduction

"... this book [Hester & Miller (1995)] equals the status of the first edition, in this reviewer's opinion, as one of the classics in the alcoholism treatment field, a must for every clinician's and researcher's library. I can hardly wait for the third edition !" (Rotgers, 1996b, p. 101.).

A focus of our concern in the present chapter is the current edition of the highly praised Hester and Millers' (1995) *Handbook of alcoholism treatment approaches: Effective alternative* 2nd ed. It contains chapters by Miller, Hester and colleagues reviewing the treatment outcome literature as well as individual chapters by additional authors providing manuals for practicing the new alternatives to the failed traditional treatments. Alcoholism counselors engaged in treating problem drinkers rather than alcoholics are the target audience.

Hester and Miller (1995) complain in their Preface that the effective alternative treatments reviewed in their book have not been adequately recognized and adopted in the treatment field which still relies on treatments with no evidence of effectiveness. Past reviews of the treatment outcome literature as well as the present one have provided Miller and Hester with impressive credentials as experts in the treatment evaluation field. Recognition of their status as experts is evidenced in part by Hester's authorship of the chapter on "Outcome Research" in, *The American Psychiatric Press Textbook of Substance Abuse Treatment* , a textbook for medical students edited by two MDs (Galanter & Kleber, 1994). Miller and Hester's reviews are obviously esteemed when even their declared opposition, the "medical model" accepts one of them as the "mavin" to present an overview of the alcoholism treatment outcome literature in a textbook for medical students.

HESTER AND MILLER'S VIEW OF THE ALCOHOLISM TREATMENT OUTCOME LITERATURE

Hester and Miller (1995) state in their Preface that they arrived at two surprising conclusions in their earlier reviews. These reviews, as well as the present one, were limited to studies with proper control or comparison groups. Their conclusions are: (a) Certain treatments were strongly supported by research results. (b) None of these treatments were in general use in the United States. Instead, the generally used treatments were 12-step programs based on the Minnesota Model for which they found no evidence of effectiveness as determined by well-controlled studies. (c) No one treatment was superior to all the others. There is an interaction between type of patient and treatment. Matching of treatment and patient is necessary. This sort of argument laid the foundation for gulling the government into supporting the $27,000,000 MATCH project that we will discuss in chapter 7.

We shall also see in chapter 7 that the effectiveness of traditional treatments evaluated in well-controlled studies is very different from that suggested by Hester and Miller. No one treatment reviewed in Hester and Miller's book appears to be consistently superior to all the others because the efficacy studies investigating treatment outcomes reviewed in their book are often poorly designed and conducted. They generally have too few subjects and therefore lack the statistical power to reliably differentiate between treatments. Most importantly, the best studies of treatment effectiveness which happen to be evaluations of abstinence oriented programs are never mentioned. No one treatment stands out in their review because the ones that stand out are ignored, never cited and discussed by Hester and Miller.

Treatment matching has become a major theme in policy and treatment proposals and Miller and colleagues have obtained very large grants to investigate matching of patients to treatments (Project MATCH Research Group, 1993). One of the major matches revisionists promote is obvious: Individuals should be able to choose whether they wish abstinence or to engage in controlled drinking. The ethical problem of allowing patients to possibly exacerbate brain damage by continuing to drink is ignored by Miller and Hester and other revisionists (Heather & Robertson, 1983; Heather & Tebbutt, 1989; Marlatt, Larimer, Baer, & Quigley, 1993; Marlatt et al., 1998). There is no indication that proper informed consent is obtained in studies providing participants a choice between treatment goals. A proper informed consent must present the possible negative as well as positive consequences of the alternative treatments available to the patient. There is also the important initial assumption that the patient has the capacity to make a considered decision based on the balancing of negative and positive consequences of alternative goals. Miller and Hester ignore the problem and by so doing they are implicitly proposing that counselors not obtain a proper informed consent. We shall return to this important issue again.

Matching is a complex issue. A person who is dependent upon their job and cannot take time off for inpatient treatment lasting 3-4 weeks, should be able to choose outpatient rather than inpatient treatment, other things being equal. Choices of this sort, however, are rapidly disappearing, since it it difficult to find inpatient treatment programs during these times of cost cutting and managed care. Outpatient treatment is cheaper. The bottom line is what counts. A major problem is that always looking at bottom lines promotes short-sightedness. It is cheaper to have outpatient than inpatient treatment, brief advice rather than counseling and rehabilitation - in the short run. This short-sighted view fails to consider the expense of relapses: the damage done to patient, family, and society, with repeated relapses that might have been avoided by an initial more intensive abstinence oriented treatment for dependent alcoholics that sticks. But we are getting ahead of our story. Let us turn to another one of Hester and Miller's erroneous conclusions:

> We found two dozen studies comparing longer with shorter treatment, residential with nonresidential programs, or more versus less intensive interventions. The results were startling. Without a single exception, the studies failed to show any advantage for the more intensive, longer, or residential approaches over less intensive and less expensive alternatives. (Hester & Miller, 1995, p. xii).

Monaghan and Finney (1996) reach a different conclusion following their systematic review of the literature. Intensity of treatment does make a difference.

Our review of the best study in the field of alcohol treatment effectiveness in chapter 7 reaches a similar conclusion. When individual patient differences are controlled intensity of treatment does make a difference, although Küfner and Feuerlein (1989) did find an interaction between severity of dependence and treatment intensity, a matching effect.

Evaluation of treatment outcomes

Chapter 2 in Hester and Miller's (1995) book titled, "What works? A methodological analysis of the alcohol treatment outcome literature", provides an evaluative review of the treatment outcome literature previously reviewed by Miller and Hester (1980, 1986) updated and with "methodological advances". Each research report evaluated by Miller et al. (1995) was rated by at least two people and submitted to the senior author of the research report for a rating and comments. Ratings were obtained for elements of quality, effectiveness, and expense, etc. Criteria for inclusion of a research report in the evaluation process were that it examined a treatment for alcohol problems, a comparison of treatments or a control condition was employed, as well as a proper research methodology such as randomization or matching, and there was at least one outcome measure of drinking or alcohol-related problems. Ratings were obtained for a variety of dimensions of quality such as statistical analyses, use of collaterals, length of follow-up, group allocations, i.e., randomization, or case control, etc. Also rated were quality control and the standardized use of a treatment manual. Use of such manuals will affect the rating of experimental efficacy studies positively and penalize effectiveness studies. Standing clinics typically do not use manuals because they presumably have experienced counselors who are capable of adapting to the individual differences and needs of their patients. Nature of contact, collaterals, objectivity of measures, treatment of dropouts and attrition, quality of follow-up, quality of statistical analyses, and nature of research site were also evaluated. Numerical scores were obtained for each measure and combined to give overall evidence scores, permitting comparisons of individual studies. Averaging the overall scores for individual studies of a particular type, a treatment modality, provided comparisons among different treatment modalities.

A final pool of 211 studies classified into 43 treatment modalities was examined by Miller et al. (1995). A few modalities could not be compared because they were based on only one or two research reports.

Methodological shortcomings

All this seems to be a rigorous basis for evaluating and comparing alcoholism treatments. However, the evaluations can only be as good as the methods employed and the assumptions on which they rest. A fundamental methodological flaw present from the outset compromises the validity of the entire review and evaluation process. Criteria for quantitative evaluations of treatment outcome and methodological rigor of each research report examined were developed by Miller and his colleagues. Ratings of each study along the various dimensions likewise were conducted by Miller and colleagues. Neither was done by an independent panel of disinterested experts.

The manner in which Miller and his colleagues conducted the review and evaluations would be equivalent to the Food and Drug Administration (FDA) asking a drug company to establish the criteria for determining the effectiveness of new drugs, including their own, and then having the drug company CEO and employees decide on the nature of the criteria for evaluation, and conduct the ratings of their drugs and those of competitors on the basis of the criteria they devised. Isn't there a real possibility that the drug company would introduce criteria favoring their own drugs? Results obtained in this way may sound good as long as the process involved is not described in detail and the drugs are not independently evaluated. If this seems to be a bad way to go about evaluating drugs, it is also a bad way to evaluate alcoholism treatments.

Critical examination of the process employed in the evaluations and the detailed examination of individual research reports suggests that the results obtained rob the review by Miller et al. (1995) of scientific value. For example, if a research report has more than one follow-up outcome interview period the method used by Miller et al. takes the highest success rate obtained as the outcome score regardless of the post-treatment interval of the various outcome interviews. In other words, if after 3 months the treatment outcome success rate is 80% and after 2 years it is 20%, the treatment outcome used in the evaluation is 80% and the research report receives a very high rating, higher than a program that has a 70% success rate after 1 year and 60% after 4 years. This does not make sense. Percent success should be the last outcome weighted by the duration of the outcome. An evaluation outcome after six months should receive less weight than one after four years. Length of the window of evaluation must also be weighted. A window of three months, i.e., the quantity and frequency of drinking, abstinence, problems, etc., during the preceding three months should receive less weight than a window of 12 months preceding the evaluation of outcomes a year after treatment. Certainly, a continuous abstinence rate or controlled drinking rate of four years should receive a higher rating than one month at the 4 year anniversary. This all seems reasonable, but it was not the manner in which dimensions of outcome were weighted by Miller et al. (1995). If they were weighted in the suggested manner, Miller and colleagues' research reports for behavioral self-control treatment (BSCT) and brief intervention programs would receive considerably lower scores than they did. Their procedure of using a short follow-up interval, usually the one providing the best outcome, enhances the apparent success of controlled drinking treatment goals, but controlled drinking outcomes tend to be short lived as we shall see.

Taylor (1987) observes that periods of controlled drinking are characteristic of the natural history of alcoholism (Schuckit, Tipp, Smith, & Bucholz, 1997). In the absence of any treatment, alcoholics and problem drinkers may go through periods where they will control their drinking and drink moderately. The problem is they cannot maintain the level of moderation. Using a short interval such as the quantity and frequency of drinking during the previous month will catch a certain percentage of alcoholic people in a moderation phase. Taylor (1987) recommends a three year interval of continuous controlled drinking as a criterion for an individual successfully engaged in controlled drinking. Such a measure differs from the usual group measure which simply reports the number or percentage of participants who are controlling their drinking for the preceding month at the 6-month anniversary, and at the 12-month anniversary and the patients constituting the percentage of controlled drinkers at the two follow-up windows need not be the same individuals.

There is an old saying of statisticians: "garbage in, garbage out". Put in bad data, no matter how sophisticated their statistical treatment, the outcome is still bad. Put another way, "you can't make a silk purse out of a sow's ear". Miller and Hester are trying to make a silk purse out of a sow's ear. It smells bad.

Another essential requirement for a valid review of treatment outcome research is that it considers a complete and unbiased pool of studies. Miller et al. (1995) did not use such a pool of research reports for their evaluation. There is a bias present that influences the number and kinds of research reports in the direction desired by Miller and Hester. What direction is that? The one that they are selling: Their own behavior therapy methods. Research reports evaluated were derived from Hester and Miller's previous data bases, and computer and manual searches of "two dozen major journals in the field". Restriction to "major" (undefined) journals in the field creates a bias towards including most behavior therapy type studies because they tend to be published in their own specialized journals, or alcohol and drug journals dominated by behavior therapists on their review boards. By no stretch of the imagination can I consider *Psychology of Addictive Behaviors* a journal where Miller and his students published several of their behavior therapy articles, a "major" journal at the time. Traditional studies conducted by investigators who are not behavior therapists are published in a great variety of different journals, including medically oriented journals and basic behavioral and neuroscience journals. For example, Miller et al. (1995) include only a single acupuncture study, which obtained positive results, in their evaluations. It was published in a specialized alcoholism journal (Bullock et al., 1987). However, another well-designed study with positive results published by the same group was not considered (Bullock, Culliton, & Olander, 1989), because it was published in a nonspecialized journal, *Lancet*, a world class British biomedical journal.

More serious is that Miller et al.'s (1995) review systematically omitted the largest and best reports demonstrating abstinence outcome rates for larger numbers of patients than all the BSCT studies combined (Feuerlein & Küfner,1989; Harrison, Hoffmann, & Streed, 1991; Küfner & Feuerlein, 1989; Smith, Frawley, & Polissar, 1991) because they were not published in specialized alcoholism journals.

Results of the biased evaluation methodology

Miller et al. (1995) state:

> what conclusions seem warranted from the cumulative evidence of these 211 controlled trials? In an earlier review, Miller and Hester (1986a) observed that although the scientific literature points to a list of treatment approaches with reasonable evidence of positive benefit, this list overlaps little, if at all, with those components commonly employed in U.S. alcoholism treatment programs. The same pattern is clearly evident in this review. Indeed, one must read halfway down Table 2.4 before encountering the first modality (disulfiram) with anything like common usage as a component of standard practice at least in the

United States. Instead, a relatively predictable combination of elements has characterized the generic 'Minnesota model' program that continues to dominate American addictions treatment: a milieu advocating a spiritual twelve-step (AA) philosophy, typically augmented with group psychotherapy, educational lectures and films, and relatively unspecific general alcoholism counseling, often of a confrontational nature (Cook, 1988).

Some programs have added components such as relaxation training, CENAPS-model relapse counseling, and family therapy... To fill in the complete set of treatment method with the least evidence of effectiveness... one need add only metronidazole, antianxiety medication, videotape self-confrontation, psychedelic medication, hypnosis...

The negative correlation between scientific evidence and application in standard practice remains striking, and could hardly be larger if one intentionally constructed treatment programs from those approaches with the *least* evidence of efficacy.

Such a gap between science and practice will not be reduced without some disciplined and demanding changes. Clinicians, like scientists, must be willing to test their cherished assumptions against hard data and to relinquish views and practices that do not stand up to the test of evidence. (pp. 32-33).

Purported efficacy of BSCT

To demonstrate the lack of validity of the evaluative review of treatment outcomes provided by Miller et al. (1995) we must examine in detail some of their highly rated individual studies. The contrast with Miller and Hester's appraisal is striking. First, however, we will consider Hester's (1995) evaluation of BSCT in the chapter devoted to the description of that ostensibly highly successful treatment modality:

Behavioral self-control training (BSCT) is a treatment approach used to pursue either a goal of abstinence or a goal of moderate and nonproblematic drinking. It consists of behavioral techniques of goal setting, self-monitoring, managing consumption, rewarding goal attainment, functionally analyzing drinking situations, and learning alternate coping skills... The client maintains primary responsibility for making decisions throughout the training.

Research shows that BSCT can be either self-directed (with a self-help manual) or therapist directed. In general, controlled outcome research has not found a difference in outcome...

In fact, the principles of BSCT may be used to pursue a goal of total abstinence... Although treatment with a goal of moderation has been controversial, researchers have extensively studied its effectiveness. BSCT appears to yield success rates comparable to treatments with a goal of abstinence. Current data suggest that moderation is most successful with clients who, at the beginning of treatment, were experiencing less severe alcohol problems and dependence. Abstinence is a more stable outcome among more severe alcohol dependent clients. (Hester, 1995, p.148).

The above statement ignores Miller et al. (1992) who could not at the outset of treatment differentiate between those who will moderate their drinking, abstain, or relapse. All were selected as fit for moderation treatment. Nevertheless, retrospective analyses of assessment information collected at the start of treatment suggested that 57% of the participants met DSM-III criteria for alcohol dependence and 66% were classifiable as alcoholics according to Jellinek's typology (Miller et al., 1992). Criteria for moderation of amount of alcohol consumed, for example, not more than 20 drinks/week with no serious side effects is unsatisfactory because of the relatively low correlation between such measures of alcohol consumption, alcohol related biomedical, social, and personal problems, and severity of dependence (Heather, 1989; Maltzman & Schweiger,1991).

Individual differences in susceptibility to brain damage as a consequence of alcohol consumption, and the individual differences in recovery from dysfunction which may be independent of susceptibility, may make it impossible to determine from questionnaires assessing frequency and quantity of alcohol consumption and negative consequences, whether or not brain dysfunction has occurred (Cala,1987). Scales of severity of dependence (Skinner & Horn, 1984; Stockwell, et al., 1979) may be a more reasonable self-report device for determining the potential for brain dysfunction (Deckel, Bauer, & Hesselbrock, 1995). Measures of brain structure and function obtained from PET, CT, MRI and fMRI, ERPs, or EEG are needed prior to participation in controlled drinking treatment programs. Also needed are studies validating scales of severity of dependence and loss of control against measures of brain function and structure. Finally, a safe amount of alcohol consumption must be matched to the individual. Effects of alcohol vary with the lean body mass of the individual, family history, amount of past consumption, individual differences in pattern of drinking, between meals or with meals, diet, and medications regularly taken, as well as other important variables (Eckardt et al., 1998). These are all ignored by Hester, Miller, and by Heather and Tebbutt (1989) in their recommendations for what ought to be the upper limit in controlled drinking.

Until Hester and Miller and other proponents of controlled drinking for problem drinkers assess brain function and dysfunction and match the individual subject with the upper limit of the amount of alcohol they may consume they are misrepresenting their treatment outcomes and placing patients at risk for more serious problems including exacerbation of brain dysfunction. They are failing to obtain proper informed consent from the participants in their experimental treatments. Their recommendations for choosing controlled drinking are unethical because they are not providing the basis for a truly informed consent.

Hester never considers the dire implications of his colleague Miller's (Miller et al., 1986, 1992) results: Approximately 60% of the people in his study - all selected initially as problem drinkers suitable for moderate drinking - were retrospectively diagnosed as alcoholics. Granted that there are problems with long term retrospective reports and analyses of reports, Miller et al.'s results suggest, again, the necessity of careful, thorough, assessment before individuals are allowed to attempt controlled drinking. In contrast to controlled drinking, abstinence does not put the patient at risk. It heeds the fundamental ethical principle of care givers: do no harm.

Hester (1995) asserts:

There are several reasons for offering an intervention with a goal of moderation. First, some clients refuse to consider abstinence without at least a reasonable trial at achieving moderation. Writers, beginning with Marty Mann (1950) have often suggested that such persons should try to control their drinking as a way of discovering whether abstinence is necessary for them. The 'Big Book' of Alcoholics Anonymous (1976) contains a number of references to moderate drinking and suggests people try it to see whether they can achieve it. Second, if you work with a client and he or she is unsuccessful in moderating drinking, you have already developed a therapeutic relationship and may be in a better position to help... pursue abstinence. Third, if the client achieves moderation you will have been successful with relatively brief treatment. Fourth... many people who moderate their drinking eventually shift to abstinence. (p.149).

Hester's arguments ignore the fact that Mary Mann (1950) and the founders of AA were not scientists and information about the high probability of brain dysfunction, often irreversible, and likely to be exacerbated by continued drinking, was not available at the time she wrote her popular book. Hester does not have the excuse of lack of pertinent knowledge in 1995 (Cala, 1987; Eckardt et al., 1980; Harper & Kril, 1990; Lemere, 1956; Muuronen et al., 1989; Volkow et al., 1992).

Another reason to consider a moderation-goal option is that you can attract and treat a broader range of drinkers with alcohol problems... within the general population there are far more problem drinkers than severely dependent alcoholics... This problem drinker population has been largely ignored or at least underserved... Less severe problem drinkers (and those who do not consider themselves alcoholics or problem drinkers) are more likely to accept services when goals other than lifelong abstinence are possible... To offer only one alternative, total abstention, is to turn away a large population in need of services. (Hester, 1995, p.149).

Hester's unsubstantiated assertion promoted by Sobell and Sobell (1995a), Marlatt (Larimer et al., 1998), and the Institute of Medicine (1990) is echoed by Rotgers (1996) in an article appearing in the magazine published by the National Association of Alcoholism and Drug Addiction Counselors. Hester and Miller are holding out the lure of financial gain to alcoholism counselors as an incentive for adopting moderation training in their programs while failing to provide safeguards protecting the health and well-being of the participants.

Grant (1996) reports evidence contradicting the assertion that an undesirable treatment goal, abstention, is preventing problem drinkers from seeking help. She obtained information pertinent to the issue of treated and untreated people in need from a national probability sample of more than 42,000 respondents. Overall, the two major barriers to alcohol treatment are unemployment and less than a high school education. They also moderate the association between severity of alcohol problems and the probability of obtaining treatment. As noted in chapter 3, Schuckit (1998) found a higher percentage of men in his prospective study diagnosed as suffering from alcohol dependence than abuse.

Hester (1995) continues:

research has noted relatively little success in teaching moderation to severely dependent alcoholics. You may find it helpful to distinguish, in your own mind, between problem drinkers and alcoholics, viewing abstinence as the only ultimately feasible goal for the latter. This distinction, though an oversimplification is generally consistent with the matching data. (p.149).

Incredible. This is the method suggested to alcoholism counselors for distinguishing between a problem drinker who will remain a problem drinker if they continue to drink, and one who may become an alcoholic. Imagine the difference in your own mind! Fals-Stewart (1997) has demonstrated that substance abuse counselors cannot discriminate between the neurocognitive impaired and unimpaired in the absence of results from a neuropsychological test battery.

In those cases where we disagree with a client's desire to pursue a goal of moderation we negotiate a contract. We agree to work with the client for six to eight weeks, providing them training in BSCT. We agree, however, that if at the end of that time the client is still having difficulty drinking moderately, he or she will consider a goal of abstinence. (Hester, 1995, p.149).

There is no understanding or concern for the health and well-being of the individual and their family and society and the potential for promoting further brain dysfunction which may be irreversible. It is all a rational interchange between two rational people. Make a contract. If it does not work, try something else. Great. How many times was the "client" driving while drunk during this trial period, missed work or other important assignments, neglected or abused significant others, spent money irresponsibly, missed school work, and continued to damage his or her brain and liver, etc.? What does the clients' family say about all this? Why are they not consulted and their informed consent obtained?

There is no information or apparent concern for carefully monitoring the behavior of the patient, contact with collaterals, employers, family members, and obtaining measures of brain structure and function. The program as described may seem reasonable to some. It must seem reasonable to Hester and to Miller. The problem is that to make it work you need to be engaging reasonable people. Problem drinkers and alcoholics are generally not reasonable, reasoning, people, at least when it comes to their use of alcohol.

Hester states:

As a weekly goal, we recommend that males and females set it at or below 12 and 7 drinks, respectively... acknowledging that there is no 'safe' level of drinking, when drinking exceeds 3 drinks per day, negative health consequences increases dramatically... finally, we encourage clients not to drink *daily*." (p.150).

Hester does not explain why he advises male patients to drink not more than 12 drinks/week and females 7 drinks/week, yet he and Miller use 20 drinks/week as the limit for moderation when classifying the results of treatment outcome studies. Remember, at one time an average of 6 drinks/day was considered controlled, moderate, drinking! (Armor et al., 1976; Sobell & Sobell, 1978).

"BSCT with a goal of moderation is, in general, less effective than purely abstinence-oriented approaches for more severely dependent clients (e.g., Foy, Nunn, & Rychtarik, 1984)." (Hester, 1995, p.154f). Hester does not attempt to explain the contradiction between the above assertion and the reported significant superiority of the Sobell's (Sobell & Sobell, 1978) moderation over abstinence groups. He describes the Sobells' study as follows:

Mark and Linda Sobell conducted what was to become the most publicized evaluation of self-control training procedures (Sobell & Sobell, 1973). In a controlled evaluation with inpatient gamma alcoholics, they reported greater improvement in an experimental group receiving moderation training than in three comparison groups in abstinence-focused treatment. Pendery and colleagues questioned the success of this treatment (Pendery, Maltzman, & West, 1982), reporting an independent review of the experimental cases. The controversy surrounding this study is complex (Marlatt, Larimer, Baer, & Quigley, 1993; Sobell & Sobell, 1984). A fair conclusion is that few of the alcoholics receiving experimental treatment sustained moderate drinking over an extended period, but they fared no worse than those receiving standard abstinence-oriented treatment. This conclusion is consistent with the findings of a subsequent study with a similar inpatient population (Foy et al., 1984)." (Hester, 1995, p.155).

It is significant that the only citations providing a basis for the asserted complexity of the controversy are to papers by the Sobells and their supporters (Marlatt et al., 1993; Sobell & Sobell, 1984). A fair and objective reviewer would cite papers on both sides of the "controversy". He could mention my allegation that the data were faked and the bases for my belief (Maltzman, 1989). He did not. His conclusion is not disinterested. It also misrepresents the results of Foy et al. (1984) who found that moderation training produced significantly poorer results after six months than abstinence. Hester is probably confusing Foy et al. and their 6-month follow-up with the long-term follow-up of the same patients by Rychtarik et al. (1987). The two groups did not differ in the Rychtarik et al. study. Since it was an "add on" design, an absence of a difference between the two groups means that moderation training had no effect. As I have noted before (Maltzman, 1994) and in other chapters in this book, the results of Rychtarick et al. have been repeatedly misinterpreted by revisionists (Graber & Miller; Institute of Medicine, 1990; Miller et al.,1987; Peele, 1988; Sobell & Sobell, 1987a, 1987b). An interesting aspect of Hester's review is that there is no mention of Caddy et al.'s (1978) three-year follow-up of the Sobells' patients, a follow-up that purports to confirm the Sobells' results.

Hester (1995) goes on to state:

Martha Sanchez-Craig and colleagues at the Addiction Research Foundation have conducted some of the best-designed studies of BSCT procedures (Sanchez-Craig, 1980; Sanchez-Craig et al., 1984). They randomly assigned less severe problem drinkers to moderate drinking or abstinence goals, with both groups receiving outpatient BSCT. Both groups improved substantially during the two years of follow-up, with no significant differences between groups over time. A small-scale replication by Graber and Miller (1987) [sic] similarly yielded no difference between groups assigned to abstinence or moderation goals. (p.155).

Hester provides an incomplete and misleading description of the Sanchez-Craig et al. study. In addition to different goals, participants received either training for abstinence or training for abstinence plus training for controlled drinking. Patients subscribing to the disease concept of alcoholism were excluded from the study whereas patients favoring moderation were accepted (Sanchez-Craig et al., 1980, p.36). Patients also received varying amounts of their designated training. It is a far more complex and confounded experimental design than recognized by Sanchez-Craig or by Hester. Its results lack external validity, cannot be generalized to clinical treatment as generally practiced in established programs. It is an efficacy study not a study of treatment effectiveness (Seligman, 1995,1996), and a poorly designed and conducted one at that.

Both the Sanchez-Craig (1980, 1984) and Graber and Miller (1988) studies suffer from a lack of statistical power due to the small number of subjects involved. Both investigators fail to determine the number of subjects needed to produce a significant effect. Sanchez-Craig's study is difficult to interpret because of the confounding of variables in her design and the probable interactions between instructions concerning goals and the participants' reactions to the treatment. It suffers further from the failure, admitted by Sanchez-Craig, to provide adequate exposure to the disease conception of alcoholism that is an integral part of traditional abstinence treatment. A major source of bias in the patient sample was the exclusion of potential participants who embraced the disease concept.

Sanchez-Craig (1980) designed her experiment in an attempt to differentiate the effects of treatment goal from the nature of the outpatient treatment received. Half the subjects were randomly assigned to the goal of abstinence and half were assigned to the goal of controlled drinking. They were informed of the goal to which they had been assigned at the start of treatment which is described as one 90-min. session/week for 8 weeks. For the first three weeks all participants received instructions in how to maintain abstinence. Abstinence goal participants continued receiving training in maintaining abstinence. In the fourth session the controlled drinking subjects were reminded of their controlled drinking goal, and instructed in controlled drinking. Subsequent sessions for the controlled drinking group consisted of similar training as the abstinence group as well as training in controlled drinking. All participants were expected to remain abstinent during the outpatient treatment phase. Nevertheless, they were instructed in how to keep a drinking diary in which they would record their alcohol consumption each day. Participants were given mixed messages by these different instructions, not an optimal procedure for attaining a treatment goal. This first paper (Sanchez-Craig, 1980) reported on alcohol consumption during treatment. Although they were instructed from the outset not to drink, both groups consumed considerable amounts of alcohol during their outpatient treatment. Groups did not differ significantly from each other in alcohol consumption and they both drank significantly less during treatment than prior to the start of treatment.

A second paper in this series (Sanchez-Craig et al., 1984) reported the results of treatment follow-up interviews concentrating on the 6-month post-treatment interview. Groups did not differ in their alcohol consumption and both groups continued to report significantly less alcohol use than during their pretreatment base level interval. Results were interpreted by Sanchez-Craig et al. and by Hester as demonstrating that abstinence and controlled drinking were equally effective as treatment goals. This conclusion does not logically follow from the nature of this complex design. Sanchez-Craig et al. used a form of add-on design where both groups received abstinence training and one group received controlled drinking training and a controlled drinking goal in addition to abstinence training. No difference between the two groups means that the controlled drinking goal and treatment had no effect above and beyond their abstinence treatment. The logic of the interpretation is the same as for the Rychtarik et al. (1987) "add on" study.

A further complication is apparent in the discussion of this second experiment. Participants differed widely in their number of treatment sessions. An aspect of the procedure not explicated in the first paper (Sanchez-Craig, 1980) is that the treatment was, "open ended in the sense that treatment was not terminated until the client achieved proficiency in problem solving and self-monitoring procedures." (Sanchez-Craig et al., 1984, p. 394). Criteria of proficiency are not described. Number of sessions ranged from 2-12 in the abstinence group and 3-11 in the controlled drinking group. Mean number of sessions is not given. If participants received only three sessions in the controlled drinking condition they did not receive controlled drinking training, since such training was not introduced until the fourth session. Sanchez-Craig et al. indicate that there was no statistically significant difference in the number of sessions received by participants in the two groups. There were no differences or interactions between groups or between pre-post treatment for various measures of social adjustment, including weeks worked, marital status, satisfaction about job, leisure activities, and physical health, etc. Unfortunately there was no control group of social drinkers with whom these results could be compared where the social drinkers were matched for age, ethnicity, gender and socioeconomic status. Results indicate that either the treatments had no effect on measures of social adjustment, certainly an important consideration as well as a cost effectiveness criterion - or there is a basement effect. Participants in the study were a select group of heavy drinkers for whom drinking had not yet progressed to the level where it interfered with their social adjustment or physical health. If this were the case, the results have limited generality for the population of problem drinkers. Since it was an efficacy study using selected volunteers who did not accept the disease concept, there is even greater doubt that it has any implications for use in the clinical treatment of problem drinkers. Finally, it must be noted that the participants in the study received a low treatment intensity, below the level likely to produce effective results (Monahan & Feeney, 1996).

Sanchez-Craig et al. (1984) are considered to have conducted an exemplary study by the Sobells (1995). It is also one of the highest rated studies in Miller et al.'s (1996) analysis of treatment outcome studies. Such ratings are not surprising in view of the interpretation placed upon the study by Sanchez-Craig et al. and others. It purports to be the first to examine the goals of controlled drinking versus abstinence and the treatment modalities of abstinence and controlled drinking training in the same study. Neither the goal nor the treatment modality made a significant difference. Controlled drinking and abstinence training purportedly were equally and highly effective. Successful outcomes were 73% and 72% for abstinence training and controlled drinking, respectively, after a 6-month follow-up. Results for the different treatment goals generally did not differ significantly at 12, 18, and 24-month followups.

Sanchez-Craig et al. (1984) conclude: "Overall, the percentage of successful clients (abstinent plus moderate drinkers) in the AB (73%) and CD (72%) group is comparable to percentages reported in studies in which selected socially stable problem drinkers were trained in controlled-drinking methods (Heather & Robertson, 1981; Miller & Hester, 1980)." (p.400).

This study by Sanchez-Craig and her colleagues poses several problems in attempting to understand the procedure employed with participants. Furthermore, the results reported by Sanchez-Craig and her colleagues are misleading. The cut-off for the classification of moderate drinking was taken as 20 drinks/week. The Abstinence treatment group (n=30) is listed as obtaining the following outcomes at 6 months: 6.7% abstinent, 43.3% moderate drinking/problem free, and 23.3% moderate drinking/with problems; 26.6% were drinking heavily with problems. Why should moderate drinking with problems be considered successful, especially since a later study shows that 20 drinks/week is too high, leads to relapse and continued neuropsychological deficits (Sanchez-Craig et al., 1995; Wilkinson & Sanchez-Craig, 1981)? For the Abstinence group the success rate is 50% once the inappropriate addition of people drinking moderately/with problems is eliminated from the success category. A similar adjustment needs to be made for the Controlled drinking treatment group, (n=29). For the latter group 3.4% were abstinent; 37.9% were drinking moderately/problem free; 31% were drinking moderately/with problems; and 17.2% were classified as heavy drinkers/with problems. Eliminating the moderate drinking/with problems subgroup leaves a 41.3% success for controlled drinking training, less than the abstinent group and considerably less attractive an outcome than the 73% and 72% represented as the results for the Abstinent and Controlled Drinking groups, respectively. Reducing these figures by another 10% due to attrition, which Sanchez-Craig et al. suggest for their original results, makes these figures even less attractive.

Sanchez-Craig et al. (1984) state:

The results of this study did not support the hypothesis that assignment to a goal of controlled drinking would produce a better outcome than assignment to a goal of abstinence. The AB and CD clients were equally successful in reducing their drinking to moderate levels during the 2-year follow-up period... However, it can be argued that controlled drinking was a more suitable goal. (p.399).

The authors argue that controlled drinking was a more suitable goal because it was more acceptable to a majority of the patients; controlled drinking subjects drank less during the outpatient treatment period; and more abstinence patients requested and received additional counseling. Sanchez-Craig et al. admit:

It may be argued that the abstinence treatment was not presented in the strongest possible manner. Although AB clients were always told that abstinence was the goal of the program, they were not told that their problem was a disease or that lifelong abstinence was essential... It is also possible that some of the tasks permitted AB clients to infer that moderation was acceptable... These procedures may have encouraged clients to assume that the therapist accepted drinking that occurred in moderation. An admission criterion was that the applicant should believe that drinking in moderation was an achievable goal... An important question to raise is why the specific training in controlled drinking did not confer an advantage to the CD clients after the completion of treatment. (p.399).

By the authors' own admission the treatment offered the abstinence group is not traditional abstinence oriented treatment. Commentators such as the Sobells do not discuss the shortcomings of their "exemplary" study. They do not comment upon the questionable procedure which exaggerates the success rate obtained by Sanchez-Craig et al. Both treatments are based on questionable ethics because they failed to inform the subjects that continued drinking at the level aspired (4 drinks/day and 20 drinks/week) could result in further brain damage and possibly further irreversible brain damage. These are the implications suggested by the results obtained by Wilkinson and Sanchez-Craig (1981).

Reviewing results from several of their studies, Sanchez-Craig and her colleagues (1995) conclude that the safe cut-off for moderate drinking is even lower. In other words, the cut-off used in the "exemplary" study is too high to avoid social problems. The newer more stringent cut-off still does not consider the risk of brain dysfunction. Considering the latter health problem, the cut-off ought to be even fewer drinks/week and per day (Sanchez-Craig & Wilkinson, 1981).

Despite the above problems including the inflated success rate obtained by including people who continue to drink "moderately" with problems, Sanchez-Craig et al. (1984) conclude: "Because the program was very successful in retaining clients in treatment and produced a satisfactory outcome for the large majority (sic) of the participants, similar programs are indicated as a measure of secondary prevention of alcohol problems." (p. 401). By Sanchez-Craig's own more current research these outcomes are unsatisfactory "for the large majority of the participants".

More recent data analyses of a one-year follow-up has lead Sanchez-Craig, Wilkinson, and Davila (1995) to conclude that:

Based on previous research, our current rules of thumb are an upper limit of 4 standard drinks on any day, no more than 3 days in a week, yielding an implicit limit of 12 drinks in a week... women are advised to set their upper limit at three drinks in any day; all clients are advised to avoid intoxication by consuming no more than one drink in any hour; and all clients should abstain if planning to drive or perform other hazardous activities, if under the legal age for drinking, if at work or returning to work, if pregnant or breast-feeding, or if on any medication. (p.823).

Even the above modification of what is moderate is rather high. These modifications obviously demand revised interpretations of the results obtained by Sanchez-Craig et al. (1984) in their "exemplary" (Sobell & Sobell, 1995) study of controlled drinking where moderate drinking had an upper limit of 20 drinks/week. Further revision in the thinking of moderate drinking advocates is needed as suggested by Sanchez-Craig et al. (1995):

Information from problem drinkers in treatment can serve to refine definitions of moderate drinking for several reasons. First, many move from "problem" status at admission to "problem-free" status at follow-up, permitting within-subject comparisons. Second, problems caused by their drinking are typically social; in North America, alcohol-related social problems tend to occur earlier in the drinking career than do physical morbidities..." (p.823).

Reference for support of the latter assertion is to Cahalan and Room (1974) which is outdated in terms of the variables employed, and misleading in that the most important health consideration, and one which appears at risk earlier than standard medical illness such as cirrhosis of the liver, is brain dysfunction. Necropsy studies by Harper and Kril (1990) show that evidence of brain damage in alcoholics appears before evidence of liver damage. As we have said before, provision of moderate drinking as an option to a patient requires a thorough neurological and neuropsychological assessment so that an adequate informed consent can be obtained from the patient. Such informed consent was obviously not obtained by Sanchez-Craig.

Self-directed versus therapist-directed treatment

Hester (1995) states:

In a series of evaluations, Miller and colleagues have evaluated alternate modes for offering BSCT to problem drinkers... [they] consistently found no significant differences in effectiveness between self-administered mode with minimal therapist contact and a therapist-directed mode of delivery, with clients in both conditions showing significant improvement at follow-ups to eight years... Longer-range follow-ups at three to eight years found increasing proportions of clients becoming total abstainers, and a consistent 10 to 15% of treated outpatients sustaining moderate and problem-free drinking outcomes (Miller et al., 1992). (p.155).

It must be remembered that Miller's BSCT studies did not have a control group that went without treatment. We have only the pretreatment base rate of the participants in the study as the basis for assessing improvement. However, the base rate ordinarily is inflated because it represents the period of extensive negative consequences of participants' drinking that led to their "voluntary" entrance into a treatment program. It is the period that "broke the camel's back" or their "hitting bottom". Pre-posttreatment change scores therefore reflect a possible regression toward the mean. Pretreatment base rate is not an effective basis for obtaining change scores, the difference between it and a posttreatment period, unless the pretreatment period is an extended one, at least a year in duration (see Küfner & Feuerlein, 1989, and chapter 7).

The statement, "longer-range follow-ups at three to eight years found increasing proportions of clients becoming total abstainers" is misleading. Even if there were increasing numbers of abstainers, these results could not be generalized because length of time between treatment and follow-up interview is confounded with experiments. Follow-ups at different post-treatment intervals were not conducted on the same participants. Each follow-up interval was conducted on different participants in different studies by Miller and his colleagues. There was no random assignment of studies or patients to studies. The 8-year follow-up was conducted on participants in a treatment study completed 8 years earlier; the 7-year follow-up was conducted on different participants in a different treatment study completed 7 years earlier, similarly for 5 and 3.5 years. Numbers of participants who were abstinent in these studies and their percentage of the total in their respective studies were 4 (10%), 7 (17%), 8 (24%), and 4 (17%), respectively (Miller et al., 1992, Table 3, p. 253). Percent abstinence in each interval was obtained by dividing the number of abstainers in each study by the number of participants in the six classifications employed, abstinent, asymptomatic, improved, impaired, unremitted, deceased, unknown. Percentages provide no evidence of a reliable increasing trend of abstinence. Even if there was such a "trend", it would be confounded with the different cohorts, and the small number of participants prohibit demonstrating a statistically significant trend. Hester's conclusion also fails to mention that the "consistent 10 to 15%... sustaining moderate and problem-free drinking" is lower than the estimated percentage of individuals of this sort who show spontaneous remission, 19% (Miller & Hester, 1980). It must also be remembered that the evaluation window employed was only 3 months. In other words, for example, 3.5 years after treatment, drinking behavior during the previous 3 months was ascertained. The percent of individuals drinking moderately after 3.5 years does not mean that they were drinking moderately for the previous 3.5 years. It means that they were drinking moderately for the previous 3 months at the 3.5 year follow-up.

In summary, BSCT procedures have been extensively studied. These studies collectively show that some problem drinkers do respond favorably to this approach, sustaining moderate and nonproblematic drinking over extended periods. Other clients, following BSCT with a moderation goal, opt for total abstinence, some with and some without additional treatment...

When clients are assigned at random to treatment programs with abstinence or moderation goals, long-term results are consistently comparable.

A final recommendation is to make BSCT procedures available as one option among many within a treatment program wishing to serve a broad range of problem drinkers. Moderation-oriented BSCT is most likely to be attractive and effective for less severe problem drinkers. We do not recommend the pursuit of a moderation goal with severely dependent alcoholics. (Hester, 1995, p.157).

The above sounds reasonable and conciliatory. There is one problem, a problem that I have emphasized before. It is a problem neglected by Hester and by Miller: valid assessment and diagnosis are lacking. At present, there is no way to know who may succeed with controlled drinking and who may fail and exacerbate their condition, unless the most careful neuroimaging scans and neuropsychological test assessments are obtained. A thorough neurological and neuropsychological assessment must be undertaken to determine whether or not the presenting individual is suffering from brain dysfunction. Alcoholism is an insidious brain disease that develops in different people varying in their susceptibiliy to alcohol induced dysfunction and the reversibility of that dysfunction. Their condition cannot be assessed by merely asking the individual which treatment they wish to try. Treatment is not a cafeteria where you can sample a variety of offerings and choose the one you really like. We are dealing with potentially permanent brain damage if the individual continues to drink when already showing signs of brain dysfunction. It is this kind of person who is at greatest risk for descending into progressively heavier drinking, lack of control, and escalation into physiological dependence, alcoholism, and brain damage and damage to others.

The only ethical approach is to conduct, or obtain from an outside laboratory, assessments of brain dysfunction. On the basis of the test outcomes, inform the prospective patient about the positive and negative consequences of one choice or the other. Even then, ethical paternalism suggests that the counselor withhold treatment for a moderation goal when there is evidence of brain dysfunction. Grounds for such a decision are that the individual has a diminished capacity to make a reasoned decision and their choice of moderation may cause irreversible brain damage.

Hester's (1995) assertion, "When clients are assigned at random to treatment programs with abstinence or moderation goals, long-term results are consistently comparable", (p.157) is misleading. It neglects the critical point that the results are comparably poor as in the long-term follow-up by Miller and his colleagues (Miller et al., 1992) and the "add-on" design of the Rychtarik et al. (1987) study which has consistently been misinterpreted.

Examination of highly rated individual studies

Table 2.4, p.18, Miller et al. (1995) shows ratings of the different treatment modalities. The three highest rated treatment modalities are: Brief Intervention, +239; Social Skills Training, +128; and Motivational Enhancement, +87. Treatment modalities with the three lowest ratings were, Psychotherapy, -127; General Alcoholism Counseling, -214; and Educational lectures/Films, -239.

The highest rated individual study of BSCT was conducted by Harris & Miller(1990). Its close examination will enable us to appreciate more fully the inadequate methodology used by Miller et al. (1995) in their evaluation of the efficacy research on treatment modalities.

Harris and Miller (1990) relied on notices in local news media to recruit participants for their study. People experiencing life problems related to alcohol were informed that they would be trained to control their drinking. Treatment was free and it was explicitly described as not intended for alcoholics. Applicants with a history of severe withdrawal symptoms, liver, or cardiovascular problems related to alcohol misuse were excluded. Harris and Miller used criteria recommended by Miller and Caddy (1977) for selecting problem drinkers and excluding alcoholics, criteria that are based on inadequate empirical evidence such as Rand Report II (Polich et al., 1980, 1981) or no evidence.

Harris and Miller (1990) planned to use 40 participants. After six months they were only able to recruit 34 people for the study, suggesting that Hester's and other revisionists' assumption about a great unmet demand for controlled drinking treatment for problem drinkers is false. Two experimental groups were employed. One received a self-directed (bibliotherapy) treatment and the other a therapist-directed treatment. The latter BSCT was based on the manual by Miller and Muñoz (1982). Self-directed BSCT followed the procedures in the manual but its participants did not meet with a therapist. Two waiting-list control treatments were also used. The self-monitoring control group was told that they would begin treatment after a further baseline period of self-monitoring. They filled out self-monitoring cards describing their drinking behavior and returned them weekly as part of the first phase of their treatment program. The untreated waiting list control group was told that they would have to wait for 10 weeks before their treatment began, receiving neither monitoring cards nor self-help manual. After a 10-week waiting period both groups of control subjects entered one or the other treatment, self- or therapist-directed.

Patients in the self-directed treatment condition were told about positive outcomes from previous BSCT studies to improve their self-efficacy. "Instructions to clients were completed... and included information intended to increase self-efficacy for success, based on our previous studies showing positive outcomes with self-help interventions." (p.84).

Several questions arise in view of the above instructions given in the past to participants: Do Miller and his colleagues now tell participants about the long term

194

failure of BSCT found in Miller et al., (1987, 1992)? Their treatment of the self-directed group involves questionable ethics. They inform subjects only of possible positive consequences of the treatment and not the negative consequences of continued drinking of 3-4 or more drinks/day (Sanchez-Craig et al., 1995), and the low probability of maintaining controlled drinking, approximately 10% in the long term (Miller et al., 1987, 1992). A proper informed consent describes the possible negative as well as positive consequences of the relevant alternative treatments. Obviously, Miller and his colleagues had not been obtaining this sort of consent. Are they now obtaining a proper informed consent?

Results of Harris and Miller's (1990) research are given in terms of self-reported weekly alcohol consumption at 10 weeks, 20 weeks, and 15-month follow-up intervals. A significant overall decrease in alcohol consumption was reported between pretreatment and 3- months post-treatment. This decrease differed among groups. There was a significant decrease in consumption in the combined self-directed and therapist-directed experimental groups versus the two waiting-list control groups. At week 20, 10 weeks after the waiting-list groups completed their treatment and 20 weeks after completion of treatment by the experimental groups, all four groups were drinking less than at pretreatment and did not differ among themselves. At 15 months there was still a significant overall decrease in alcohol consumption as compared to intake with no significant differences among the groups.

An outcome classification of, abstinence, controlled drinking, and improvement was used for evaluations at 10 weeks, 20 weeks, and 15 months. *Abstinence* was defined as refraining from drinking during the evaluation period as confirmed by collaterals; *controlled drinking* was defined as not exceeding 20 drinks/week on the average or a particular average estimated blood alcohol concentration produced by a typical drinking episode and no disconfirmation of subjects' self-reports by their collaterals. *Improved* was defined as failing to meet the criteria for controlled drinking but reporting a 30% or more decrease in weekly number of drinks not disconfirmed by collaterals. All other participants were classified as not improved. Evaluation windows were the drinking behavior during the prior 6 weeks at week 10, the prior 10 weeks at week 20, and the prior 3 months at month 15.

A major difficulty with Harris and Miller's (1990) study is its evident lack of statistical power for between-group analyses due to the small number of subjects involved, seven or eight per group. Only significant overall decreases in alcohol consumption compared to the pretreatment baselevel are statistically significant. Such a result does not provide grounds for Harris and Miller's conclusion that self-directed and therapist-directed treatments are equally effective. Nevertheless, this is their conclusion. They are, "proving the null hypothesis", a criticism directed by Heather (1989) against BSCT and other brief intervention studies:

The methodological problem applies mostly in the alcohol area but is potentially applicable to other addictive behaviours. The highly influential study by Orford & Edwards (1977) and the series of studies by William Miller and his colleagues on controlled drinking treatments are of this type... The problem consists in the fact that this interpretation [treatment groups are equally effective] is quite erroneous and is an example of a classic error in the logic of hypothesis testing, known as 'proving' the null hypothesis. The point is... that the null hypothesis of no difference between groups cannot be proved. If an experiment fails to find any significant differences between two sample groups, it cannot be concluded that the experiment provides evidence that the populations from which the samples are drawn do not differ; all that can be legitimately concluded is that the experiment provides no evidence that they *do* differ, a quite different deduction. One implication of this is that, if the experiment were repeated, perhaps with a larger or more representative sample, a significant difference might emerge. (Heather, 1989, p. 364).

Put in a slightly different way, these experiments are designed to test the null hypothesis, the hypothesis that the experimental treatments do not differ. The hypothesis can be contradicted by finding a significant difference in alcohol consumption between the groups. However, the hypothesis of no difference cannot be proven because if no difference is found, an infinite number of factors may be responsible, including the possibility that the two treatments do not differ because they both are ineffective. To disprove the latter interpretation, it would be necessary to have a control group receiving no treatment which did not differ in outcome from the experimental treatment groups. Harris and Miller's study lacks such a control group. In the absence of a control group, the hypothesis that the treatments are equally ineffective cannot be disproven. Harris and Miller draw an inappropriate conclusion from an inadequately designed experiment.

Another difficulty with the Harris and Miller's (1990) research report is their inflated positive outcome produced by use of their inappropriate measure of improvement (Riley et al.,1987). Positive outcomes reported by Miller and his colleagues are not simply the sum of participants who remain abstinent and those who engage in controlled drinking for which the principal criterion is an average of approximately 20 drinks/week. Harris and Miller's (1990) positive outcome measure also includes participants who are improved. "Cases failing to meet criteria for controlled drinking but showing at least a 30% reduction in weekly SECs [standard ethanol content, 1/2 oz] ... were rated as *Improved*." (p.88). Thus, an individual drinking 90 drinks/week prior to entering treatment who reduces consumption to 60 drinks/week after treatment will be rated improved and categorized along with abstinent and moderate drinking participants as a positive outcome, a procedure inflating the percent positive outcomes and apparent effectiveness of the treatment. Harris and Miller simply indicate the percent participants who met the criterion of "improvement" (Table 2, p. 88).

The 30% improvement measure as well as the pre- post-treatment change scores take advantage of a possible atypical increase in consumption and/or negative consequences of drinking occurring during the course of alcohol and other drug misuse which leads to involuntary or voluntary seeking of treatment. In short, the pretreatment baseline is inflated, especially if the pretreatment baseline is relatively brief. Participants are not really "getting better"; they are returning to their more typical level of misuse. Individuals in the improved category of the initial follow-up should have been tracked over time to determine the stability of their improvement. For example, there are three participants who were categorized as improved in the Waiting List control group at the 10 weeks interview. There are three people in this same group listed as improved after 20 weeks. Are they the same or different participants? Harris and Miller (1990) report that 71% of the participants had a positive outcome (abstinent, controlled drinking, improved) after 20 weeks and 62% had a positive outcome after 15 months. These results and others by Miller and his students are the grounds for the widely acclaimed conclusion that positive BSCT outcomes range from 60-80%. Omitting the "improved group" from the category of positive outcomes yields a very different picture. Including only abstinence and moderate drinking as positive outcomes yields a success rate of 38% for 20 weeks and 32% after 15 months. These are results hardly worth boasting about, especially in view of the small number of participants and the relatively short follow-up intervals and brief evaluation windows.

Another shortcoming in their study is that Harris and Miller (1990) failed to describe, much less analyze, gender and ethnic differences. Equal numbers of women and men participated in the experiment but results are not provided by gender and statistical analyses using gender as a between-group variable are not provided. In view of the small number of participants there is little likelihood that there would be a statistically significant difference between genders, but at least we should be informed of the results by gender. Harris and Miller should not have ignored this opportunity to investigate matching of treatments and gender. Does treatment method interact with gender and with the gender of the therapist in therapist led BSCT? Leaving these subgroups unexamined within the treatment subgroups also increases the variability within groups, increases the error variance and decreases the likelihood of obtaining statistically significant differences between treatment groups.

Ethnicity of the participants was unfortunately not reported. If ethnicity of the participants differed, then ethnicity should also have been analyzed statistically and examined for possible interactions with treatments and therapist. Ethnicity x treatment interactions, indicating a match between ethnic groups and treatment, was a powerful effect in a study by Spinrad (1993) on techniques for increasing disulfiram compliance. A treatment x ethnic groups interaction could well occur among Harris and Miller's (1990) treatment conditions. A more carefully controlled study with a much larger number of participants of different ethnicities would be needed to determine whether treatment x ethnic matching occurs. On the other hand, a large investment of time and money in this research is not the wisest decision as indicated by the failure to obtain evidence of the efficacy of BSCT in the long term (Miller et al., 1992) and the failure of the MATCH (Project MATCH, 1997, 1998) project discussed in chapter 7.

There are few grounds for the glowing depictions of the scientific status of BSCT methods for treating problem drinkers in view of the above serious shortcomings in the study by Harris and Miller (1990), the highest rated BSCT study, shortcomings that are characteristic of the other BSCT studies by Miller and his colleagues as well. Any remnants of a basis for exaggerated claims for BSCT should be dissipated completely upon serious examination of the long term outcome of these studies by Miller et al. (1987, 1992) (see chapter 1).

Another caveat is necessary concerning the Harris and Miller (1990) results. Their study suffers from a difficulty common to all controlled drinking studies. A relatively brief, and in their case, variable evaluation window was employed. When it is reported that the 15 month follow-up showed that 15% of the participants were engaged in controlled drinking it does not mean that 15% of the participants had been engaged in controlled drinking for the entire 15 months since participating in the treatment program. It means that approximately 15 months after treatment participants were asked to report their drinking during the previous 3 months. At the 20 week interview they were asked to report their drinking during the prior 10 weeks and at the 10 week interview point they were asked to report their drinking during the prior 6 weeks. Engaging in controlled drinking, or showing a reduction in drinking, "improvement", for several weeks or even three months, does not reliably predict controlled drinking at a later time (Küfner & Feuerlein, 1989; Miller et al., 1992; Pettinatti et al., 1982). Heavy drinkers, problem drinkers, and alcoholics may wax and wane in their alcohol consumption. They are not always drunk the first thing in the morning, remaining drunk all day every day. They may moderate their drinking level for weeks or even months, but very few can maintain it for years (see chapter 7).

Harris and Miller conclude:

It is noteworthy that our self-directed BSCT group showed the largest absolute improvement in weekly consumption, estimated BAC peaks, and mood states, as well as the highest compliance rate with self-monitoring. This is also consistent with our earlier studies... There is a striking difference in responses between this group, given a self-help manual and instructed to work on their own, and two groups waiting for treatment. A clear practical implication is that in clinical settings with a waiting list, clients may be better served by getting them started with an assessment and self-help program, rather than having them merely wait for treatment... The cognitive set of a 'waiting list' may impede natural recovery processes that are activated when people are assessed, given minimal intervention and self-help instructions, and told to pursue change on their own. (p.89).

These speculative recommendations for treatment are unsupported by statistical evidence of reliable differences between individual groups. Classification differences are the consequence of a difference between two or three people. During the first 10 weeks three people showed "improvement" in the waiting list control (33% positive outcome) whereas in the self-directed BSCT condition, 1 person was abstinent, 1 person engaged in controlled drinking and 4 showed improvement, for a total positive outcome of 67%. This large percentage difference is based on 3 people, providing no statistical, "scientific", support for the exaggerated claims by Harris and Miller.

Perhaps the study by Harris and Miller (1990) with its inadequate methodology, small sample size, and unsupported claims was an anomaly. We shall therefore turn to an examination of another BSCT study (Graber & Miller, 1988) also with a high methodology rating by Miller et al. (1995) and results ostensibly supporting BSCT. Examination of another research report may help the reader decide whether or not Miller's BSCT really merits serious consideration as an "alternative treatment".

Graber and Miller (1988) randomly assigned participants to either controlled drinking or abstinence treatment goals. A total of only 24 subjects participated, with five women in the Abstinence treatment condition and two in the Controlled drinking condition. Ethnicity was not specified. Participants were solicited through the media and received six weekly individual sessions on behavioral self-control techniques. Nine graduate students and three undergraduate psychology students served as therapists after receiving three months of specialized training. Intensity of their training, e.g., number of hours/day, is not specified.

Follow-up interviews occurred after 3 months for the first interview and as part of Miller et al.'s (1986, 1992) long-term follow-up, again at 3.5 years. An evaluation window of 12 months was used in the latter interview. Collateral reports were obtained at each interview period. Results from this study were less impressive than prior BSCT studies according to Graber and Miller (1988). Using an average of 20 drinks/week without impairment symptoms as a criterion of controlled drinking, only 17% were engaged in controlled drinking after 3 months and 13% after 3.5 years. Abstinence rates were not much better, 25% after 3 months and 17% after 3.5 years. Once again, overall positive outcomes are inflated as the result of the addition of the third classification, "improved but impaired".

Graber and Miller (1988) attribute the relatively poor outcomes, a total of 63% positive outcomes after 3 months and 29% outcome after 3.5 years, to the fact that this sample was more severely alcohol dependent than previous samples. They ascribe this difference in severity of drinking problems to the fact that their advertisments soliciting participants for this study did not emphasize that controlled drinking would be administered to problem drinkers as distinguished from alcoholics.

An alternative interpretation not considered by Graber and Miller is that their poor treatment outcomes were due to the young and inexperienced therapists employed in the study, nine graduate students and three undergraduates with three months training. Despite the above shortcomings in the Graber and Miller (1988) report, it received a top rating of 16 on methodology by Miller et al. (1995). We may conclude that the Harris and Miller (1990) study is not an anomaly. Poor methodology, use of the 30% improvement classification which includes symptomatic drinking inflating the short-term success rate, and the small number of participants in each of the groups in these studies, do not form an adequate basis for considering BSCT an efficacious "alternative treatment".

Hester and Miller claim that Miller and his colleagues have consistently found no significant difference in a self-administered, self-directed, form of BSCT and a therapist-directed form, suggesting a great economic advantage of the former since these treatments are equally efficacious. However, as Heather (1989) has observed, Miller and his colleagues are proving the null hypothesis in their interpretation of these studies. The small number of subjects in the different treatment conditions do not provide sufficient power to demonstrate that the two treatments are differentially efficacious. That they are efficacious at all is questionable in view of the disappointing long term treatment outcomes (Miller et al., 1986, 1992) and the absence of a nontreated control group. The nagging question remains: How much better off would these people have been if they had received traditional abstinence treatment instead of these poorly designed and conducted efficacy studies?

Importance of a control group

An interesting study by Stimmel et al. (1983) is ignored in Miller et al.'s (1995) evaluation of treatment outcome studies. This omission is surprising for several reasons. First, it was cited earlier by Miller (1990, 1992) as evidence that there is no difference between abstinence and moderation oriented treatment goals. Second, it compared controlled drinking treatment using behavior therapy methods with abstinence treatment using traditional methods and, a rarity, included a no-treatment control group. Approximately 100 participants in a methadone treatment clinic who were active alcoholics were randomly assigned to the three groups. Stimmel et al. (1983) found no significant difference between the two treatment methods. Most importantly, Stimmel et al. found that the treatment groups did not differ significantly from the no-treatment control group. All showed some improvement over their pretreatment baselevel. Stimmel et al. caution that their results cannot be generalized to other populations for several reasons, including the small sample size, approximately 30 patients/group and their methadone treatment for heroin. Nevertheless, their results underline the importance of having a no-treatment control group. Stimmel et al. demonstrate that no difference between treatment groups may mean that neither had an effect, a possibility overlooked by Miller.

Harm reduction as secondary prevention

Improving treatments by analyzing what works and what does not is an important task. Devising new and more efficient behavioral treatments, discovering new pharmacotherapies and improving compliance are all worthy endeavors, but all will still be insufficient even if eventually successful. Effective prevention methods must be developed to adequately address the problem of alcoholism. This will require far more funding than currently allocated for this difficult and complex problem. In approaching the problem there is one direction I can recommend not taking: so-called harm reduction as promoted by Marlatt and his students (Dimeff, Baer, Kivlahan, & Marlatt, 1999; Marlatt et al., 1998).

Some 15 years of funding secondary prevention of drinking on a college campus has supported the harm reduction nee controlled drinking efficacy research of Marlatt and his student colleagues. Their research has culminated in a purported means of solving the problem of excessive drinking on college campuses as represented by a research project conducted on the campus of the University of Washington (Marlatt et al., 1998). A manual has been published providing a step-by-step description of how to implement this questionable program (Dimeff et al., 1999).

Despite the claims for a new means of preventing college students' alcohol problems the study has no ecological validity, has no value as a means of dealing with problems of excessive drinking on college campuses. A program requiring assessment of incoming students who volunteer for the service cannot meet the needs of all the heavy drinkers matriculating in a college or capture those who develop a problem after their first semester on campus. Using a monetary reward for completing the initial assessment and for participating in the subsequent study Marlatt et al. (1998) only captured half the matriculating class. The 25% with the highest levels of alcohol consumption and problems were recruited from the sample assessed and randomly assigned to a brief intervention or control group. A representative comparison group was also assessed.

A follow-up two years after the intervention indicated that the treated students reported 3.3 alcohol related problems in the previous 6 months as compared to 4.7 problems by the untreated control group. The difference between groups is statistically significant. Both groups showed a significant decline in problems since their college matriculation. Average drinking declined to 3.6 drinks/occasion by the treatment group as compared to 4 drinks/occasion by the nontreated control group. "Only" 70% of the high risk participants who received the intervention treatment reported drinking as much as 5-6 drinks on at least one occasion during the previous month as compared to 78% in the nontreated control group. In other words, only 70% of the students at risk were getting drunk at least once a month after treatment as compared to 78% who were not treated. In comparison, 42% of the normative representative cohort were binging. The intervention produced an 8% decrease as compared to the control group of excessive drinkers. The normative student cohort was drinking approximately at the unacceptably high binge rate found on the average college campus (Wechsler, Dowdall, Moeykens, & Castillo, 1994). Half the binge drinkers on campus, presumably, were not enticed into the project by a monetary incentive and allowed to continue drinking at their previous high rate.

Is this success? Seventy percent of the treated heavy drinking subjects still getting drunk at least once a month? Marlatt and his colleagues think so. They published a manual (Dimeff et al., 1999) so that other colleges can adopt their method and Marlatt is now advising NIAAA on how to reduce drinking on college campuses. Treated students still have an average 3.6 problems each semester and 70% of the treated students are still binging. More than 40% of the freshman cohort is binging - and ignored. These results for the intervention and control participants are for students captured for the study as paid volunteers, less than half the entering freshman class. Does it seem reasonable that colleges will now adopt this procedure, paying students at risk to enter a brief intervention which leaves 70% of these high risk students still binging and more than 40% of the untreated remaining student body binging? By definition, a decrease of 8% is harm reduction. But I do not believe that college administrators would think this is an effective approach to the problem of excessive drinking on their college campus when it leaves 70% of the group at risk still binging with 3.6 problems approximately each semester and the remainder of the freshman cohort binging at the unacceptable national rate.

The Marlatt et al. 1998 study has additional shortcomings that have not been addressed. The initial assessment asked students to report on drug use. These results are not described. Whether use of other drugs increased or decreased as a result of the intervention focused on alcohol consumption and alcohol problems is not considered by Marlatt and his colleagues.

Another serious shortcoming is evident in the Marlatt et al. (1998) harm reduction project: Neuropsychological assessments were not obtained at baseline or follow-up. What affect does the heavy drinking, and continued drinking have on the brain function of these students? Evidence suggests that neurobiological brain function is maturing until at least the age of 21 years, and there is an important spurt in maturation of frontal lobe function between years 17-21 (Hudspeth & Pribram, 1992). What affect does drinking an average of 3.6 drinks/occasion and 5-6 or more at least once/month, the drinking rate of the treated students, have on the brain function of a young person still maturing? Marlatt's harm reduction for college drinkers is nothing of the sort. In all likelihood it is a form of harm induction. It must be treated as such until it can be demonstrated that the level of drinking attained after "harm reduction" treatment does not increase brain dysfunction and cause brain damage which may or may not be reversible. I believe it is unethical to promote such a treatment program when critical information concerning its possible harm has not been gathered. It is contrary to the first principle of research: nonmaleficence.

Finally, it must be remembered that the participants in the harm reduction project are minors. They are below the legal age for drinking. Marlatt and his colleagues ignore this ethical and legal problem. They send the message that the university condones breaking the law as long as you drink a little less. What affect does this have on the attitudes of students toward the law in general and their character development? Why is this not an issue that is addressed by ethicists on the Institutional Review Board (IRB) for the university and by university administrators? Does NIAAA condone teaching minors to break the law and approves drinking rates for minors with unknown and potentially deleterious consequences for neurobiological development?

Marlatt's harm reduction program is unethical because it does not inform the student of the possible damage to brain function occurring if they continue to drink. It is condoning and reinforcing the students' behavior in breaking the law with no attempt to determine the effects on the attitudes of the participants. "Harm reduction" for minors may be producing far more serious psychological and neuropsychological problems than it is reducing. One of the most disturbing aspects of all of this is that the investigators seem oblivious to the serious implications of their work, as do the adminstrators of NIAAA and the University of Washington.

It is not the case that Marlatt's harm reduction is the only approach to prevention. Evidence suggests that the most effective way to approach prevention must be multifaceted and community based (Williams & Perry, 1998, Williams, Perry, Farbakhsh, & Veblen-Mortenson, 1999). Prevention of drinking by young people in the community as well as on campus must include policy changes and the adherence to policy. To work, community prevention programs must have the involvement of parents, schools, and leaders in the community. The same approach must be implemented on college campuses. Instead of a leaking band aid such as "harm reduction" colleges need to engage in the difficult work of changing the social environment, behavioral norms, so that drinking by minors is unacceptable, and heavy drinking by anyone is unacceptable. Accomplishing this task requires hard work and cooperation from all segments of the campus community, students, faculty, staff, college administrators, as well as parents, alumni and people in the surrounding community.

Conclusions

Based on our examination of Hester and Miller's (1995) evaluation of the alcoholism treatment outcome literature we conclude the following: Hester and Miller's claim that there is no evidence showing the efficacy or effectiveness of traditional treatment programs geared towards abstinence in alcoholics is based on a biased sample of old and inadequate treatment studies and the failure to review all publication sources (see chapter 7). Their claims for the success of behavior therapy for training problem drinkers to engage in controlled drinking or to abstain are based on studies suffering from a variety of one or more shortcomings, inadequate designs, small samples, poor procedures, and misinterpretations of the obtained results. Moos (1997) provides a brilliant, witty, and incisive criticism of the shortcomings in the kinds of efficacy studies under consideration. There is no point in beating a dead horse. I will only reiterate a few points.

Miller and Hester's biased and limited pool of studies captured for their evaluations omitted the largest and best designed studies of alcoholism treatment outcomes. Omissions include studies of traditional treatments with abstinence as a goal appearing in books, book chapters, and journals not within their narrow sampling net. These studies will be reviewed in chapter 7.

The gold standard of treatment studies purports to be a clinical trial, an efficacy study which employs random assignment of subjects to treatments thereby randomizing all extraneous variables (Seligman, 1995). It ideally uses a nontreatment control group. The idealized version of the clinical trial has not been realized in alcohol studies, neither by a study such as the one conducted by Harris and Miller (1990) nor the multimillion dollar MATCH project considered in chapter. 7.

Finally, Hester, Marlatt, et al. (1998) Miller, Heather (Heather & Tebbutt, 1989) the Sobells and other proponents of controlled drinking or harm reduction are insensitive to the ethical implications of their promotion of controlled drinking for problem drinkers and the "self-determination" hypothesis: Patients have the right to choose their treatment goal, abstinence or controlled drinking. A proper informed consent, one that treats patients as autonomous agents, provides information concerning available alternative procedures and the positive and negative consequences of each. An essential form of information for people seeking treatment for alcohol misuse who are offered controlled drinking is knowledge of their state of brain function and the consequences for that state entailed by continued moderate, controlled, drinking which must be defined explicitly. Remember that not too long ago controlled drinking was defined as an average of 6-drinks/day with not more than 10 on a typical day with a restriction that no more than 3 dependency symptoms occur (Armor, Polich, & Stambul, 1976, 1978). If controlled drinking is to be offered to problem drinkers as an alternative treatment, they must first have a thorough neuropsychological and neuroimaging assessment of brain structure and function.

Offering controlled drinking treatment in the absence of information provided the patient concerning their potential for brain damage and the likelihood of relapse is unethical and contrary to the implications of federal regulations. Such practices violate the basic ethical principle of health service providers: Do no harm: nonmaleficence.

Ethical principles are social in nature. Significant others, such as close family members, should be consulted about treatment goals and participate in the decision making process with patient and provider. Approving controlled drinking for a problem drinker is of great concern to family members, not only because of their concern for the patient, but also for their own well-being. It is unfortunate that advocates of controlled drinking and harm reduction ignore the need for harm reduction to significant others and the public at large.

7 ABSTINENCE DOES WORK

Controlled clinical trials provide support for a finite number of strategies, including aversion therapies, behavioral self-control training, monitored disulfiram, social skills training, behavioral marital therapy, stress management, and community reinforcement. What these strategies have in common, aside from their support in the scientific literature, is the fact that they are rarely used in current U.S. treatment practice. In contrast, the typical components of current treatment programs have in common a lack of empirical evidence for effectiveness....

A serious reader of the available scientific literature on alcoholism treatment would be led to approaches that differ radically from present standard and state-of-the-art programs. Treatment methods currently in use have been shaped more by historic accident and economic considerations than by systematic research. There is every reason to believe that if treatment practices were changed to conform more closely to the available evidence, we could be much more effective in reducing the incidence and effects of alcoholism. (Miller, 1990, pp. 260, 262).

The purpose of the present chapter is to review the research literature refuting the above oft repeated claims by Miller and other revisionists that there is no scientific evidence supporting the use of so-called traditional treatment programs. In the United States traditional programs characteristically follow the "Minnesota Model." Such programs are a blend of 12-step principles developed by the AA fellowship and current clinical practices, a blend originating at Willmar State Hospital and Hazelden in Minnesota, hence the label, "Minnesota Model".

Table 7.1 lists the approximate average hours/week 13 different midwestern treatment programs following the Minnesota Model allocate to different activities. It should put to rest the notion that the Minnesota Model treatment program is nothing but didactic lectures and the recitation of 12-step principles. Data shown in Table 7.1 were collected by a joint project of the Illinois Hospital Addiction Treatment Administrators' Forum (IHATAF) and State Farm Insurance Companies (Farrar, 1990). It gives some idea of the variety of treatments used, including such contemporary treatments as relapse prevention and family therapy, although they are not necessarily a variation of behavior therapy or cognitive behavior therapy. Wallace et al. (1988) describe the different treatments that had been used in the inpatient program at the Edgehill Newport treatment center. Again, they include current clinical modalities. Treatment in different facilities vary in amount of time allocated to each modality, its contents, and quality just as different hospitals

Table 7.1 Average hours/week spent in formal therapeutic activities in 13 different Minnesota Model treatment programs

Activity	Mean and standard deviation
Didactics	35 (16.7)
Individual Therapy	9 (5.0)
AA Group	17 (7.3)
4th Step	6 (10.6)
5th Step	1 (1.5)
Exercise	8 (9.3)
Family therapy	4 (15.5)
Group Therapy	29 (15.5)
Assertiveness Trng	2 (1.9)
Release Planning	1 (0.9)
Peer Confrontation	4 (5.9)
Work Therapy	5 (7.2)
Relapse Prevention	4 (8.0)
Relaxation Trng	3 (4.1)
Other	2 (4.8)

Note. From Farrar (1990).

specialize and are better in some areas such as cancer as compared to cardiovascular diseases. There is no monolithic Minnesota Model relying solely on didactic lectures and the 12 steps of AA. Although all share a core of common elements, an emphasis on the 12 steps of AA, they provide current treatment modalities as well. Amount of time devoted to different modalities and the skill with which they are employed will undoubtedly vary from facility to facility, but that is true of all treatment facilities and treatment modalities.

There are many negative results in the treatment outcome literature. Negative results such as failure to obtain a difference between two groups or a difference from baseline, may be due to an infinite number of reasons. That traditional treatments may really be ineffective must be considered a possibility. It must be remembered however that there may be highly significant differences among different traditional treatment programs. Traditional treatment facilities may differ in a variety of ways including intensity of the treatment program, individual components employed and their effectivness, experience and skill of the alcoholism counselors, extent to which the family is counseled and integrated into the program, intensity of the after-care program, and one of the most important variables of all, the kind of patient admitted. Are the patients first admissions, chronic alcoholics with a long history of treatments, street people with no social supports, polydrug users as well as alcoholics, suffering from comorbidity, socially stable middle class professionals, etc.? A thorough evaluation of treatment effectiveness requires a multi-site study in which the different treatment programs can be analyzed as one of the variables as well as the processes involved in the treatments. Most neglected of all, physiological state variables need to be assessed if we are to obtain an adequate understanding of the variables underlying treatment success.

Before turning to an examination of large multi-site evaluation studies we will consider results from studies that involve a single treatment program with a feature rarely found in treatment outcome studies, use of a comparison group with no index treatment (Smith, 1985, 1986). A second feature of these successful studies is that I have never seen a discussion of their results by Miller, Hester, or any other reviewer of alcoholism treatment effectiveness in the United States including the purported authoritative Institute of Medicine (1990) report.

Three studies by D. I. Smith (1983, 1985a, 1985b, 1986) conducted in Australia illustrate some important methodological issues in the evaluation of treatment outcomes. Evidence of the effectiveness of "traditional" treatment programs was obtained in two studies whereas evaluation of the effectiveness of a third program revealed a striking treatment failure. All three evaluations employed a matched comparison group. The one treatment failure (Smith, 1983) was conducted with hospital inpatients matched with a comparison group that only received detoxification. There were 145 non-aboriginal males in each of the two groups matched on a large number of demographic and personal dimensions. A 2-year follow-up was conducted employing a large number of dependent variables assessing social adjustment, alcohol consumption and alcohol related behavior. On almost all of the measures the treatment group was neither significantly better nor worse than the control group that received only detoxification. Smith attributes the poor outcome to absence of an adequate after-care and re-entry program.

That we cannot generalize the treatment outcome results of one poorly run abstinence oriented treatment program to all traditional treatment programs is apparent from the results of the next two program evaluations conducted by Smith and the studies in Germany and the United States that follow.

RESIDENTIAL TREATMENT OUTCOMES

A study of women

This first study (Smith, 1985b) helps fill a void since there is relatively little information on treatment effectiveness for women. In part this lack has been due to the fact that most of the early treatment outcome research was conducted in VA Hospitals with its overwhelmingly male patient population. A second reason is that there were relatively few women in public treatment facilities and results for women were not differentiated from the majority men. It is therefore particularly unfortunate that Smith's (1985b) study has been omitted from the Hester and Miller (1995) reviews of the treatment outcome literature.

Smith (1985b) studied two groups of women, 43 patients in a residential treatment program and a matched comparison group of 35 women who went through the same detoxification center but did not immediately enter the index treatment. Participants were matched on a large number of demographic and background variables. One significant difference appeared in the matching variables. Drinking was initiated at an earlier age on the average by participants in the treatment than the comparison group.

Participants in the treatment group were recruited from a voluntary agency which operates a residential AA programme for up to 42 people. The 'staff' consisted of four recovered alcoholics whose only financial reimbursement was free board. Each morning after an early breakfast, Monday to Saturday inclusive, the twelve-step AA programme is studied, one step per day. All residents then participate in a work programme until noon and have the afternoons free of organised activities, with the exception of AA meetings on Wednesday and Saturday afternoons. On arrival at the Lodge each person is required to sign a contract which specifies that she will participate in all AA activities, pay her board of $42 (Aust.) in advance and leave immediately should she consume any alcohol. Residents are encouraged to stay a minimum of six weeks. Reality therapy (Glaser, 1965) is an integral part of the programme. (Smith, 1985, p. 315).

Of the 48 women in the treatment group, 43 (90%) were interviewed. Two were deceased. Thirty-five (73%) of the comparison group were interviewed. One was deceased and eight (17%) declined to be interviewed. Follow-up interviews occurred after approximately 10 months for the control group and 14 months for the treatment group. A correction was applied to pertinent measures to adjust for the time difference.

Results showed a striking difference in outcome. Significantly more women from the treatment than the comparison group reported complete abstinence during the follow-up interval, 79% versus 3%. Treatment as compared to comparison group participants drank significantly less alcohol in the week prior to the interview and in a typical week and had a significantly lower blood alcohol level at the time of the follow-up interview. Group differences were not limited to alcohol consumption. Women receiving treatment were employed for more weeks in the follow-up period as well as during the 30 days prior to the interview and had significantly fewer mental and physical problems than the comparison women. Treatment women had no drunk days on the job during the past 30 days versus 2.86 days for the comparison group. Their number of admissions to hospitals during the follow-up period was significantly fewer, 0.28 versus 0.72. Rehospitalizations for detoxification during the follow-up period were 0.00 for treatment women versus 0.56 for comparison women.

Of the 48 women in the treatment group, 35% stayed for the recommended six weeks, 32% stayed for less than six weeks and 33% stayed for seven or more weeks. Significantly fewer women who left before six weeks remained abstinent than women who stayed longer. Women who stayed longer than seven weeks did not show a higher abstinence rate than those who remained six weeks. Only one of the women in the treatment group who relapsed during the follow-up stayed in residence the full six weeks. Only one woman in the comparison group remained abstinent throughout the follow-up period.

A possible criticism of the quasi-experimental design of Smith's study is that the two groups differed in their motivation to change. Women in the treatment group were more motivated. They sought additional treatment following detoxification whereas the comparison group did not. The readiness for change hypothesis is contradicted by information Smith gathered from the comparison group indicating that a total of 88% of the comparison group had received treatment some time during their drinking career. He found that 71% of the comparison women participated in at least one other treatment program during the follow-up period. An additional six (17%) of the women participated in a treatment program in the year before their detoxification, suggesting that there was little difference between the two groups in their motivation to change.

It is apparent that the majority of efficacy studies obtain insufficient follow-up information when they fail to determine the extent to which their subjects have been or are participating in other intervention programs than the target treatment. Important information of this kind is lacking in the behavior therapy studies conducted by Miller and others reviewed in chapter 6.

A study of men

Smith (1986) described a similar evaluation of residential treatment effectiveness for men and a matched comparison group receiving only detoxification. Treatment and comparison groups each contained 137 men at the start of the study. Approximately 75% of the men in each group were interviewed approximately 15 months following treatment. Abstinence rates for the entire follow-up interval were 62% versus 5% for the treatment and comparison groups, respectively. Treatment as compared to control group men had a significantly lower blood alcohol level at the time of the follow-up interview. Significant differences, as was true of the women, were found on a large range of social living and adjustment measures. For example, treatment men were employed 50.99 weeks in the follow-up period as compared to 32.83 weeks for the comparison group; dollars spent on alcohol during the follow-up period, 6.33 versus 22.02 for the treatment and comparison groups, respectively; times drunk on the job during the previous month, 0.22 versus 3.33 for the treatment and comparison groups, respectively. An interesting finding is that before the study 33 of the men in the treatment group attended 89.67 AA meetings whereas 35 men in the comparison group attended 101.10 meetings. During the follow-up period, 73 men in the treatment group attended 66.25 meetings whereas 37 men attended 23.62 meetings in the comparison group.

A considerable number of men in the control group participated in AA prior to their inclusion in the study. Follow-up period data also indicated that many of the control-group men attended AA meetings but did not remain abstinent... These findings raise the question as to whether participation on a nonresidential basis in AA is sufficient treatment for persons with advanced alcohol problems. It is not inconceivable that the effectiveness of the... program is at least partly due to its residential nature as it enables people to literally sort themselves out free of the pressures of daily living. By contrast, if one's only treatment is nonresidential AA meetings this opportunity for readjustment is not available as the pressures of daily living return the instant a meeting is finished. The view that people with advanced alcohol problems need a period of residential treatment followed by after-care is not new, but [this] evaluation study does appear to be the first time it has been shown to be effective. (Smith, 1986, p.47f).

A somewhat different interpretation of the effectiveness of residential treatment is that, at least in part, it provides time for the recovery of brain function in the absence of the stress and strains of daily living in their old environment or in a new unprotected one. As was true of women, men who left residential treatment before the recommended 6 weeks relapsed more frequently then the men who stayed at least 6 weeks. The former had more admissions to public hospitals and more mental and physical problems.

Smith (1986) found that 71% of the comparison group men participated in a treatment intervention during the follow-up period and an additional 15% had received some form of intervention for alcoholism during the year prior to the index treatment. Men in the treatment group showed similar results in that 77% received additional treatment during the follow-up period and 9% had received treatment for alcoholism during the year prior to the start of the index treatment. These results indicate that both comparison and treatment groups of men were motivated to change and that the intervening event responsible for the differences between the two groups at the follow-up period most likely was the index residential treatment.

Smith (1985) reported the results of a further analysis of a subgroup of men who had some contact with the police during the year preceding the index treatment. He found that 47% of the treatment group received a conviction for drunkenness or disorderly conduct and 48% had at least one drunk-driving arrest. For men in the comparison group 48% received drunkenness or disorderly conduct convictions and 40% were arrested for drunk-driving. His analysis was limited to the 43 men in the treatment group and 25 men in the comparison group who had one or more of the above contacts in the month prior to the target treatment.

Results for this subgroup in terms of drinking behavior were highly significant as was true of the groups as a whole. Fifty-three percent of the treatment group were abstinent for the entire follow-up period as compared to 0.0% for the comparison group. The groups also differed in the amount of alcohol consumed during the week prior to the follow-up interval, during a typical week during the year and in the amount of money spent on alcohol. Of particular interest, given the history of these two subgroups, the treatment group had significantly fewer convictions for drunkenness and disorderly conduct then the comparison group. Both groups showed a decrease in drunk driving convictions. An important, difficult, and neglected problem was not investigated, the incidence of family abuse before and after the index intervention.

Smith (1986) emphasizes that the positive results found in his studies of residential treatment do not necessarily generalize to all residential treatment programs. Smith's evaluation of treatment effectiveness for a 12-step oriented treatment program for men and for women as compared to matched comparison groups shows highly significant differences in a wide range of social adjustment variables and abstinence rate in favor of the traditional treatment. It does not follow that all traditional treatment programs are equally as effective. It does show that the program at Serenity Lodge was highly effective, contrary to the myth propagated by Miller, Hester, and others that there is no evidence that traditional treatment works. Results of the kind obtained by Smith, despite the limitations in design, compare favorably with the highly rated behavior therapy studies we reviewed in chapter 6. Smith's studies raise several questions: Why are residential treatment programs of the kind described not more common in view of their apparent effectiveness? Why are not federal funds supporting research on such projects rather than projects based on the shaky research base formed by behavior therapy studies?

KÜFNER AND FEUERLEIN'S MULTI-SITE OUTCOME STUDY

I will now describe results reported in a major study of alcoholism treatment programs in the Federal Republic of Germany (Feuerlein & Küfner, 1989; Küfner & Feuerlein, 1989). It will be reviewed in some detail because it is one of the best treatment outcome studies I have read and has been ignored in reviews of the alcoholism treatment outcome literature in the United States. Its results contradict Miller's statements opening this chapter.

A basic aim of the Küfner and Feuerlein (1989) study was to try to answer the question: "what features of in-patient rehabilitation treatment for alcohol dependence lead to what results in what patients?" (p.1). A detailed answer requires determining the characteristics of patients and treatments and their interactions that lead to improved treatment outcomes. It is the study of patient/treatment matching, which makes it all the more disconcerting that this major report has been ignored given the great interest expressed in matching in recent years.

Küfner and Feuerlein assumed at the outset that alcoholism is the consequence of a multifactor network and that the consequence, alcohol dependence, is a disease. It is apparent that their basic assumptions influenced the large number of different kinds of variables they examined. Unfortunately, they apparently failed to administer a neuropsychological test battery which could have provided a rich source of information with respect to prognostic factors and might help explain some of the interactions obtained.

METHOD AND PROCEDURES

Subjects

Results are reported for 1410 consecutively admitted alcoholics (73% men) in 21 different inpatient treatment facilities. The gender ratio corresponded to the ratio for inpatient treatment in the Federal Republic of Germany. Approximately 90% were diagnosed as alcoholics, 5% as problem drinkers, and 5% unclassifiable. According to Jellinek's system, approximately 67% were gamma alcoholics, 24% were delta and episodic drinkers, 4% were alpha, and 4% were beta, the latter two classifications constituting problem drinkers. A total of 89% were physically dependent, defined as showing withdrawal symptoms, and 79% reported loss of control over their drinking. Seventy percent of the men and 58% of the women had liver disease; 71% of the patients had received some kind of previous treatment. A personality inventory indicated that patients at intake were significantly above the norm in nervousness, depression, and emotional lability.

Treatment facilities

Treatment centers ranged in size from 10-169 beds. There were 479 treatment staff members in the 21 centers, full or part-time. Neither the physicians nor psychologists had specialist training in treating addictions. A majority of the social workers and nurses who had an active role in treatment did have special training in addiction treatment. General treatment orientation of the centers were: depth psychology/psychoanalysis, 4 facilities; humanistic psychology, 5 facilities; eclectic, 11 facilities; behavior therapy, 1 facility. Financial support for the treatment facilities stemmed from universities, the state, private sources, and charities. Support for the research was provided by The Federation of German Pension Institutions.

Treatment modalities provided by the various facilities include: individual therapy, group therapy, work therapy, occupational therapy, alcohol information, life plan and values, ward group, and sport and physiotherapy. All 21 facilities provided group therapy and sport and physiotherapy; only six provided individual therapy with an average of 39 min/week. Fifteen facilities provided work therapy for the greatest amount of time, 16 hrs/week followed by group therapy for approximately 6 hrs/week. Relapse prevention, social skills training, or other behavior therapy modalities were not provided. Achievement of the goal of abstinence was emphasized in all programs.

Dependent variables

Data were collected at admission for treatment and follow-ups 6, 18, and 48 months after discharge from treatment. Interviewers and research staff were not members of the treatment staffs. Treatment outcomes were assessed in terms of measures of alcohol and other drug consumption, social adjustment, physical health, personality, ward outcomes and life events. Data on sick leave, inpatient treatment, and retirement were obtained from health and pension insurance agencies. Measures of alcohol consumption for the 6- and 18-month follow-up interviews included three categories: (a) total abstinence, (b) improved, defined as daily consumption of less than 60 g alcohol for males and 30 g for women (4 drinks for men and 2 for women) with no signs of physical or psychological problems as a consequence of the alcohol consumption, and (c) unimproved, defined as all other cases.

Four different categories of drinking behavior were established for the 48-month follow-up: (a) abstinent versus relapsed in the entire 4-year period; (b) abstinent, improved, or unimproved according to the classifications described above for the 6- and 18-month follow-up periods; (c) the same categories of abstinent, improved, and unimproved with improved now defined as "*either* abstinent after a relapse period of at most 1 month and no in-patient treatment due to alcohol abuse, *or* 'social drinking', no signs of pathological drinking and no in-patient treatment for to [sic] alcohol abuse." (Feuerlein & Küfner, 1989, p. 146); (d) abstinent, improved or unimproved according to the criteria of classification (b) but only covering the last 6 months, i.e., using a 6-month evaluation window.

Approximately 150 treatment variables were defined by measures derived from semi-structured interviews. Variables included: (a) length of treatment, short term (6-8 weeks), medium term (4-5 months), long-term (6 months), (b) size of facility, (c) staffing of facility, (d) treatment method(s), group therapy, therapeutic community, family involvement, etc., (e) general orientation, e.g., behavior therapy versus psychodynamic or religious orientation, (f) admission criteria, (g) therapeutic atmosphere assessed by staff and patients.

Abstinence was the treatment goal of all the facilities regardless of general orientation or treatment methods. None of the facilities considered controlled drinking a goal of their treatment. Validity and reliability of the basic data, the self-reports of the patients, were assessed in a number of ways:

1. Self-reports for a given patient obtained at each of the follow-ups were compared with subsequent reports for the same period. In case of a discrepancy the most unfavorable report was employed in the statistical analyses.
2. Wherever possible, self-reports were compared with information from independent objective sources such as records of sick leave, hospitalizations and inpatient treatment obtained from pension and insurance agencies.
3. Self-reports of the patient were compared with impressions of the interviewer during the interview.
4. Self-reports were compared with reports by family members and significant others where available.
5. Original self-reports from the 48-month follow-up interview were compared with additional control interviews obtained from 93 patients comparable in gender and prognosis to the sample as a whole.
6. Some patients at any given follow-up were interviewed by telephone, others by written mail-in questionnaire and still others by face-to-face interview. Patients generally received a different mode of interview at each of the follow-ups. Results showed that type of interview was not a significant factor.

Sample characteristics

Eighteen percent of the initial sample refused to participate in the study. Percent refusals varied considerably among facilities. One hundred additional unselected patients were added to the study in the order of their admission. Divorce rate among patients was 55%; 23% were unemployed or unemployed for more than 3 months; 2% were homeless; 38% were drinking at admission; 34% were abstinent for at least 4 weeks prior to admission; average daily alcohol consumption was 199 g for men (14 drinks) and 151 g (11 drinks) for women. Eighteen percent had no alcohol related medical diseases; 17% had experienced delerium tremens; 37% had been treated in a psychiatric hospital; 22% had been treated in an alcohol or other drug facility; 24% had received psychotherapy.

Inclusion in the study required alcohol as the primary drug misused. Many other drugs, legal as well as illegal were used. Primary dependence upon another legal or illegal drug resulted in exclusion from the study. Inpatient treatment only as a short-term crisis intervention was also a criterion for exclusion.

RESULTS FOR 6-MONTH FOLLOW-UP

Alcohol consumption

Data are reported for 85% of the 1410 patients who volunteered for the experiment on admission to inpatient treatment. Those who dropped out of therapy, n = 231, are included in the analyses of treatment outcomes. Reasons for dropping out of treatment were assessed by therapists as follows: approximately 22% relapsed with alcohol; 4% relapsed with legal drugs; 32% lacked motivation; 16% were discharged for disciplinary reasons; it was a personal decision for 52%; 20% had other reasons such as somatic diseases which required hospitalization. Multiple reasons for dropping out resulted in a total greater than 100%. Number of relapses among facilities varied from 0 - 26%. There were no relapses of any kind in one facility, neither from alcohol nor legal and illegal drugs. Seven patients (0.5%) died after discharge. Their data are excluded from this and all other follow-up evaluations. Sixty-seven percent of all patients remained abstinent for the entire 6 months following treatment, 69% of the men and 60.5% of the women. Eleven percent, 10% of the men and 14% of the women, were classified as improved, may be considered engaged in controlled drinking. Twenty-two percent, 20% of the men and 25.5% of the women were not improved. If patients who are missing and died are considered as relapsed, then 57% are calculated as abstinent for the first 6 months following treatment.

Social and personal adjustment

Twenty-one percent were unemployed at follow-up versus 23% at admission; 8% had new partners; 11.5% regularly took potentially addictive legal drugs. Consumption of illegal drugs was rare.

Changes in patients' personalities as measured by various scales were generally in the direction of normalization. There were significant mean decreases in nervousness, spontaneous aggression, excitability, inhibition and emotional lability. Scores increased for sociability, calmness, extraversion, and masculinity and self-assertiveness. Reactive aggressiveness did not change. Complaints decreased significantly.

Many details of results are not summarized here because of the excessive length required for the task. Some of these, such as treatments received during the follow-up period since the index treatment, will be reviewed after discussion of the subsequent follow-ups. Others, such as the specific details of outcomes from interviews versus written questionnaires will not be considered other than to note the important overall conclusion that there were no significant differences among methods of obtaining self-report data. Similarly, changes in attitude and personality during and following the course of treatment will not be considered. Interested readers may find information on these and other variables in the book by Küfner and Feuerlein (1989). Because I do not discuss a particular variable or kind of variable, it does not necessarily mean that it was overlooked or ignored by Küfner and Feuerlein.

RESULTS FOR 18-MONTH FOLLOW-UP

Eighty-four percent of the original 1410 patients were interviewed at the 18-month follow-up. Thirty-seven, 3%, of the patients died during this follow-up interval.

Alcohol consumption

Fifty-three percent were abstinent for the entire 18-month follow-up interval, 55% of the men and 47% of the women; 8.5%, of the patients had improved, 9% of the men and 8% of the women; 38% showed no improvement. Using a 6-month window, evaluating drinking during the interval 6 months prior to the 18-month interview, showed that 63% were abstinent.

An interaction occurred between treatment outcome and duration of treatment. For the entire 18-month follow-up, long-term treatment yielded a 60% abstinence rate, whereas 45% were abstinent with medium-term, and 54% were abstinent with short-term treatment. Remember, that short-term in the present study conducted in Germany consisted of 6-8 weeks of inpatient treatment, medium-term treatment was 4-5 months and long-term treatment was 6 months. Bases for the interaction will be considered later in this section.

Patients with a previous hospitalization for drug use had a lower rate of abstinence, 39%. Three percent of the abstinent patients were regularly taking legal drugs such as sleeping pills, tranquilizers, and pain killers. Use of illegal drugs was low. Hashish, the most commonly used illegal drug, was used by 1.5% of the alcohol abstinent patients.

Patients with a secondary diagnosis of abuse of legal drugs had a similar rate of abstinence from alcohol as those with no drug misuse diagnosis. However, patients with a secondary diagnosis of dependence on legal or illegal drugs had lower rates of abstinence, 45% alcohol abstinence; 27% were abstinent from alcohol and all other legal and illegal drugs. Twenty-five percent attended self-help group meetings regularly in the 18-month period. Their abstinence rate was 72.5% compared to the overall rate of 53%.

Data from the health and pension insurance agencies indicated an overall reduction of 56% in number of sick-leave days. Days of in-patient medical treatment were reduced by 51%. Days unfit for work showed a decrease of 64%, from 118 to 43 days. Average number of days sick-leave for abstinent and relapsed patients were 34 and 47, respectively.

Social and personal adjustment

There were no appreciable changes in marital status during this follow-up period; 17% were unemployed, a decrease from the first follow-up interval. There was a continued trend towards normalization of scores on personality scales. Abstinent and relapsed patients were significantly different on all scales except extraversion.

RESULTS FOR 48-MONTH FOLLOW-UP

Eighty-one percent of the original sample were interviewed at the 48-month follow-up; 92 had died during the interval. Forty-six percent were abstinent for the entire 4-year interval since discharge from the index treatment facility, 48.5% of the men and 41% of the women. In addition, 2.6% were in the improved category of controlled drinking; 42% had not improved, 40% of the men and 46% of the women.

Considering results from a 6-month evaluation window prior to the 48-month follow-up interview, 66% were abstinent, 65% of the men and 70% of the women; 4% were improved, 4% of the males and 2% of the females; 30% were unimproved according to the criteria of classification (b), 31% of the men and 28% of the women. Examining outcomes of the patients who dropped out of treatment prior to completion of the program, 23% were abstinent during the entire 48-month follow-up. Only 62% of the drop-outs were interviewed as compared to 81% of the entire sample. Patients who relapsed and received additional inpatient treatment during the 4-year follow-up period yielded the following results: 35% were abstinent as compared to 73% who did not require additional inpatient treatment. Seven percent of the sample abstaining from alcohol for the entire 48-month period used other legal or illegal drugs.

Social and personal adjustment

Divorces rose from 17.5% to 24% whereas the number of patients living with their parents declined, 11% at admission versus 6%. Increased employment rate was related to abstinence. Seven percent of the patients employed at admission to treatment and abstinent at the 6-month follow-up were unemployed at the 48-month follow-up. In contrast, 23% of patients employed at admission to treatment who had relapsed at the 6-month follow-up were unemployed at the 48-month follow-up.

Data obtained for a sample of patients, n=297, from health and pension insurance agencies showed a 64% decrease in days of sick leave at the 18-month follow-up interview for the entire period since treatment. Patients who were abstinent during the entire period had significantly less days of sick leave than those who relapsed.

Sixty-three percent of the patients gave the investigators their consent to obtain information from health and pension insurance agencies concerning their days of sick leave and additional in-patient treatments. Data for 651 patients were obtained covering the 2-year period prior to their index treatment as well as for a 2- year evaluation window prior to the 48-month follow-up. There was a 55% reduction in mean sick leave for the 2 years immediately following treatment versus the 2 years prior to entering treatment, and a 43% reduction in sick leave for the second 2-year block following treatment versus the pretreatment period. Comparable reductions in days of inpatient treatment were also observed. There was some reduction in number of days of sick leave and inpatient treatment for people who relapsed, 71.7 days pretreatment versus 51.5 posttreatment days; the decrease in combined days lost to illness was greater in the abstainers, an average 73 days in the pre-treatment period versus 7 days posttreatment. Abstinence pays off in more ways than one.

Stability of drinking measures

Seventy-seven percent of the patients who were abstinent in the first 6-months, n = 628, were continuously abstinent for the full 48-months; 14% were classified as unimproved and 3% were classified as improved in the 6-month evaluation window preceding the 48-month follow-up interview. Fifty-two percent of the patients classified as *unimproved* at the 6-month follow-up, n = 130, continued in their relapsed state for the entire 48 months; 31.5% were abstinent in the 6-month window preceding the 48-month follow-up and 2% were improved for that 6-month period. Only 3%, 2 patients of those classified as improved in the first 6-month interval, n = 7, continued controlled drinking for the entire 48-month follow-up; 7% were improved during the 6-month evaluation window preceding the 48-month follow-up interview, 38% were abstinent, and 55% were unimproved. These results demonstrate that controlled drinking is not a stable state as compared to abstinence. Almost as many people engaged in moderate controlled drinking at six months were relapsed at the 48-month follow-up interview as people who were relapsed within 6 months following treatment. Only two patients in an original sample of 1410 diagnosed alcoholics were able to continue moderate drinking in the long term. In contrast, 77% of those abstinent in the first 6 months maintained their abstinence for the entire 48 months.

PREDICTING TREATMENT OUTCOME

Küfner and Feuerlein have an extensive discussion of the methods and results of their analyses of prognostic variables predicting treatment outcome. Two classes of variables were studied, (a) general factors that are independent of any particular treatment such as patient characteristics and experiences occurring prior to entering treatment, and (b) specific factors that are dependent upon a particular treatment, such as treatment duration and staff and patient rated atmosphere.

All individual difference patient variables were taken as possible predictors of treatment outcome. Men and women were analyzed separately. Reliability was assessed by randomly dividing the total patient sample in half. Only variables that were statistically significant in both halves of the patient sample were accepted as prognostic factors. Outcome criteria for which dependent variables were devised included, drinking behavior, work, interpersonal relations, satisfaction with work and with partner, and life complaints. Abstinence rate was the principal dependent variable.

Patient Variables Predicting Outcome

Patient prognostic variables were obtained from admission and discharge data. Abstinence from alcohol at the 18-month follow-up was taken as the basic dependent variable. Selection of the 18-month follow-up interval rather than the 6- or 48-month follow-up was a compromise. Greater stability of the dependent measure is reflected at 18 months than 6 months and there has not been sufficient opportunity for life events independent of treatment to play an overwhelming role in influencing long-term outcomes as may be the case for the 48-month follow-up.

Prognostic factors derived from admission data

"Having only one place of work in the last 2 years" was the general prognostic factor with the greatest effect size for men. It was followed by "no previous treatment in an addiction unit" and "no history of suicide attempts". Fewer general prognostic factors were significant for women then for men. Items on a self-assertiveness scale had the highest prognostic value. Drinking less than 625 g of pure alcohol/week was a significant prognostic factor. "Previous treatment in an addiction unit" was also predictive of an unfavorable outcome for women. Having had a previous inpatient treatment indicates that the odds of long-term abstinence are lower than for people who had no previous inpatient treatment.

Multivariate analyses showed that the general prognostic factors predicting treatment outcome variance were independent of the length of treatment, with one exception. Number of suicide attempts by men interacted with length of treatment. Prognostic variables were combined into prognostic indices and discriminant analyses conducted on these indices for men and for women using abstinence as the outcome criterion. Sixty-four percent of the men and 67% of the women were correctly classified. Social stability factors appeared to be better general prognostic factors for men than for women. Correlations were low for both genders and relatively small amounts of variance in the outcome measure could be predicted.

Prognostic factors derived from discharge data

Additional information was derivable from discharge data not available at admission. These included demographic information about the patient reflecting events occurring during treatment such as divorce, participation of significant others in the treatment program, and dropping out of treatment.

For men, dropping out of treatment, relapse during treatment, and relatively little involvement of significant others in treatment were unfavorable predictors of outcome. Dropping out and a low complaints score were unfavorable predictors for women. Most of the significant factors showed a main effect on outcome independent of treatment duration.

Prognosis for outcomes other than abstinence was also examined for criteria of employment/unemployment, satisfaction with work, satisfaction with partner relationship, and complaints as an indicator of physical well being. Multiple correlations of a prognosis index developed for abstinence was similar for abstinence, work situation, and work, approximately 0.30. Multiple correlations of specific sets of predictors combining information from admission and discharge produced multiple correlations as high as 0.64 for men and 0.63 for women for complaints score.

Age as a prognostic factor

Age did not appear as a general prognostic factor. However, clinical experience and the research literature led Küfner and Feuerlein to examine age in relation to abstinence/relapse in greater detail. Abstinence rates among the youngest men and women, age under 24, were low, although the number of patients was also small. For men, n=10, 37% were abstinent. For women, n=3, 23.1% were abstinent. For the mid-range in age, 35-44, men, n = 196, showed an abstinence rate of 56.6%; 47.7% of the women in the same age range, n=61, were abstinent. Men, age 55+, n=22, showed an abstinence rate of 68.8%. Women in the same age range, n=7, showed an abstinence rate of 46.7%. Combining men and women, in the age range below 25 years, n=40, revealed that 32.5% were abstinent. Combined men and women age 25+, n=1078, showed that 54.0% were abstinent. A chi-square test of abstinence as a function of age was highly significant.

A revisionist might argue that these data are very misleading. According to Rand Report II (Polich et al., 1980), controlled drinking works better for young men and abstinence works better for older men. Miller and Caddy (1977) recommend controlled drinking for young but not older people. Küfner and Feuerlein's results in terms of abstinence, revisionists may argue, are therefore very misleading for young people; a higher rate of abstinence in the older than the younger age group appears to support their contention.

Fortunately, Küfner and Feuerlein analyzed age in three levels and drinking outcome in terms of the three categories, abstinent, improved (controlled drinking), and unimproved. For men, ages -30, 31-49, and 50+ abstinent rates were 49.3%, 56.1%, and 62.1%, respectively. Improved (controlled) drinking rates for the same age groups were 5.9%, 9.4%, and 8.0%, respectively. It is apparent that a higher percent of the older men are improved (engaged in controlled drinking), as well as abstinent at the 18-month follow-up. Women show the same trend. Abstinence was more frequent in the combined two older groups as compared to the youngest group, as was true of the percent engaged in controlled drinking, improved. Percentages for the combined three age groups were 36.2%, 49.0%, and 47.2% abstinent and 4.3%, 8.5%, and 8.1% improved, respectively.

These results contradict implications of Rand Report II and Miller and Caddy's (1977) recommendation based on them. As I have noted, Welte et al. (1983) also failed to corroborate the results reported in Rand Report II (Polich et al., 1980). The most likely interpretation is that the results in Rand Report II were the consequence of chance, especially in view of the fact that the result in question, an interaction of age and outcome, was the consequence of an interaction which was not predicted.

Küfner and Feuerlein found that a variety of prognostic indicators favored the older male groups over the younger, including home ownership, living with a spouse/partner, and employment. Low alcohol consumption prior to admission for treatment and a higher "social decency score" were the only two prognostic indicators that favored older over younger women.

On the basis of personality variables obtained at admission, it was found that the youngest age group of men differed significantly from the older groups as well as the norms for the following personality scales: more aggressive, more depressive, more inhibition, more emotionally labile, less calm, more open, more extraverted, less yielding, fewer guilt feelings and less "socially decent". There was movement towards normalization on the part of some young men on the following scales: aggression, emotional lability, calmness, openness, yielding, guilt feelings, social decency, and a lower total complaints score.

In other words, young alcoholics tend to be sociopathic. Whether the sociopathy is primary or secondary cannot be determined from Küfner and

Feuerlein's data. Their results and interpretation tend to be in accord with that of Cloninger and his colleagues (Sigvardsson, Bohman, & Cloninger, 1996).

TREATMENT VARIABLES PREDICTING OUTCOME

Treatment facilities, a total of 21 different centers, are the units of analysis in the examination of specific prognostic factors. Potential biases due to patient differences among facilities were controlled by stratifying patients as high or low prognosis within each facility. Analyses correlated a facility's treatment variables with its abstinence rate and compared treatment variables in the most and least successful facilities.

Abstinence rates for the good prognosis group were predicted by the following variables: "higher minimum age limit for admission (21 years); regular individual therapy; broad spectrum of therapeutic techniques; therapeutic response to unpunctuality; flexible control for drugs sent in by post; and intensive involvement of relatives." (Feuerlein & Küfner, 1989, p. 152). The following predicted successful outcomes for the poor prognosis group: "segregation of men and women; information and discussion groups for life planning; extended waiting list for admission." (p. 152).

Length of treatment

In view of the commonly expressed belief that length of treatment makes no difference (Miller & Hester, 1995; Vaillant, 1995), having the large and well-conceived study by Küfner and Feuerlein address this issue is of considerable moment. However, two problems must be kept in mind. (a) Treatment durations studied by Küfner and Feuerlein are considerably longer than those usually examined in North America and Great Britain. (b) Patients were not randomly assigned to the short- medium- and long-term treatment programs.

Results obtained by Küfner and Feuerlein are complex due to interactions between subject prognosis and treatment duration. Differences in prognostic indicators among patients at the three types of treatment facilities varying in duration of treatments must be controlled to examine the independent effects of the treatment facilities. Several different approaches were used to circumvent the effects of different kinds of subjects receiving different treatment durations. One method was to create more homogeneous subgroups within each facility by stratifying subjects as good or poor prognosis on the basis of a variety of demographic and personality variables. Stratification was within each gender.

No significant correlation was found between abstinence and length of treatment for men as a group. Significant relationships were present within subgroups of men stratified by prognosis. In other words, there were significant interactions indicating matching effects. Short-term treatment had an unfavorable outcome for men with a poor prognosis as evidenced by an abstinence rate of 8% receiving short term versus 40% for poor prognosis men receiving long-term treatment. Medium-term treatment seems unfavorable for men with a good prognosis, as seen by an abstinence rate of 59% versus 75% for good prognosis men in medium versus long-term treatment. It is apparent that prognosis, good versus poor, interacted significantly with treatment duration.

In contrast to Miller and Hester's (1995) assertion that there is no evidence that length of treatment makes a difference, Küfner (cited in Feuerlein & Küfner, 1989) reports that of 27 studies examining length of treatment that he reviewed:

16 found positive effects with longer treatments, 9 found no differences, and two found negative effects of longer treatments. Together these results on the whole support the provision of longer treatment. However, they also indicate that generalizing about length of treatment is not a very useful exercise, as one must always bear in mind the likelihood that length of treatment and patient variables are interacting... The oft-cited finding of Orford and Edwards (1977), that a single individual counselling session is at least as effective as quite lengthy out-patient treatment (average 9.6 contacts) cannot be applied to inpatient treatment. (Küfner & Feuerlein, 1989, p. 276).

Neither can Orford and Edwards' (1977) generalization be applied to outpatient treatment since it is proving the null hypothesis. Orford and Edwards failed to provide an adequate number of counselling sessions to produce a differential effect (Monahan & Finney, 1996; see later discussion in this chapter).

Treatment Facilities As Variables

Two strategies were employed in assessing the effectiveness of treatment facilities. First, a center's treatment variables were correlated with its overall abstinence rate and for the rates of the good and poor prognosis subgroups within the facility. A second strategy was to compare the variables of the most and least successful treatment facilities, controlling for the response rate, gender differences, and overall prognosis index of the centers. Again, it must be kept in mind that the treatment facilities are being compared on the basis of the outcomes determined only at the 18-month follow-up. Average abstinence rate of positive prognosis subgroups was 67.5% and for the negative prognosis subgroup, 41.8%. The range among facilities was 42.9% - 88.9% for the positive prognosis subgroup and 28.1% - 58.8% for the negative prognosis subgroup.

Characteristics of successful treatment facilities

Life planning was an important treatment variable in relation to abstinence for the poor prognosis patient in successful as compared to relatively unsuccessful treatment facilities. Another significant variable for the negative prognosis patient, somewhat surprisingly, was length of waiting list. An interpretation of this result is that a waiting list serves as a selection device for motivation. Segregation of men and women seemed to be beneficial primarily for the men.

Among the good prognosis patients, variables that seemed to be predictors of abstinence were: use of regular individual therapy, use of a broad spectrum of therapies, and an attitude on the part of the staff that attaches importance and promotes the involvement of family and significant others in the patients' treatment.

Regular individual therapy was the only variable that had a significant effect for the positive prognosis subgroup, negative prognosis subgroup, and the combined groups. All eight variables previously mentioned account for 63% of the variance in abstinence rates among treatment facilities but only 6% of the variance among the total patient group.

Length of treatment

Length of treatment for the purpose of the present analyses was defined as the planned length of treatment for a given facility not the length of time individuals spent in treatment. The latter definition is confounded with relapses and termination of treatment for different reasons.

Ignoring all patient variables, treatment centers categorized into long-, medium-, and short-term facilities showed significant differences in abstinent rates, 60.4%, 52.4%, and 49.5%, respectively. A relatively poor outcome for the medium-treatment facility is gender specific. Mean abstinence rates for men in the short-, medium-, and long-term treatments were 54.9%, 46.6%, and 61.6% respectively. Men in the medium-term facility also had the lowest rate of abstinence in drop-outs from their program. Examination of the results for each of the facilities in the medium-treatment group indicated that the poor outcome was not peculiar to one extreme facility. To avoid biased treatment outcomes due to patient selection, facilities were matched by controlling for subjects' prognostic factors summarized by the prognostic index developed by Küfner and Feuerlein. Multivariate analyses were used to statistically control for patient differences in prognostic indices.

Summarizing the outcome of several different methods of analyses and transformations, treatment length interacts significantly with gender and prognosis. The majority of men profit most from long-term treatment. Poor and good prognosis men have significantly higher abstinence rates following long-term treatment. Short-term treatment provided the best abstinence rate for good prognosis women. "Among women, length of treatment showed no significant effect after allowing for prognosis index. This is probably due to the low case numbers, as the differences in abstinence rates are as great as among the men" (Küfner & Feuerlein, 1989, p. 196). Number of cases in question is 21, the number of facilities, not the number of patients.

Interpretation of the effects of length of treatment is a complex problem. Time is an abstract concept. What matters is what fills the time. What sorts of treatments, therapies, social learning skills and family interactions have an opportunity to occur and flower is what matters. Of the eight variables that were found to relate significantly to abstinence, three accounted for most of the variation in outcome. The multiple correlation between these eight variables and length of treatment was 0.88. The multiple correlation between the three most influential variables and treatment length was almost as great, 0.85. Three variables account for more than 70% of the variance in treatment centers: "involvement of significant others", regular "individual therapy", and "segregation of men and women".

"Short-term" inpatient treatment in this study and generally throughout The Federal Republic of Germany was 6 - 8 weeks. Long-term treatment was 6 months. There is a matching effect, an interaction between duration of treatment, given the durations studied by Küfner and Feuerlein, and gender and prognosis. None of these issues are addressed by Hester and Miller (1995) and other revisionists despite their insistence that matching is a critical problem. Apparently they never considered length or intensity of treatment a variable that may require matching.

AFTER-CARE IN THE FOLLOW-UP PERIOD

Self-help groups

Abstinence rates in relation to attendance at self-help groups, primarily AA, were 71.6% by patients who attended meetings regularly, 51% for those with no attendance and 48.1% for those with irregular attendance. If regular and irregular attenders are combined, their joint abstinence rate, 55%, is still significantly greater than the abstinence rate for nonattenders.

A more analytic examination of the relationship between attendance at self-help groups following treatment was undertaken by categorizing after-care into three 6-month follow-up intervals and matching for attendance during the first 6-month interval. Of those patients who were abstinent during the entire first 6-month period and who attended self-help meetings on a regular basis during the second 6-month interval, 84.1% were abstinent in the third 6-month interval. Those who attended irregularly or not at all during the second 6-month interval had an abstinence rate of 75.2% in the third 6-month period, a significant difference. A similar analysis was conducted of patients who relapsed during the first 6-month interval and who did or did not attend self-help meetings regularly during the second 6-month interval. In the third 6-month interval, 49.1% of regular attendees were abstinent in contrast to a 20.7% abstinence rate for those who attended on an irregular basis or never. Similar analyses were conducted on men and on women separately with corresponding results.

This imaginative analysis of self-help group attendance during after-care shows that regular attendance is even more important for those who relapse after treatment than for those who do not. In part the difference is due to a ceiling effect in the abstinent group. As a group they are doing well. Further increases in the abstinence rate are difficult to achieve because there is relatively little room remaining for improvement. There is much more room for improvment in the relapse group. Küfner and Feuerlein's analysis suggests that there is a causal relationship between attendance at self-help meetings and remission and not just a correlation between the two which is all that can be concluded in the usual examination of attendance at AA meetings and sobriety (Vaillant, 1995). One cannot ordinarily determine whether former patients are attending AA because they are sober or that they are sober because they are attending AA meetings. Küfner and Feuerlein's creative analyses disentangles the direction of the effect. Additional evidence supporting the interpretation that attendance in AA meetings and degree of involvement in the 12-step program facilitates abstinence and mediates the success of formal treatment is reported by The VA Comparative Outcome Study (Humphreys, Huebsch, Finney, & Moos, 1999).

Individual therapy

Following inpatient alcoholism treatment patients sought individual and group therapy on an outpatient basis as well as self-help groups. In the case of individual therapy, there was no difference in the third 6-month period as a function of attendance for those who were abstinent in the first six month period. Regular attendance for individual therapy versus irregular/nonattendance during the second 6-month interval resulted in abstinence rates of 77% and 78%, respectively. For those who relapsed during the first 6-month period, regular attendance versus irregular/nonattendance in individual therapy did make a difference in the third 6-month period, 63% versus 22% abstinence, respectively.

Once more, there is a ceiling effect apparent in the abstinent group which would limit their room for improvement. Such was not the case for the people who relapsed during the first 6-month period. Individual therapy for them made quite a difference. However, the number of patients in some of these subgroups is relatively small and therefore the results must be accepted with caution. Only 19 patients were in regular attendance for individual therapy and 231 were in irregular/nonattendance. Comparable numbers were involved in the group therapy analysis.

Group psychotherapy

Effects of group psychotherapy were analyzed for the abstinent patients and those who relapsed in the same "causal-analytic" fashion as for attendance in self-help groups and individual psychotherapy. Patients were matched in the first 6-month after-care interval as abstinent or relapsed, differentiated in the second 6-month period as in regular attendance versus irregular/complete nonattendance, and assessed for abstinence in the third 6-month period. For the 738 patients abstinent in the first 6-month period who regularly attended group therapy in the second 6-month interval, 89% were abstinent in the third 6-month period. Of the 708 patients who irregularly or never attended group psychotherapy in the second 6-month period, 78% were abstinent in the third period.

For the 248 patients who relapsed in the first 6-month interval, differences between those with and without regular attendance in group therapy are greater. Of the 12 patients who relapsed during the first 6-month period and who regularly attended group therapy in the second 6-month period, 75%, were abstinent during the entire third 6-month period. In contrast, of the 236 patients who relapsed during the first 6-month period and who did not regularly attend group psychotherapy in the second 6-month period, 22.5% were abstinent during the third 6-month period.

Prognosis and after-care

Küfner and Feuerlein observe that in addition to the positive effect on abstinence of participating in self-help groups, the patients with a good prognosis were more likely to regularly attend meetings than patients who entered treatment with a poor prognosis. Apparently good prognosis patients are more realistic following completion of treatment about their risk for relapse than the poor prognosis patients. They therefore attend self-help group meetings more diligently than the poor prognosis group. An implication of the difference is that the poor prognosis group suffers from greater frontal lobe dysfunction than the good prognosis group. The poor prognosis group is therefore less capable of planning for the future and suffers from less self-control than the good prognosis group. This hypothesis is readily testable by means of neuropsychological testing and neuroimaging of frontal lobe structure and function.

Drop-out rates

Küfner and Feuerlein reported an overall treatment drop-out rate of 17.1%, relatively low compared to rates in the United States, but typical for similar inpatient treatment programs in Germany. The drop-out rate from the two treatment arms of Project MATCH (1997) was twice the above rate. Drop-out rates varied considerably among the treatment centers studied by Küfner and Feuerlein, ranging from 4.5% - 31.6%. Drop-out rates are higher in the English speaking countries averaging approximately 25% for inpatient treatments which are shorter than the inpatient treatments evaluated by Küfner and Feuerline. Their short treatment progams reported only 7.5% drop-out. Drop-out rates for outpatient treatment centers are much higher according to Küfner and Feuerlein, approximately 50%-60%.

Dropping out of treatment is generally regarded and often treated as a failure. Küfner and Feuerlein found that the abstinence rate of their drop-outs was 30% at the 18-month follow-up as compared to a 57.1% abstinence rate for patients who completed their treatment. In a later section in this chapter we will consider an original approach to the drop-out problem taken by Harrison, Hoffman, and Street (1991).

Motivation to change has become an active area of research in the United States in recent years. Emphasis is placed upon inducing the proper motivation for change or matching the stage of motivation with the treatment approach (Miller & Rollnick, 1991). Küfner and Feuerlein on the other hand find low or no correlation between measures of attitude toward treatment and change and treatment outcome. However, there is the possibility of significant interactions between various measures of motivation to change and treatment length for some subgroups, but these possible interactions are not discussed in detail in publications concerned with motivation to change. Küfner and Feuerlein (1989) provide an extended appendix of outcomes from statistical analyses which can be examined for further information on motivation to change.

TREATMENT OUTCOMES FROM PRIVATE TREATMENT FACILITIES IN THE UNITED STATES

The existence of reasonably high success rates for select private abstinence oriented treatment programs in the United States has been a well kept secret by revisionist reviewers who dominate academic publications in the field of alcoholism studies (Fingarette, 1988b; Institute of Medicine, 1990; Miller,1988; Miller & Hester, 1980, 1985; Miller, Leckman, & Tinkcom, 1987; Miller et al., 1995). There have been a few exceptions (McClellan et al.,1993). We described some of the results from private treatment centers in chapter 1 reported by Benchmark, a treatment evaluation service conducted by Hazelden (Gilmore et al., 1986) and by Smith et al. (1991).

Two studies from the 1970s and early 1980s will not be considered here in detail. One received attention and support far beyond the quality of the research warranted; the second received far less attention than its relative excellence warranted. One fit the needs of the revisionists, the other did not. The former is the Rand Report I (Armor et al.,1976, 1978) and II (Polich et al.,1980, 1981) and the second is *Easy does it* by Laundergan (1982), an assessment of treatment outcome for approximately 3,000 patients treated at Hazelden from the latter part of 1973-1975. I will not discuss the Rand Reports because their extraordinary weaknesses have been reviewed in chapter 1 and elsewhere (Blume, 1977; Laundergan, 1982; Wallace,1989a, 1989b, 1990). I will not discuss Laundergan (1982) because the studies based on the CATOR registry have superseded it as an evaluation of treatment outcome from the private sector due to CATOR's size and methodological advances.

Studies from the CATOR registry

CATOR (Comprehensive Assessment and Treatment Outcome Research) was founded out of the growing concern for documentation of treatment effectiveness. Seven programs in the Minneapolis-St. Paul metropolitan area collaborated to design data-collection instruments and study procedures... In time, other programs entered the fee-for-service registry system. After 10 years CATOR had collected intake data on more than 50,000 adults from 80 programs in 29 states, and 6,000 adolescents from 28 programs in 15 states.

Treatment programs in the CATOR registry use standardized data-collection instruments to collect information on each admission at intake and discharge. Each patient fills out a detailed background questionnaire. Patients are asked for consent to follow-up, and approximately 90% of the patients agree to the interviews after treatment...

All individual patient data are... confidential. Treatment center data are also confidential; only the designated official at each participating treatment program receives reports on the program. As part of their contract with CATOR, participating programs agree that their data can be aggregated and analyzed for the purpose of general treatment population and outcome studies. It is this compilation of vast amounts of data over time, from a variety of sources, with centralized follow-up procedures and exact standards for data analysis that lend credibility to CATOR findings. (Harrison et al., 1991, p.1169).

Results from a sample of 9,000 participants from inpatient programs and 1,000 participants from outpatient programs have been presented by Harrison et al. (1991). Numbers of cases studied, success rates, and sophistication of the detailed analyses of pertinent variables far exceeds any reported outcomes for controlled drinking training efficacy or brief intervention studies. Nevertheless, abstinence results reported by CATOR are not cited by Marlatt et al. (1993) or Hester and Miller (1995) and other reviewers including the Institute of Medicine (1990). These studies are not mentioned much less considered effective ways of producing harm reduction.

Harrison et al. (1991) report that participants in inpatient as compared to outpatient programs tend to have greater severity of alcohol and drug use, more severe emotional, social, and vocational problems, including more attempted suicides, depression, and a history of antisocial disorders. Inpatients also tend to be older with fewer social supports than outpatients. Placement into either an inpatient or an outpatient treatment facility is subject to a number of considerations. Daily alcohol or drug use with symptoms of dependence suggests that inpatient treatment with its greater contact hours with staff, isolation from variables contributing to usage, and greater intensity of treatment would be desirable. Other indicators for inpatient treatment include, multiple drug use along with alcohol misuse, a history of withdrawal symptoms, and evidence of severe alcohol dependence. Lack of a social support system, including absence of a spouse and family suggests the need for a social network and personal contact provided by an inpatient or a residential setting. Dual diagnosis, depression with the threat of suicide, schizophrenia and other conditions requiring medication and observation to ensure safety of the patient suggests inpatient treatment is preferable if possible. Other factors determining a choice of inpatient versus outpatient treatment are distance, disruption of family, care of children, loss of work, availability of the facility, and third-party payments. Insurance coverage may currently be the major determinant of the kind and intensity of treatment obtained by a patient.

Following a review of the literature of inpatient versus outpatient treatment differences Harrison et al. (1991) conclude:

> studies that compare intake characteristics of inpatients and outpatients consistently report among inpatients a higher prevalence of factors generally associated with a poorer prognosis. In spite of initial differences showing inpatients to be sicker than outpatients, nonrandomized studies consistently show no differences in outcome at follow-up... But similar recovery rates for inpatients and outpatients do not prove that the treatments they receive are equally effective. Similar outcomes for the two groups may mean merely that less impaired drug and alcohol abusers respond to outpatient treatment about as well as more impaired drug and alcohol abusers respond to inpatient treatment. No conclusions about the relative efficacy of the treatments can be drawn from such studies, unless patient subgroups are matched for intake characteristics and analyses conducted for interactions between patient variables and treatment type. None of the studies reviewed reported such an analysis. (p.1168).

Comparisons of inpatients and outpatients

A comparison of approximately 9,000 inpatients and 1,000 outpatients show a number of characteristic differences along with some similarities. Males outnumber female patients 3:1 in both kinds of treatment facilities. There is a greater proportion of inpatients over the age of 50 whereas outpatients have a greater proportion of patients under age 30. A differential factor here may be the extent of social support, less for the older than the younger patients. Although the number of symptoms of alcohol misuse are similar in inpatient and outpatients, symptoms of illicit drug use are not. Average number of cocaine symptoms for inpatients and outpatients are 4.4 versus 2.4 and all other drugs combined, 3.0 versus 1.5, respectively. Although the number of symptoms of alcohol misuse are similar in the two groups, inpatients show symptoms reflecting greater dependence than outpatients, delerium tremens, drinking to avoid withdrawal symptoms, binge drinking, etc. On the other hand, outpatients report a higher proportion of driving-while-intoxicated (DWI) arrests as an immediate factor contributing to their entering treatment. Inpatients are more likely to report working while impaired by alcohol use and are more likely to report previous treatment for alcohol or other drug misuse. More inpatients have attempted suicide than outpatients and have been treated for depression and other emotional disorders more often. Histories of antisocial behavior occur proportionately more often in inpatients who report more recent arrests for criminal offenses whereas outpatients report more frequent recent arrests for drunk driving. Inpatients also have a higher proportion of recent medical care than outpatients and were more likely to have been hospitalized during the previous year for detoxification, alcohol or drug treatment, and other illnesses or injuries. They were also receiving more outpatient psychiatric and medical care than outpatients.

INPATIENT TREATMENT OUTCOMES

Treatment outcome results are based on a sample of 5,075 patients from 19 treatment facilities in 13 states studied during 1986-1988. They represent 84% of the sample admitted to these treatment centers.

Treatment completion

Characteristics at admission of patients who failed to complete treatment either because they were discharged for noncompliance or because of their own volition were compared with the patients who completed their treatment. Noncompleters were not analyzed further in terms of their reasons for noncompletion. Men and women were equally likely to complete treatment. Various measures of socioeconomic status and social stability were significantly related to completion. Antisocial or criminal behavior were related to dropping out, especially for individuals who had two or more arrests during the year prior to admission aside from traffic violations. Patients with heavy drug use in addition to alcohol misuse were at risk for dropping out. Patients with minimal symptoms of dependence were likely to drop out as well as individuals with severe symptoms who denied the seriousness of their condition.

Twelve percent of the patients completing treatment refused to consent to follow-up interviews. Analysis suggests that variations in consent are not due to subject variables so much as variability among facilities. A number of nonsignificant trends and significant effects which account for small portions of the variance were obtained. There was a significant tendency for a negative relationship between consent and socioeconomic status, contrary to the usual finding in public facilities that the poorest, the street people, are most likely to refuse or cannot be found for follow-up. People who used cocaine or other drugs aside from marijuana yielded a lower consent rate.

Most of the attrition was related to contact bias. It was easier to contact married or widowed patients than single, separated or divorced people. Contact rates were lower for people on welfare, disability assistance, an unemployed member of a minority, and living in a city rather than a rural community. Higher usage of cocaine and other drugs is generally found in urban than rural areas. Antisocial behavior, a history of arrests for criminal offenses, particularly recent arrests, also predicts noncontact. Harrison et al. (1991) recognize that this sort of contact bias tends to create a more positive treatment outcome. Number of risk factors are misleading because they are not necessarily independent, tending to cluster in individuals. Harrison et al. attempt to account for possible sample bias due to attrition by extrapolating results to patients lost to follow-up.

Treatment outcomes

Some of the results Harrison et al. report for a 12-month follow-up of approximately 1,900 completers of inpatient treatment who were interviewed at 6- and 12-month follow-ups are as follows: 72% were abstinent from alcohol and all other drugs for the entire first 6 months; 63% were abstinent for the entire year; 87% were abstinent at least 6 of the 12 months and 75% were either totally abstinent or suffered a relatively brief relapse. Outcome varied with several factors: 71% of inpatients with alcohol misuse only were abstinent the entire year; 52% of inpatients with marijuana misuse with or without alcohol misuse were abstinent for the year; 50% of inpatients with cocaine misuse regardless of other drug misuse were abstinent for the year.

INPATIENTS: CORRELATES OF ABSTINENCE

Family involvement

Harrison et al. (1991) raise an important problem in their examination of the relationship between family involvement and treatment outcome. Most treatment programs now require family involvement in the treatment process. Küfner and Feuerlein (1989) report that a counselor's attitude favoring involvement of significant others in the treatment of their patients is an important correlate of successful treatment outcomes. However, requiring family involvement may be a negative factor for certain patients. Patient refusal to have family involvement in their treatment may be a healthy decision at times, reflecting an attempt on the patients' part to deal with problems of sexual and physical abuse within their family.

After-care

Treatment program sponsored after-care was not utilized by all patients for a variety of reasons, personal choice, lack of availability, lack of transportation, etc. Treatment outcome was correlated with intensity of after-care involvement. An abstinence rate of 84% was obtained by patients involved in after-care for the full year as compared to 72% for those involved 6-11 months and 54% for those involved less than 6 months in after-care.

Peer support groups

An abstinence rate of 76% (n = 943) was obtained by those engaged in weekly meetings of a peer support group such as AA, 62% (n = 115) for those who attended several times a month, decreasing to 51% (n = 519) for those who did not attend at all. Attendance in support groups, in most cases AA, was related to significant improvement in abstinence rates. We must remember, again, that these kinds of results demonstrate a correlation between AA attendance and improvement in abstinence rate. Küfner and Feuerlein's (1989) analyses suggest more clearly that the relationship is a causal one as do the results reported by Humphrey et al. (1999).

Risks for relapse

Most patients, relapsed and abstinent, cite dysphoria as a major obstacle to recovery, boredom, anger, fear, etc, conditions noted by Ludwig and Stark (1974) as correlates of relapse. Harrison et al. (1991) found that relapsers, (n=707), had significantly more complaints than abstainers, (n=1211), concerning marital or relationship problems, stress from family problems, financial problems, craving for alcohol or other drugs, not really wanting to quit, and the belief that they were really not dependent. Ten percent of the abstainers voiced the latter complaint as compared to 25% of the patients who relapsed.

There is a common problem in retrospective reports of factors contributing to relapse. Are the reports accurate depictions of conditions leading to relapse or are they a description of the consequences of relapse? Using prospective and retrospective reports, Hall et al. (1990) found that patients' retrospective reports confused the dysphoric consequences of relapse and its causes. Harrison et al. (1991) conducted further analyses of their data to address the potential dangers inherent in retrospective reports. Their analysis is similar to Küfner and Feuerlein's "causal analytic" procedure. They compared inpatients abstinent during the first and second 6-months following treatment with patients who were abstinent the first 6 months who relapsed during the second 6-month interval. Relapsed patients had significantly more dysphoric complaints during the first 6 months of abstinence than the abstinent patients had during that same period. Reported risk factors preceded the occurrence of relapse rather than followed as a consequence of the relapse. These results suggest that the abstinence outcome rate could be increased if treatment addressed the kinds of problems voiced significantly more often by the eventual relapsers, 59%, especially the feelings of dysphoria, as compared to abstainers, 33%. Although dysphoria was the most common complaint expressed by the relapsers, it also was the most common complaint expressed by the abstainers.

Why did the abstainers who voiced the same complaints not relapse whereas the relapsers did? There must be factors differentiating relapsers and abstainers in addition to reported feelings of anger, loneliness, or depression, including the basic physiological processes producing the dysphoric feelings expressed in verbal reports. Interactions among dysphoric complaints and their possible partial correlations with other variables influencing inpatient outcomes need to be examined to institute an effective and efficient relapse prevention program.

by the authors of the first Rand Report for minimizing their large attrition rate (Armor et al., 1976) and the lack of concern by uncritical supporters (Marlatt, 1983; Mendelson & Melo, 1985) of the Rand Report I because of its purported evidence for controlled drinking.

HAZELDEN TREATMENT RESULTS

Hazelden, a private treatment facility with a research and education arm, is one of the origins of the Minnesota Model, the integration of 12-step principles and clinical psychology. A study of patients treated at this facility between 1989-1991 as well as a description of its treatment program is therefore worth reviewing (Stinchfield & Owen, 1998). A sample of 1083 patients was recruited from among 1128 admitted to Hazelden during the index period. Their average age was 39 years; approximately 95% were white and 32% were female. A majority were full- or part-time employed and had graduated high school; 31% were college graduates. Using DSM-III-R criteria, 94% were diagnosed as suffering from alcohol abuse or dependence; 58% met the diagnostic criteria for marijuana abuse or dependence. Average length of stay was 28 days with a range of 1-49 days. A subgroup of 62 patients received further extended care averaging 122 days. Following their discharge patients and family members were encouraged to attend meetings of 12-step oriented self-help groups.

Residential treatment was provided in separate units for men and women. Group therapy was the largest component of the treatment, 80%-90%. Individual therapy provided an opportunity to review progress, treatment issues, and highly sensitive experiences that might be inappropriate for group sessions. Lectures, group discussions, homework assignments, and attendance at self-help groups were integral parts of the treatment. Individualized treatments were developed with an emphasis on the 12-steps and group affiliation as the agent of change. Matching of patients with treatments occurred through groups focused on specific problems or patient characteristics such as women, incest and dual disorders. A family program was provided for family members and a family conference was arranged near the end of treatment with the patient, counselor, and family members. Weekly after-care sessions were scheduled for at least 10 weeks following discharge from treatment.

Patients were mailed a follow-up questionnaire at 1, 6, and 12 months following discharge. A collateral also received a questionnaire after 12 months. A telephone follow-up interview was given if the questionnaire was not returned in three weeks.

Results for the 12-month follow-up showed that complete abstinence from alcohol and all other drugs since discharge was attained by 53% of the participants. An additional 35% reported that they were not using as much as prior to treatment. Analyses of pre- and posttreatment use of alcohol and other drugs showed a significant decrease in all drug use, alcohol, marijuana, cocaine, sedatives, stimulants, opiates, etc., except for one, inhalants. Its use did not decrease significantly because of a basement effect. Use prior to treatment was so low there was no room to show a significant decline. Good agreement was obtained between collateral and patient reports. More than half the patients reported improvement in their relations with their significant others and in their physical health. A contact bias was evident in that 75% of the patients who returned their questionnaires were abstinent as compared to 45% who required a follow-up telephone interview. Since their results are based on a follow-up response from 71% of the sample, Stinchfield and Owen (1998) suggest that their results represent the upper limits of outcome success. People lost to the follow-up probably had poorer outcomes.

AVERSION CONDITIONING AS PRACTICED AT SCHICK SHADEL HOSPITALS

An extensive study of aversion conditioning made use of the CATOR registry to develop a comparison group (Smith, Frawley, & Polissar, 1991). Some of its results were briefly described in chapter 1. We will now consider its rather striking results in greater detail, as well as the results of a larger more recent study (Smith & Frawley, 1993) and a third study that differentiates between the treatment outcomes for chemical aversion and faradic or electric shock aversion (Smith, Frawley, & Polissar, 1997). Results for both kinds of aversion therapy are combined in the first two studies by the Schick Shadel group.

Rather than attempting to control individual differences among patients receiving aversion conditioning versus patients receiving traditional treatments by means of multivariate analyses of prognostic variables, Smith et al. (1991) matched 249 patients treated in a Schick Shadel hospital with patients from the CATOR registry. Patients were matched on 17 different variables from pretreatment baseline measures selected as likely prognosticators of treatment outcome. There was an additional requirement that the 6-month follow-up rate be comparable in the two groups. Such matching was possible because of the large CATOR registry. Baseline matching variables included gender, age, marital status, education, amount of full time work in past year, work problems, marijuana use, cocaine use, prior treatment, psychiatric hospital treatment, last alcoholic use, and detoxification.

Aversion conditioning as employed at Schick Shadel hospitals is part of a multimodal treatment that includes more than simply submitting patients to classical conditioning with an aversive unconditioned stimulus. It involves, if necessary, detoxification from alcohol and all other drugs followed by 10 days of treatment involving alternate days of conditioning, either chemical aversion or faradic shock, and interviews under sodium pentothal. Behaviorally oriented (Smith, 1980) daily group counseling is furnished as well as individual and family counseling. Educational programs provide information on drugs, and there is an individualized treatment and continuing after-care plan. Theoretical orientation is based on a biobehavioral disease concept of alcoholism. Treatment received by the comparison patients from the CATOR registry follow the Minnesota Model. None employs aversion conditioning.

Not all participants at Schick Shadel hospitals receive chemical aversion conditioning. Older patients and those with biomedical conditions precluding nausea and vomiting, an integral part of chemical aversion conditioning, receive faradic aversion conditioning instead, electric shocks to the wrist. Results obtained with faradic and chemical aversion conditioning are not differentiated in the present study. They are in a later study (Smith et al., 1997). Results for faradic aversion conditioning are especially interesting because electric shock in the hands of other investigators (no pun intended) has generally been a failure (Cannon & Baker, 1981; Cannon, Baker, & Wehl, 1981). Reasons for the difference in results will be discussed following a review of treatment outcomes.

Family counseling, after-care, and return reinforcement during after-care are also part of the Schick Shadel treatment program. Each of these components may have important effects on treatment outcomes. Another noteworthy aspect of the Schick Shadel program is that it is relatively brief, only 10 days of inpatient treatment following detoxification. After completion of the 10 day treatment program the patient is discharged and is scheduled to return after 1 month and again after 3 months for 2-day reinforcement treatments. These provide aversion treatment, an interview under sodium pentothal, counseling, and a review of the continuing care plan individually designed for each patient.

Results

As in the CATOR study outcomes described by Harrison et al. (1991), treatment evaluations were conducted by a team independent of the Schick Shadel treatment group. Treatment outcome was assessed in terms of abstinence defined as total continuous abstinence during the time interval specified, i.e., 0-6 months, 7-12 months, and 0-12 months. Results for the three intervals were, 85%, 86%, and 79% abstinence for Schick Shadel and 72%, 74%, and 67% abstinence for the comparison group. These are rather striking results, continuous abstinence for the entire year by 79% of the Schick Shadel patients and 67% for the comparison group. Between-group differences are statistically significant. Two features are noteworthy, the high rate of success for the aversion conditioning multimodal treatment provided by Schick Shadel and the relatively high success rate for traditional Minnesota Model treatment programs in the private sector.

Polydrug use is common among inpatients, as we have seen in the CATOR report by Harrison et al. (1991). Rates of abstinence from all drugs for the three evaluation periods for the Schick Shadel patients were, 79%, 77%, and 69%, respectively. For the comparison group, abstinence rates from all drugs were, 70%, 73%, and 65%. Only the difference between treatment groups obtained for the first six month interval is statistically significant. Rates of 69% and 65% continuous abstinence for a year from all drugs including alcohol, again, are striking. These rates are more than twice as high as those reported for the MATCH PROJECT (Project MATCH Research Group, 1997) for alcohol alone. Participants were not randomly assigned, but does anyone really think that the results are due to chance or spontaneous remission, the product of uncontrolled observations not worth mentioning in reviews of the literature and handbooks for counselors?

Forty-two Schick Shadel patients and 44 comparison group patients were lost to the 12-month follow-up. Drop-outs had a lower rate of abstinence at the 6-month follow-up in both groups as compared to those that were found at 12 months. Considering the 12-month abstinence rates for completers excluding the drop-outs at six months, included in the above results, abstinence rates for all drugs for the completers was 83% and for alcohol alone it was 89%. Abstinence rates for the completers in the comparison group were 73% and 79% for all drugs and for alcohol only, respectively. It is noteworthy that the MATCH project (Project MATCH Research Group, 1997, 1998) only presents results for completers of treatment.

Reinforcements During After-care

Patients in the Schick Shadel program are asked to return one month following treatment discharge for two days to receive a session of aversion conditioning, a sodium pentothal interview, and counseling. Patients are asked to return again after 3 months post-treatment discharge for another two days of treatment. Percent abstinence for alcohol alone and for all drugs is significantly related to compliance. For those who returned for both reinforcement sessions, 75% were continuously abstinent for all drugs and 86% were abstinent for alcohol alone. Percent abstinence among people who came to neither reinforcment session was 47% for all drugs and 47% for alcohol. There were 176 compliers and 16 noncompliers. Intermediate results were displayed by the remainder who came for one reinforcement session.

After-care support groups

Participating in support groups following treatment including AA, Schick Shadel-sponsored groups, and church groups was correlated with increased abstinence rates in the index and comparison groups. For example, patients in the Schick Shadel group who did not attend AA meetings during the first six months had an abstinent rate for all drugs of 77% during months 7-12 as compared to an 84% abstinence rate for those attending on a weekly basis. For patients in the comparison group, nonattendees during the first 6-months post-treatment period had an abstinence rate of 54% in the second 6-month follow-up period as compared to the weekly attendees who had an abstinence rate of 81% for all drugs for months 7-12.

Comparison of chemical and faradic aversion

A later report compared the subgroups receiving either faradic or chemical aversion conditioning (Smith et al., 1997). Participants were the same as described in the earlier report. Thirty-two patients received faradic and 212 received chemical aversion. After attrition, 20 participants receiving faradic aversion and 142 receiving chemical aversion remained for the 1-year follow-up interview. Percent abstinence from all drugs for one year was 80% for faradic aversion and 66% for the chemical aversion group, a nonsignificant difference. Aversion conditioning was used only for alcohol in this study with counseling for other drugs.

Further analyses showed that the faradic aversion group was older, had fewer unmarried participants and more prior treatment. Controlling these factors did not modify the results. Returning for posttreatment reinforcement increased rate of abstinence with both forms of aversion conditioning.

ANOTHER SCHICK SHADEL STUDY

Another treatment outcome study (Smith & Frawley, 1993) has been reported on a sample of patients from four different Schick Shadel facilities, n=600, but with no matched traditional treatment group. Telephone interviews by an independent research organization were obtained from 71.2% of the sample. An independent interview was obtained from a collateral of 42% of the patients. Charts of noncontacted patients were reviewed for documented relapses so that there was some form of follow-up of all 600 patients. Interviews occurred from 12-20 months following completion of treatment, mean = 14.7 months. A majority of the patients were white males who were married and employed. All met the DSM-III-R criteria for alcohol dependence. More than half the patients, 52.5% were using one or more drugs in addition to alcohol. Marijuana, 25%, and cocaine, 15%, were the two most frequently used additional drugs.

Results

A 14-month alcohol abstinence rate was reported by 69% of the total sample. The 14-month abstinence rate for patients reporting cocaine abuse prior to treatment was 65%. Patients reporting marijuana abuse prior to treatment had an alcohol abstinence rate of 68% for 14 months. Patients who had no other drug problem than alcoholism had a 14-month alcohol abstinence rate of 72%.

Some of the patients who had been abusing cocaine and marijuana agreed to have aversion conditioning for these drugs as well as for alcohol. Of the 75 patients who had received aversion conditioning for cocaine, their 14-month abstinence rate for cocaine was 76%. For the total sample of patients receiving aversion conditioning for marijuana abuse, n = 47, 73% had a 14-month abstinence rate.

There was no difference in alcohol abstinence as a function of type of aversion conditioning, chemical or faradic, or in a few cases both. The latter occurred when an individual started with chemical aversion conditioning and for medical reasons or personal preference was switched to faradic aversion.

Prognostic indicators of abstinence

As before, two variables were related to increased abstinence, (a) reinforcement treatments following completion of inpatient treatment and, (b) after-care attendance in support groups. Nearly half the patients attended support groups; more than one hundred each attended AA meetings and Schick Shadel sponsored groups. Smaller numbers attended church sponsored groups and others received some form of professional counseling. Some people attended more than one kind of support group. A comparison of the participants that attended support groups, n=232, with those attending no support group meetings, n=195, showed total abstinence rates of 68% and 49%, respectively. Once again, it was found that after-care support group attendance is a significant correlate of treatment success.

A second predictor of abstinence in the Schick Shadel treatment program is the number of post treatment reinforcements received. People who received no reinforcement showed a total abstinence rate of 29% as compared to 51% for 1 reinforcement, 69% for 2 reinforcements and 80% abstinence for those who received more than 2 reinforcements. These abstinence rates cover the entire 12-20 month follow-up period.

Craving

The best predictor of abstinence was the loss of urges or craving (Smith & Frawley, 1993). Following treatment patients were asked to respond to a questionnaire: whether they lost all urges, lost all uncontrollable urges, or still have urges to drink or use drugs. Participants who reported that they lost all urges showed an abstinence rate of 90% as compared to 57% for those who said they lost uncontrollable urges and only a 6% abstinence rate for those who reported that they still had urges. In turn, persistence of craving was inversely related to the number of post-treatment reinforcements received.

Conclusions

Treatment results obtained by the Schick Shadel group with the conditioned aversion method, especially with faradic conditioning are striking for several reasons: (a) Their high abstinence rate obtained by faradic as well as chemical aversion conditioning appears to be the most effective treatment program available; (b) inhibition of craving by faradic as well as chemical aversion is striking, and (c) the complete disregard of these results by alcohol treatment practitioners as well as research investigators is deplorable. Aversion conditioning especially by the faradic method demands further experimental study. An explanation for the discrepancy between the success rate attained by the Shick Shadel group in contrast to other investigators and suggestions for research that may resolve the apparent conflicting results follows.

An interpretation of faradic aversion conditioning and a research proposal

Results from the Schick Shadel aversion conditioning treatment program are striking and in some respects surprising. First, a 10-day treatment program with two subsequent reinforcements was significantly better than a matched comparison group of participants in more extended Minnesota Model treatment programs. Both groups' treatment outcomes are markedly superior to results obtained in the MATCH project and in behavior therapy efficacy studies (see chapter 6). Second, patients receiving faradic aversion conditioning did at least as well as patients receiving chemical aversion conditioning although it must be recognized that different kinds of patients received the two types of treatment and results from a relatively small number of patients receiving faradic aversion conditioning were involved. Third, small efficacy experiments have not had corresponding success, especially with faradic conditioning (Cannon & Baker, 1981; Cannon et al., 1981; Miller, Hersen, Eisler, & Hemphill, 1973).

Chemical aversion conditioning as a treatment for alcoholics was introduced many years ago based on Pavlovian classical conditioning principles. Subsequent research indicates that there is a biological basis for the rapid development of powerful taste aversions. An association between taste and nausea develops more quickly, is more robust, and may develop after a longer temporal interval than the familiar conditioning of an external stimulus and response. An extensive body of research demonstrating this "Garcia effect", conditioned taste aversion (Garcia, McGowan, & Green, 1966; Gustavson, Garcia, Hankins, & Rusiniak, 1974), provides a reasonable experimental and theoretical basis for use of chemical aversion conditioning in alcoholism treatment.

Faradic aversion conditioning using electric shock appears to be a different story. It has met with repeated failure in efficacy studies and generally has been discarded by behavior therapists as a viable treatment (Hester & Miller, 1995; Wilson, 1978). A perplexing problem is the marked discrepancy between results of faradic aversion conditioning in the Schick Shadel treatment program and experimental attempts by other investigators to treat alcoholism with electric shock. The answer may be that other investigators have not replicated the Schick Shadel program in all its aspects including the conditioning procedure it uses.

As previously observed, the Schick Shadel treatment program has several unique characteristics. It uses sodium pentothal interviews and conditioning on alternate days and calls back its patients twice for after-care conditioning sessions, sodium pentothal interviews, and counseling. Faradic aversion conditioning as a component in the treatment package is especially interesting because it along with sodium pentothal interviews could be given on an out-patient basis to a wider range of patients than possible with chemical aversion conditioning. It also appears to be an effective treatment for other drugs of abuse as well as alcohol.

Perhaps aversion conditioning of both kinds, chemical and faradic, are ineffective and it is the sodium pentothal interviews that produce the striking therapeutic outcome. It is logically possible that all or most of the effectiveness of the Schick Shadel treatment program is due to its counseling interviews while under sodium penthothal. In the sodium pentothal interview the patient can describe their motivation, craving for alcohol or other drugs and other problems more freely than in the usual counseling session. Sodium pentothal is a fast acting barbiturate with a short half life. It quickly inhibits anxiety induced while the patient is relating their experiences in an unusually relaxed and pleasurable state. However, it is unlikely that sodium pentothal interviews are the entire basis for the effectiveness of chemical aversion conditioning, since a high degree of success was reported for the conditioning procedure prior to the introduction of sodium penthothal interviews (Lemere & Voegtlin, 1950).

Examination of the details of the faradic conditioning procedure used in efficacy studies shows that investigators have not replicated the Schick Shadel conditioning procedure quite aside from the absence of sodium pentothal interviews. Cannon and Baker (1981) describe their faradic conditioning procedure based on one used by Vogler, Lunde, Johnson, & Marti (1970), as follows:

> On each trial, the subject lifted the glass, sniffed the beverage, and swished a mouthful. Shock was usually initiated as soon as a subject tasted an alcoholic beverage, and it remained on until the beverage was spit into an adjacent basin... The occurrence and intensity of the shock varied unpredictably across trials to increase shock aversiveness and promote resistance to extinction. (p. 23).

A similar faradic conditioning procedure was used by Miller et al. (1973) who also obtained negative results. Faradic shock aversion used at Schick Shadel treatment facilities is fundamentally different. The patient is provided with an array of alcoholic and nonalcoholic beverages. Forced choice trials are initially given where the patient is asked to reach for an alcoholic beverage, smell, taste, and spit it out. From 1 to 8 unpredictable shocks occur during the behavior sequence. After several forced trials the patient is instructed that they have a choice between alcoholic and nonalcoholic beverages. In the latter free choice trials the patient will continue to receive intermittent shocks until choice of a juice results in cessation of shock or the avoidance of shock entirely if juice is initially selected. Each conditioning session consists of several forced and free choice trials (Chapman & Smith, 1972; Jackson & Smith, 1978; J. W. Smith, personal communication, April 4, 1999).

Major differences between the two conditioning procedures are apparent. Free choice trials interspersed among forced choice trials was not the procedure used in studies obtaining negative treatment outcomes (Cannon & Baker, 1981; Miller et al., 1973). The latter studies used a partial reinforcement escape conditioning procedure with an alcoholic beverage. One consequence is that the more unpredictable shock treatment used by Schick Shadel on forced choice trials is a more stressful conditioning situation than the one used in other studies. Stress induced by unpredictable shock induces the release of endogenous opioids (Lewis, Cannon, & Liebeskind, 1980), whereas the relatively predictable stress used by Cannon and Baker and other investigators using shock aversion conditioning may not have the same effect. Free choice trials in which choice of juice terminates or avoids shock forces the participant to orient to an alternative beverage thereby activating the mesocorticolimbic system component of the OR. Participants are thus conditioned to orient to an alternative beverage in a stressful situation facilitating inhibition of ORs to alcohol. At the same time the stressful unpredictable shock temporarily increases endorphin levels, reducing the need for alcohol. All this is part of a package of behavioral treatments provided in the multimodal Schick Shadel program.

Chemical and faradic aversion may be equally and highly effective not only because they are part of the same treatment package in which common components may contribute to a comparable outcome, but we suspect because they both produce changes in the biological state of the alcoholic. Chemical aversion has the apparent advantage of relying on the biological preparedness of the Garcia effect, an evolutionary disposition for nausea to be readily conditioned to taste and smell. It may be more important in the long term that chemical aversion activates the HPA system and the release of beta-endorphins. Chemical and faradic aversion conditioning as used in the Schick Shadel program are effective in large part by sharing the same basic biological mechanism: stress induced release of endogenous opioids. Aversion conditioning also involves dopaminergic activated orienting to alcohol which is extinguished by nonreinforcement and the conditioning of an incompatible biological state in chemical aversion and orienting to nonalcoholic beverages in faradic aversion. A critical component in Schick Shadel faradic aversion conditioning is the free choice situation where choice of a nonalcohol beverage avoids or escapes shock, forcing the individual to orient and taste an alternative beverage. This choice component is missing in other electric shock aversion conditioning studies. Just as a choice situation promotes acquistion of alcohol dependence (see chapter 3), a choice situation in which a nonalcoholic beverage is chosen promotes extinction of the dependence.

Research designed to demonstrate the efficacy of faradic aversion conditioning and sodium pentothal interviews with a representative patient sample would be especially useful. It could provide an effective short - only 10 day - outpatient treatment program applicable to a diverse population and a variety of different drugs. It would require a 2 x 2 factorial design in which half the participants receive faradic aversion conditioning according to the Shick Shadel protocol and half receive the usual forced choice escape conditioning procedure with alcohol as the only beverage presented. Half of each of these two groups would receive interviews under sodium pentothal and half would receive interviews following injection of a placebo.

Since it costs nothing to fantasize, I suggest that the proposed research project should have two aims: (a) Evaluate the effectiveness of components of the Schick Shadel faradic conditioning treatment; and (b) evaluate the effects of the criteria for "moderate drinking" recommended by Heather and Tebbutt (1989) and related criteria in use. The necessity of follow-up assessments provides an opportunity to evaluate the use of "moderate" drinking criteria promoted by behavior therapists. At the same time as an evaluation of a potentially useful treatment program is conducted, for the first time an adequate evaluation can be obtained of the effects of "moderate" drinking levels on brain structure and function. A large sample of participants would be employed to provide a sufficient number of individuals who engage in controlled, moderate, drinking following treatment. During the pretreatment and follow-up periods MRI, fMRI or other neuroimaging procedures and neuropsychological tests could be administered as well the usual measures of alcohol consumption, liver function, social adjustment and quality of life. It would be possible, finally, to determine whether the "moderate" drinking levels proposed by Heather and Tibbutt (1989) and other such criteria (Harris & Miller, 1990) used in treatment efficacy studies are safe - and ethical.

Neuropsychological assessments of frontal lobe functioning and measures of brain structure and function by MRI and fMRI must be obtained in an initial assessment prior to the start of treatment, at discharge, and at follow-ups at 6-month intervals for at least four years. Where possible, blood, urine, or saliva should be sampled and assayed for levels of hormones, neurotransmitters, and their metabolites and ingestion of other licit and illicit drugs. Rather than relying solely on verbal reports modern biotechnology must be applied whenever possible to assess therapeutic change. Only then will this serious disease, alcoholism, be treated in the manner its seriousness requires, but always remembering that it is a human being who is being treated not a behavioral symptom, the discriminated operant of elbow bending.

COMPARISON OF INPATIENT VERSUS OUTPATIENT TREATMENT BY WALSH ET AL.

One of the myths promoted by Hester and Miller (1995) and others is that inpatient and outpatient treatments do not differ. As we have seen, Harrison et al. (1991) describe some of the difficulties in attempting to compare inpatient and outpatient groups. Such groups differ in a variety of dimensions. One relatively large single site study does avoid these problems in part by randomly assigning participants to inpatient and different outpatient treatments. The study has some design problems as we shall see, but the effort was enormous and the results interesting and worth reviewing.

Walsh et al's. (1995) extensive study comparing inpatient versus outpatient treatment was a major organizational and community effort made possible through the cooperation of a large union, the employer, a large corporation, and some 10 local hospitals. The study was conducted in conjunction with the employee assistance program (EAP) in a General Electric plant of 10,000 employees.

Individuals could participate in the study if, as an employee at the plant in question, they entered the EAP because they manifested alcohol related problems that interfered with their work. Exclusions were for the following reasons: it was not the first time an individual entered the EAP; severity of their alcohol problems required immediate hospitalization and medically supervised detoxification; a recent history of delirium tremens (DTs) and seizures or the imminent appearance of DTs would require medical attention; they posed an immediate danger to themselves or to others; they needed immediate psychiatric care; they would be difficult to follow-up because they were likely to be jailed or fired in the immediate future. Of the 371 employees who came to the attention of the EAP in the time frame of the study, 128, 35%, were ineligible for the study due to the above and related exclusionary criteria. The remaining 65%, 243 men and women, were recruited for the study, given a breathalyzer test that showed a blood alcohol level less than 0.2%, judged competent to give an informed consent and for whom a written informed consent was then obtained. A total of 227, 93%, provided their informed consent and were randomly assigned to one of three treatment groups. Staffs of the EAP program and research team were independent. Participants were assured that nothing revealed to the research staff would affect their treatment or their job.

Mean age = 33, white, 90%, men, 96%, comprised the sample studied. During the month preceding admission into the study they averaged 6.3 drinks/day, and approximately 20 drinking days/month. Twenty-one percent reported that they were drunk daily and an additional 45% were drunk weekly during the previous month. Approximately 90% were classified as alcoholic according to the short form of the Michigan Alcoholism Screening test (SMAST) (Selzer, Vinokur, & van Rooijen, 1975); 56% were classified as alcohol dependent according to DSM-III criteria. Other drug use during the past 6 months was common, cigarette smoking, 75%, marijuana, 59%, and cocaine, 39%.

Subjects were randomly assigned to the following three groups: (a) Compulsory hospitalization, n=73. Ten different hospitals provided inpatient treatment of approximately three weeks duration, although the great majority, 83%, were treated in one of two hospitals. (b) Compulsory AA only, n=83; participants were given an escort to daily meetings of AA if possible, or at least three meetings a week for at least one year; (c) Choice, n=71; participants in this group were involved in the planning of their own treatment. It was felt that the choice approach would enhance the self-efficacy of the patient and facilitate patient-treatment matching. Participants in the Choice group were not required to regularly attend AA meetings or enter a hospital for inpatient treatment. They were free to engage in no treatment program as long as they remained sober on the job, performed their job in an acceptable manner and reported to the EAP on a weekly basis. Twenty-nine participants in the Choice group voluntarily entered a hospital for inpatient treatment; 33 elected AA meetings; 3 selected outpatient psychotherapy, and 6 elected to abstain from any form of treatment or participation in a support group. Subjects in all three groups were required to participate in a year of after-care following their stay in the hospital, frequent AA meetings for one year, or the choice of treatment, respectively. After-care involved a year of job probation, attendance at AA meetings at least three times a week, and mandatory weekly checks with the EAP.

Staff of the EAP were authorized to recommend supplementary hospitalization for any participant who was not succeeding with their randomly assigned treatment. Such a decision was made on the basis of information collected by the staff of the EAP not the research staff. Criteria for additional treatment were enumerated in advance: intoxication at work, unexcused absenteeism in conjunction with imminent job termination due to alcohol related problems, and infringement of company rules and policies. Participants who received additional hospital treatment were retained in their original assigned group for purposes of statistical analyses. Such a procedure clouds the interpretation of some of the results, as we shall see.

Data were collected from interviews at the time of admission into the study and 1, 3, 6, 12, 18, and 24 months following admission. Three interviews were also conducted with spouses or significant others and the job supervisors. Trained research interviewers conducted all interviews blind to group assignment and independent of the staff of the EAP.

A structured 90-minute interview was used to obtain information designed to construct 12 composite variables describing job performance and 12 variables describing drinking and related behaviors. Information was also obtained related to job, family, and health histories, and current and past drinking and other drug use. Possible medical and psychiatric disorders were assessed with interview schedules based on DSM-III. Interviews with job supervisors assessed the participants' work performance, disciplinary actions, and drinking or intoxication on the job. Additional information was obtained at follow-up intervals from records of the EAP, hospitals, insurance-carrier claims, and the computerized plant payroll.

RESULTS

All 227 participants were followed-up through company records of job performance and time to additional treatment for drinking related problems. Ten to 14% of each group was lost to any one interview. The lowest percentage of subjects included in any one interview was 84%.

Job performance

There were no significant group differences in job performance. Significant improvement occurred on a variety of job performance measures in all three groups. For example, job warnings decreased from 33% at intake to less than 5% at each of the follow-up interview points.

Drinking outcomes

A total of 46 subjects, 23%, reported continuous abstinence at each interview point for the entire 24 months of the study. The three treatment groups differed significantly on eight of the twelve measures of alcohol consumption. The hospital group had a significantly higher rate of continuous sobriety for the 24 months than each of the other two groups which did not differ significantly from each other. Forty-three percent of the total sample was rehospitalized for additional treatment sometime during the two years of follow-up; hospital group, 23%; choice, 38%, and AA 63%. The hospital group was significantly superior to the other two groups and the choice group was superior to the AA group.

Walsh et al. (1991) report that at an exit interview, 41% of the participants reported that they were abstaining from alcohol; 23% reported continuous abstinence for the 24 months. Supervisors or significant others confirmed the reports of 85% of the abstainers. Average daily drinking was reported to be 1.5 drinks, down from the 6.3 reported at admission; average number of drinking days in a month decreased from 19.8 to 3.1. Proportion of participants classified as alcohol dependent decreased from 56% at admission to 14% at completion of the study. Walsh et al. (1991) conclude:

> We found no differences among the three groups in any job outcome, including being fired. All three groups evidently brought their drinking problems under sufficient control at work for group differences in job performance to be rendered statistically insignificant. But compulsory hospitalization with AA follow-up addressed drinking problems significantly more effectively than did compulsory AA alone. Results of choice were intermediate between the two. The relatively low rate of relapse in the hospital group was an unexpected finding.
>
> This study had limitations that should be borne in mind. First, a larger sample would have bolstered our confidence in the absence of differences in job outcomes and permitted fuller investigations of differences among subgroups of the choice group and interactions between subjects and treatments. Second, because the study spanned seven years, a cohort effect in the workers enrolled and in historical events might have influenced the outcomes. The randomization process should have distributed these influences evenly among the three groups, and in several analyses we found scant evidence of cohort effects at followup. (p.780).

Treatment costs

An estimate of inpatient treatment costs during the 24 month follow-up period was obtained for the three groups, assuming inpatient costs of $400/day. It is a limited analysis of cost effectiveness since it did not consider time lost from work, outpatient psychotherapy received by participants in the choice group, and medical costs aside from alcoholism treatment. However, it is the simplest figure to calculate. It was found that the AA group averaged $1200 less per person than the inpatient treatment group, and the choice group was almost identical to the AA group yielding a figure that amounts to a 10% savings in inpatient costs. This relatively small difference is due to the relatively large number of relapses requiring hospitalization in the AA and choice groups. Sixty-three percent of the participants randomly assigned to the AA group eventually needed hospitalization. Results for the choice group were almost identical to the AA group for the same reason, relapses requiring hospitalization. Despite the limited assessment of costs these results suggest that what may appear to be a less expensive treatment initially may cost more in the long run because of relapses.

Cost effectiveness results as well as the high rate of relapse in the two groups not receiving inpatient treatment suggest that Walsh et al. should have attempted to analyse the subgroups within the AA, choice, and inpatient hospitalization groups who did or did not receive inpatient rehospitalization, in terms of the various performance and consumption variables. Absence of differences in job performance may be due to the hybrid nature of the two outpatient groups; more than half received some inpatient treatment. What was their job performance and drinking before and after the rehospitalization? In other words, a fine-grained analysis of the subgroups within each of the three randomly assigned groups, although involving relatively small numbers of subjects, could have been informative.

It is apparent that inpatient treatment has an important role, especially for individuals with severe alcohol dependence, which may be an oxymoron. All cases of alcohol dependence are a serious matter. It is also apparent that inpatient treatment is more cost effective than it appears once the long term including relapses is considered, a problem that needs to be analysed in greater detail. Superiority of inpatient to outpatient treatments as found by Walsh et al. on a variety of important variables, cannot be generalized to all inpatient versus all outpatient treatments. However, it is equally clear that the unqualified generalization promulgated by Miller, Hester and other revisionists, that there is no evidence that inpatient treatment is better than outpatient treatment is contradicted by the results reported by Walsh et al. (1991).

Several aspects of the Walsh et al. (1991) study must be kept in mind. There was random assignment of the subject pool to inpatient and outpatient conditions with certain restrictions. Severe cases of alcoholism, those requiring medical attention for detoxication or dual diagnoses were not randomly assigned but sent directly to inpatient hospital care. Exclusions from the study as well as the obtained results indicate that there is an essential need for inpatient treatment that is not a matter of choice. People with severe dependence on alcohol or other drugs and severe comorbid psychopathology need inpatient treatment, intensive treatment in a safe environment. Second, the circumstances of the Walsh et al. study are relatively unique. It was conducted with the cooperation of a large industrial corporation, a union, and hospitals.

All segments of our society should be as farsighted and thoughtful! On the other hand, obtaining volunteers from media advertisements, the recruitment method employed by Miller and others conducting clinical trials, is also relatively unique and has limitations with respect to the type of participant suited for such treatment. Still larger studies of the sort pioneered by Walsh et al. are needed so that more detailed analysis of subgroups can be conducted. There is a need for studies with a greater ethnic and gender mix of participants. Different kinds of outpatient therapies need to be studied such as behavioral self-control and problem solving skills and compared with inpatient multimodal traditional treatment. Type of treatment and inpatient versus outpatient treatments are confounded in the Walsh et al. study. A similar study needs to be conducted with multimodal traditional treatment provided to inpatients and outpatients. With a larger sample of subjects and treatment facilities the effectiveness of individual treatment facilities could be examined as well as the type of treatment. Finally, the participants in this study were all employed, functioning problem drinkers and alcohol dependent (56%) individuals. Nevertheless, inpatient treatment yielded significantly more abstinent participants than found among employees randomly assigned to treatment choice and AA alone. Offering a choice of treatment to participants did not result in superior outcomes, contrary to the proposition that choice, autonomy, promotes self-efficacy and treatment success (Rotgers, 1996a; Sobell & Sobell, 1995b).

TREATMENT INTENSITY AND TREATMENT GOAL

Monahan and Finney (1996) avoid many of the biasing effects found in the Miller et al. (1995) review by conducting a more comprehensive computer search of data bases between 1980-1992 than attempted by Miller et al. At the same time Monahan and Finney limited their search to more recent studies likely to have employed current treatment methods. They still find problems in using all relevant studies because many do not adequately describe their participants, treatment methods, or number of participants entering treatment. Studies also fail to employ common outcome measures.

Abstinence rate at the 3-month follow-up was the basic outcome measure Monahan and Finney (1996) used in their analysis because the majority of studies had at least this one measure and follow-up interval. Treatment conditions were examined rather than independent studies, in contrast to Miller et al. (1995). Examining treatment conditions rather than entire studies permitted Monahan and Finney to analyze reports which had only one group of patients, provided that they had at least one relevant measure of a pretreatment subject characteristic as well as the appropriate outcome measure. Pretreatment measures of social stability, either information on marital status or employment, were a requirement for inclusion of a study in the review.

Results were synthesized for 150 treatment conditions obtained from 100 different studies. Conditions assessed were: (a) treatment goal, either abstinence or controlled drinking; (b) treatment intensity; (c) availability of antabuse or similar medications; (d) involvement of family members or significant others in treatment; and (e) use of behavioral techniques such as social skills training, aversion therapy, relapse prevention, or community reinforcement. Research design characteristics examined were: (a) exclusionary criteria, whether severely impaired patients were excluded or not; (b) definition of abstinence employed, whether complete no-drinking was the criterion or whether slips were allowed; and (c) length of the follow-up evaluation window and the follow-up rates. Examination of the effects of different treatment conditions on post-treatment abstinence rates was accomplished by statistically controlling patient and design characteristics by multiple regression techniques.

Treatment intensity

Treatment intensity effects were one of their most interesting and important findings. A variety of studies and reviews have concluded that more intense treatment is no more effective than less intense treatments and, since they are related, inpatient treatment is no more effective than outpatient treatment for most patients (Annis, 1986; Hester & Miller, 1995; Miller & Hester, 1986). We have already seen that this kind of generalization is meaningless unless treatments are matched in terms of prognostic characteristics of patients or patients are randomly assigned to treatments. When these controls are employed the generalization that amount of treatment and inpatient versus outpatient treatment is of no consequence is contradicted (Küfner & Feuerlein, 1989; Walsh et al., 1991). The range of intensity of treatments provided is a variable of considerable importance. This variable is usually ignored in brief interventions that fail to find a difference between treatments of different intensity. Hence short treatments or advice is as effective as longer treatments (Orford & Edwards, 1977).

Monahan and Finney (1996) averaged the number of days of treatment in high-intensity settings such as inpatient settings, residential and day-hospital settings, and in outpatient settings. They then estimated the number of hours/day in each of these kinds of settings. Not all settings provided the necessary information but for those that did, high-intensity treatment programs averaged 148 hours of treatment whereas low-intensity treatment settings averaged 14 hours of treatment.

Intensity of treatment and treatment goal were found to be significant treatment characteristics. High intensity treatment settings produced abstinence rates 15 percent higher than low intensity settings. Treatment intensity was a significant variable regardless of facility type, private or public. Monahan and Finney (1996) discuss the discrepancy between their results and claims by other investigators such as Hester and Miller (1995) that treatment intensity does not make a difference. For one thing, Monahan and Finney did not limit their analyses to studies that compared two or more treatments differing in intensity within the same study. "By focusing on treatment condition abstinence rates rather than paired comparisons, we were able to incorporate studies that did not explicitly compare higher-intensity with lower-intensity treatments." (p. 801).

Another difference in Monahan and Finney's (1996) synthesis of results as compared to earlier analyses is that they had a wider range of intensity in their studies than had been examined in previous surveys. Their sample of high-intensity treatments provided an average of 148 hours of treatment as compared to an average of 14 hours for low intensity treatments, 10 times as many hours of treatment, considerably greater than the classic studies of advice versus 9.6 hours of treatment (Orford & Edwards, 1977). The average number of hours in the less intense group of studies, 14, which yields significantly poorer outcomes than the high intensity treatments, is greater than the number of hours of treatment provided in the MATCH project (1997), 12 and 4 which were even less in practice due to drop-outs. Project MATCH's treatment intensities were an unfortunate choice given the information on reliable differences in treatment outcome as a function of treatment intensity reported by Monahan and Finney (1996).

Treatment goal

Treatment goal also makes a difference. Statistically controlling for other variables, programs with an abstinence goal averaged 26 percent higher abstinence rates than treatments with alternative goals. Family involvement and the use of behavioral elements were not related to treatment success. Family involvement results appear surprising because Küfner and Feuerlein (1989) found family involvement to be an important variable. It is difficult to compare Monahan and Finney's (1996) synthesis of results from many independent treatment programs with Küfner and Feuerlein's results obtained from far fewer and possibly more homogeneous programs. There may have been greater variability in how families were involved in programs studied by Monahan and Finney than in Küfner and Feuerlein's study. A more analytic approach is needed to assess differences among programs and the nature of family involvement in such programs. Flexibility is essential in that family involvement may have negative impact on treatment success for a patient who had suffered physical or sexual abuse from a family member who is now actively involved in their treatment program.

"Facility type was a significant predictor of abstinence rates... Controlling for the other predictors, private programs reported abstinence rates that were an average of 10 percentage points higher than rates reported by public treatment programs" (Monahan & Finney, 1996, pp. 798-799). It is possible that any number of variables not incorporated in Monahan and Finney's synthesis may be responsible for the obtained result, including unexamined patient characteristics. It is also possible that private sector facilities simply provide better treatment due to more and better trained counselors and a more effective program. A serious shortcoming in many studies is the lack of information concerning the workings of the treatment facilities, nature of the interactions of staff and patient, satisfaction of the patient at the beginning and completion of treatment, etc., the kind of information that could be obtained using one or more of Moos' (Moos & Humphrey, 1974) social climate scales. It is a pity that such scales and others (Finney, 1995; Moos, 1997a) are not a standard part of an assessment battery administered on intake and completion of treatment in all treatment programs.

PROJECT MATCH

Project MATCH (1993, 1997, 1998) was the largest and most expensive clinical trial of alcoholism treatments ever funded by the NIAAA, $27,000,000. It appears to have come about as a consequence of revisionists' successful promotion of two false propositions: (a) There is no evidence that traditional treatments work, and they are too long and expensive. (b) There is no one treatment that is effective for everyone with alcohol problems. There has to be matching of treatments to patients. Present traditional treatments force every one into the same mold.

The above propositions and their implications lead to the conclusion that the most cost effective way to deal with alcohol problems is to employ the research confirmed behavior therapy methods such as brief interventions, behavioral self-control, social skills training, and motivational enhancement. A clinical trial of these methods would provide proof of the above propositions. A condition resembling traditional treatment should be included in the trial to placate traditionalists and to demonstrate its inadequacy.

Results obtained by Project MATCH were described by its spokespersons as follows:

Overall, Project MATCH participants showed significant sustained improvement in increased percentage of abstinent days and decreased number of drinks per drinking days, with few clinically significant outcome differences among the three treatments in either treatment arm... However, outpatients who received 12-step facilitation were more likely to remain completely abstinent in the year following treatment than outpatients who received the other treatments...

The Project MATCH patients probably did well because the treatments were of high quality and well delivered, according to Thomas F. Babor... principal investigator for the Project MATCH Coordinating Center: 'The striking differences in drinking from pretreatment levels to all followup points suggest that participation in any of the MATCH treatments would be associated with marked positive change.'

The Project MATCH findings may surprise but should not dismay those who foresaw a revolution in alcohol treatment delivery based on patient-treatment matching, said Dr. Gordis [Director of NIAAA]. 'These findings are good news for treatment providers and for patients who can have confidence that any one of these treatments, if well-delivered, represents the state of the art in behavioral treatments.' (NIH News Release, nd).

Methodologically, Project MATCH is the largest and most sophisticated study ever conducted on alcoholism treatment efficacy. Participants were randomly assigned to treatments; different teams conducted treatment and research; sources of subject attrition were determined; collateral sources including physiological measures confirmed validity of reports; and extensive measures of preassessment status were obtained. Its external or ecological validity, its generalizability to regular treatment facilities and its substantive contribution to possible improvement in the treatment of alcoholics and problem drinkers is another matter. Its results make no contribution to treatment effectiveness or theory. Such an outcome was predictable from the studies reviewed in this and the previous chapter. Let's see what results were obtained by Project MATCH and why the disappointing outcomes contrary to the claims of establishment spokespersons, were predictable.

Three treatment modalities were selected as the independent variable against which matches with clients were studied: Cognitive Behavioral Coping Skills Therapy (CBT), Motivational Enhancement Therapy (MET), and Twelve-Step Facilitation (TSF). They were delivered over a 12-week period. Weekly sessions were conducted with CBT and TSF whereas MET was delivered in four sessions, the 1st, 2nd, 6th and 12th weeks. Duration of each session in the three treatment modalities was not specified. If we can assume that they were each 1 hr in duration, the intensity of treatment is less than the average, 14, for the low intensity treatments that yield significantly poorer abstinence outcomes then high intensity treatments (Monahan & Feeney, 1996). On the average, approximately two-thirds of the sessions were attended. Patients received follow-up assessments every three months during the first-year follow-up.

The two principal measures of treatment outcome employed were: "percent days abstinent (PDA) and average number of drinks per drinking day (DDD)." (p. 8). Subjects were recruited at nine clinical research units (CRUs) each one responsible for several treatment facilities in the region. Five were outpatient CRUs and four were after-care CRUs. Since there was no random assignment to outpatient and after-care treatments, these were conducted as two independent experiments or arms of the project. There was random assignment of participants to the three treatment modalities within each of the project arms but not between arms.

Participants

Inclusion criteria for the participants in the outpatient arm of the study were: DSM-III-R diagnosis of alcohol abuse or dependence with alcohol as the principal drug misused; drinking during the 3 months immediately preceding participation in the study; minimum age of 18 with at least a sixth grade reading ability. Exclusion criteria were DSM-III-R diagnosis of current dependence on a sedative/hypnotic drug, stimulants, cocaine or opiates; intravenous drug use in previous 6 months, a danger to self or to others, criminal justice jurisdiction interfering with study participation, acute psychosis or organic impairment, social instability as indicated by uncertain residence and lack of a reliable collateral, and involvement in another treatment plan except for self-help groups during the 12 weeks of the index treatment. MATCH excluded patients suffering a dual diagnosis, comorbidity, polydrug dependence, and those lacking social stability and education. It excluded low social and economic status people with a poor prognosis. Of those included, 95% of the participants in the outpatient arm and 98% in the after-care arm met DSM-III-R criteria for alcohol dependence. Remaining participants met criteria for alcohol abuse.

Participants in the after-care arm of the study met the same criteria as the outpatients. In addition they completed at least a 7-day inpatient or day-hospital program other than detoxification and were referred for after-care treatment by the staff of the previous intensive treatment program.

All participants had to be within reasonable commuting distance of the outpatient or after-care facility and be willing to submit to random assignment to the treatment modalities. The outpatient arm of the study recruited 952 participants, 72% male and the after-care arm recruited 774 patients, 80% male. As the CATOR (Harrison et al., 1991) study found, outpatients tended to be younger, less dependent on alcohol, received fewer prior treatments, and were more socially stable then the after-care patients. Ethnicity and religion of the participants are not reported and presumably were not analyzed.

Recruits for the two arms of the study came from initial samples of more than 2,000 each, screened by CRUs, excluding people clearly ineligible due to dependence on other drugs in addition to alcohol. Of those eligible for the study, the largest single group declined to participate because of inconvenient location of the treatment facility or lack of transportation. As a result of attrition from the original sample of potential participants, less than half of the eligible participants were randomized within each of the two arms.

Following the initial screening, participants provided informed consent and participated in three intake sessions in which they received a battery of questionnaires. Included were evaluations of drinking behavior, previous treatments, and neuropsychological testing. All interviews were audiotaped. Urine and blood samples were obtained. Participants randomly assigned to treatment modalities within each of the two arms did not differ significantly on any of the pretreatment baseline assessment measures. Following initial assessments were 12 weeks of treatment, weekly meetings for the TBS and CBT groups and 4 meetings of the MET groups. All treatments were conducted individually. Subjects were recruited and participated in the study over a 2-year period.

During the first year each of the five assessments given at 3-month intervals included a group of sessions determining daily drinking estimates and the negative consequences of alcohol use. Information was obtained from collaterals and laboratory tests were conducted designed to monitor alcohol use and corroborate self-reports. Results were obtained from more than 90% of the participants at each assessment.

Treatments

Each of the three treatments was based on a specially prepared manual and training protocol. Eighty therapists were trained and certified to administer one of the treatments. All sessions were videotaped and 25% of all sessions were monitored by supervisors. Therapists selected were dedicated to the treatment they would provide.

Social learning theory was the basis for the CBT treatment which emphasized coping skills and relapse prevention. Alcoholism as a spiritual and medical disease was the basis for the TSF treatment which was designed to promote attendance in AA meetings and related activities. Motivational psychology was the basis for the MET treatment designed to promote motivational change and the redirection of "internal resources".

Completion rates for the treatments in the outpatient and after-care arms were 68% and 66% respectively. No information is provided concerning possible follow-up of noncompliant participants or participants who failed to complete treatment. Factors contributing to noncompliance or failure to complete treatment were not determined. Rates of noncompletion by treatments within each arm are not presented, unfortunately. A later follow-up provides some information on completions within outpatient treatments (Longabaugh, Wirtz, Zweben, & Stout, 1998). Absence of information on treatment completion rates for each treatment modality and the type of patient who failed to complete treatment makes interpretation of the results obtained for the different treatment modalities somewhat ambiguous.

RESULTS: 1-YEAR FOLLOW-UP

After-care treatments

Adjusting for 10 matching characteristics at pretreatment baseline resulted in a small but significant treatment x time effect. There was also a CRU x treatment interaction, indicating that the success of particular treatments varied with the CRU. Participants in the TSF group showed an increased PDA toward the end of the 1-year follow-up. There were no differences in DDD. The MATCH Research Group concluded that in the light of the significant interactions, there were no clinically significant differences in after-care treatments. In the absence of a control group that did not receive an experimental treatment one might also conclude that there were no significant effects of the three experimental after-care treatments.

Outpatient treatments

Among outpatient treatment conditions, 24% of TSF participants achieved total abstinence for the 12-month follow-up period as compared to 15% and 14% abstinence rates for the CBT and MET groups, respectively. Analysis of a second drinking measure, three days of heavy drinking, showed that TSF did significantly better than the other groups with 53% not meeting the criterion of heavy drinking for three successive days as compared to 49% and 48% for the MET and CBT groups, respectively; TSF participants also had a longer period of time before the first drink than the other two groups.

After-care matching

There were no significant patient attribute x treatment interactions (ATI) in the PDA measure for any of the primary matching hypotheses, contradicting the major hypothesis of the study. There was an attribute x treatment x time interaction. Meaning-seeking patients receiving TSF had more abstinent days than when they received CBT or MET during the later follow-up intervals. In terms of DDD, a typology x treatment x time interaction was significant. Type B subjects treated with CBT and TSF as compared to MET participants improved over follow-up intervals.

Outpatient matching

There was only one significant attribute x treatment interaction for the PDA measure. It involved psychiatric severity. The lower the patients' psychiatric severity score the greater the PDA when treated with TSF as compared to CBT. There was also a significant quadratic trend component to the interaction of these two treatments and psychiatric severity. A post hoc analysis of patients with no psychiatric symptoms showed that TSF was significantly better than CBT in terms of PDA. There was no significant difference in PDA between the two treatments at the high end of the psychiatric severity inventory contrary to the original hypothesis. Finding that patients without psychiatric problems did significantly better with TSF than CBT was not anticipated by the MATCH Research Group.

Patients with low motivation to change receiving MET as compared to CBT were abstinent more days in the later follow-up intervals. Participants with high motivation to change did equally well in either treatment program.

Overall results: 1-year follow-up

Overall results were disappointing. Only 35% of the participants receiving after-care were abstinent for the entire year. No measures independently assessing the effects of the preceding inpatient or day-hospital treatment were obtained. In the outpatient arm only 19% were abstinent for the entire year.

Matching results: 3-year follow-up

A 3-year follow-up of Project MATCH participants was limited to the outpatient arm of the study (Project MATCH Research Group, 1998). A 3-month evaluation window was employed. Performance during months 37-39 following completion of treatment was assessed. Cost-saving was given as a consideration in limiting the follow-up to the outpatient arm as well as the purported greater clinical generalizability of the brief outpatient interventions. Another probable reason was the realization that the after-care arm would not yield interpretable evidence supporting matching hypotheses after three years, since it did not yield such effects after one year.

Briefly, only two matching effects were obtained in the outpatient arm. Participants high in anger did better in MET than in the other two treatment groups whereas those low in anger did better in CBT and TSF than in MET. The significant matching effect for psychiatric severity found in the 1-year follow-up did not persist. Personal attributes such as readiness to change and self-efficacy accounted for some of the variance in drinking outcomes.

It was also found that those who had a social network supporting drinking did significantly better in TSF than in the other two treatments. These results are considered in detail in a second publication (Longabaugh et al., 1998).

The matching hypothesis tested was that TSF and MET would interact with a social network supporting drinking. Questionnaires determined the patients' social network and whether or not its members drank and approved of the patient's drinking. The matching hypothesis predicted an interaction between treatments and high and low social network support of drinking. No difference in treatment outcome should be present with low social network support of drinking. A difference in treatment outcomes should be apparent when there was high social network support of drinking.

No significant effect was found in the after-care arm. The predicted interaction did occur in the 3-year follow-up of the outpatient arm. No difference was obtained between treatment outcomes at the end of the treatment period or after the 1-year follow-up. Categorizng the patients above and below the median for social network support of drinking showed that the effect occurred primarily among those patients with high social network support for drinking. Longabaugh et al. (1998) found that participating in AA, a practice fostered by TSF, mediated the superior outcome obtained by TSF in both the measures of percentage of abstinent days and drinks per drinking day. Unfortunately, results are not reported for the percentage of patients in each treatment group abstinent during the three month evaluation window as a function of AA participation and social network support of drinking. In general, TSF and participation in AA served as a buffer against the influence of membership in a social network promoting drinking.

Overall results: 3-year follow-up

Overall, only 29% were abstinent during the three month evaluation window, months 37-39. Best overall abstinence results were again obtained by TSF, 36%, as compared to CBT, 24%, and MET, 27%. Unfortunately, Project MATCH failed to report the percentage of people continuously abstinent for the entire 3-year follow-up. They also failed to report what proportion of the 19% continuously abstinent during the 1-year follow-up were abstinent during months 37-39.

The Project MATCH Research Group (1998) describe their overall results as follows:

A high rate of abstinence was noted within the first year posttreatment, and this was sustained after two more years. Almost 30% of the outpatient sample was totally abstinent in months 37 to 39, comparable with abstinence rates reported in other long-term follow-up studies [Polich et al., 1980; Taylor et al., 1985]. Subjects who did report drinking were nevertheless abstinent two-thirds of the time, on average, in the 90 days prior to the 3-year interview, an improvement in abstinent days of about 150% over the 90-day baseline period. When drinking, they drank an average of between 6 and 7 drinks per occasion, down from nearly 11 at the time of their intake into the study, representing a considerable improvement over baseline. Although the design of the matching study focused on interactions and therefore did not include a no-treatment control group, it is unlikely that the drinking reductions reported herein, by more than 800 alcoholics, were solely the result of natural progression. If the reasons for these apparently successful outcomes can be identified, they would provide a basis for enhancing treatment effectiveness. (p. 1309).

What does it all mean?

How do we know that the "high rate" of abstinence (19%) in the 1-year follow-up is "sustained" when no information is provided indicating that the patients constituting the 19% are contained within the 30% found in the 3-month window used for the 3-year follow-up? Participants were not assessed over the three year interval, only the final three months. I do not consider 19% a high rate of abstinence, especially when compared to results obtained in studies reviewed earlier in the present chapter. Furthermore, a 3-month evaluation window is too short. Schuckit et al. (1997) found that during the course of alcohol dependence approximately 36% of individuals without formal treatment exhibited at least one 3-

month period of abstinence. Such variability is not uncommon in diagnosed alcoholics. Reliable assessment of treatment effects requires a longer evaluation window than 3 months.

The argument for not needing a control group is questionable. A reason for much of the improvement was probably regression toward the mean. Abstinence rates are compared with Rand II (Polich et al., 1981) and the follow-up of subjects in the Orford and Edwards (1977) study. Neither study is noted for its internal validity nor the quality of treatments delivered. Why not compare the MATCH results to the results for the thousands of patients in the CATOR registry (Harrison et al., 1991) or Küfner and Feuerlein's (1989) study? The latter report long term results: 48% continuous abstinence for the entire 4-year interval since discharge. Why did the Project MATCH Research Group not give the abstinence rate for their entire 3-year period rather than a 3-month window? How does the 1-year 19% abstinence rate in the outpatient arm compare to the 70-80% continuous abstinence rates for 1-year reported for Schick Shadel and the Minnesota Model treatment programs in the CATOR registry? It is difficult to accept the MATCH (1998) Research Groups' evaluation of their result as, "a high rate of abstinence" (p. 1309). Even the low abstinence rates reported are misleadingly high because approximately one-third of the patients failed to complete treatment and apparently were not followed-up.

Compared to treatment results obtained by some current traditional multimodal treatment programs in the United States and in Germany, MATCH is an abysmal failure. I do not consider the outcome highly successful when the majority of participants who completed treatment are still drinking and at an average of more than 6 drinks every third day. Drinking at this rate may cause brain dysfunction, in addition to other medical complications in the majority of the participants (Cala, 1987; Eckardt et al., 1998) as well as numerous social problems (Sanchez-Craig et al., 1995). Furthermore, no information is provided on the one-third of the participants who did not complete treatment, a group unlikely to have attained even the modest level of success reported for those who completed treatment. Additional efficacy studies matching specific treatments to specific individual differences and characteristics are pointless. Reasons for this conclusion are obvious: (a) the failure to confirm any matching hypothesis in the after-care arm and, (b) the high rate of abstinence obtained by some multimodal treatment programs and Schick Shadel in contrast to the results obtained in Project MATCH.

Absence of any matching effect in the after-care arm suggests that the prior intensive treatment, in most cases probably multimodal traditional treatments, accomodated the individual differences that behavior therapists believe need matching to specialized treatments. Given the high rate of success found in traditional treatment programs in the CATOR registry and the Schick Shadel treatment program, there is little variance remaining that could be accounted for by individual differences in anger, self-efficacy, readiness to change, typology, drinking network, etc. These are all addressed in the effective traditional programs reviewed earlier in this chapter. Amount of time a particular individual spends in one treatment modality in a traditional program rather than another can be adjusted to meet specific needs or characteristics of that individual. For example, the high incidence of sexual abuse among women can be addressed by participating in groups focused on this problem and in individual therapy. Men as well as women suffering from physical and/or sexual abuse as well as other traumas would find no help from these specialized behavior therapy efficacy treatments. Treatment for their problems is not in the manual that counselors must follow. All of the above suggests that much of the kind of matching problems proposed and studied by revisionists is an artifact of their brief single treatment modality efficacy studies.

The most striking effect obtained, one which has received scant attention from the Project MATCH Research Group as far as I can determine, is the overall superior abstinence outcome obtained in the after-care as compared to outpatient arm of the study: 35% continuous abstinence versus 19% abstinence, respectively, for the 1-year follow-up. Unfortunately, the after-care arm participants were not followed up at three years except in a study that examined variables in only two sites and which will be reported elsewhere (Project MATCH Research Group, 1998). It is a pity.

Overall results obtained in the two arms contradict the assertions of Miller and other revisionists that in- and outpatient treatments, and high and low intensity treatments do not differ. Excuses for not comparing the two arms are that, (a) such a comparison was not the purpose of the project, and (b) participants were not randomly assigned to the two arms. However, there are acceptable ways of comparing the two arms, for example using multiple regression analysis to adjust for initial differences. A second approach is to compare patients in the after-care and outpatient arms matched on the basis of the baseline measures following the example of Smith et al. (1991). Either approach would probably heighten the difference between the two groups. Patients in after-care had been discharged from inpatient and day-hospital care prior to the MATCH project whereas people in the outpatient arm did not have prior inpatient treatment. As we have seen in the report by Harrison et al. (1991) and the descriptions of the participants in MATCH, inpatients and therefore those in the after-care arm tend to be older, more severely dependent, report more prior treatments, and are less socially stable, than oupatients, characteristics that predict a poorer outcome for the after-care arm, other things being equal. Despite the handicap, other things were not equal. After-care patients had two advantages over the outpatients who received the same set of experimental treatments. After-care patients all received more treatment, received greater treatment intensity, and probably in the majority of sites, it was traditional multimodal treatments.

Factors working to the advantage of the after-care group were the very ones that Miller and other revisionists have repeatedly asserted do not make a difference. Obviously they did. The Project MATCH Research Group did not wish to study these factors. That was not the purpose of the Project. Creative scientists take advantage of serendipity, unanticipated unusual occurrences and hunt down their causes. The Project MATCH Research Group chose not to engage in that adventure. It is unfortunate. They ignored the most important variable revealed in their study: the effect of intensity of treatment. After-care patients received a greater amount of treatment which resulted in superior overall outcome and accommodated different patient attributes.

The Project MATCH Research Group (1998) suggest future research:

The present findings do not rule out the possibililty of discovering other client treatment matching effects that may be clinically meaningful. Such matching studies might involve therapies not used in Project MATCH, such as family therapy, group therapy, or a combination of elements from the MATCH therapies, such as support for AA involvement (TSF) and enhancing self-efficacy (MET). Other studies might entail combining elements of psychotherapies, such as coping skills therapy or motivational counseling with medications found to be effective... Consideration should also be given to designing matching studies for client populations excluded from Project MATCH, such as those with comorbid drug dependence. (p. 1410).

Strange, but these suggestions begin to sound like a multimodal Minnesota Model treatment. Note, however, that the Project MATCH Research Group still fails to consider a critical variable that needs to be investigated in the context of effective treatments: intensity of treatment.

The VA Comparative Outcome Study

Moos, Finney, Ouimette, and Suchinsky (1999) have conducted a major treatment outcome study on approximately 3000 patients in Veterans Administration (VA) Hospitals. One of many interesting findings was that abstinence rates increased with amount of inpatient care and intensity of outpatient after-care. Patients in 12-step programs had significantly better outcomes at the 1-year follow-up than patients receiving cognitive behavior (CB) therapy or an eclectic blend of the two treatments. Study participants were not excluded because they were dependent on other drugs or suffered from psychiatric problems or lack of social stability as in the MATCH project. Although VA programs are generally from 21-28 days, many patients receive less intensive treatments, permitting the investigators to examine treatment outcomes as a consequence of treatment intensity. Their finding that increased intensity is followed by more successful outcomes is in accord with the analysis of Monahan and Finney (1996) and contrary to Miller's dictum that intensity of treatment does not make a difference.

Given the great diversity of patients and the relative absence of exclusionary criteria, the VA population seems ideal for examining patient treatment matching, for example, the interaction between kind of treatment and severity of psychiatric symptoms. No such interaction was obtained. The 12-step program provided overall greater percent abstinence for alcohol and other drugs at the 1-year follow-up, 45%, versus 36% for CB treatments, and 40% for the eclectic blend of the two treatments.

Possible proximal processes responsible for the outcomes obtained by the 12-step and CB treatments were examined by Finney, Moos, and Humphreys (1999). Indices were developed for the different processes presumably related to the theories underlying the two kinds of treatments. Cognitions and behaviors that may serve as proximal processes for 12-step treatment outcomes include belief in the disease model, acceptance of the attribution of an alcoholic and/or addict and striving for an abstinence treatment goal. Related behaviors include attending 12-step meetings such as AA, NA, and CA, having a sponsor, reading 12-step material and having friends in 12-step programs. Proximal processes contributing to treatment outcomes in CB treatments include self-efficacy, expectancies of reinforcment and outcome, and coping and cognitive appraisal.

Results showed that although significantly correlated with outcome measures, indices of the above processes account for only small portions of outcome variance. Finney et al. (1999) conclude that, "these findings suggest that the theories on which 12-step and CB treatment are based are not sufficiently comprehensive" (p.542). I suggest that the lack of comprehensiveness and the inability to predict with a higher degree of accuracy is due to the absence of appropriate physiological measures of catecholamines, serotonin and the endorphins.

Superiority of the 12-step treatment outcome for alcohol and other drugs as compared to CB was mediated by the degree of involvement in 12-step fellowships (Humphreys et al., 1999). I suspect the effect occurred because the social affiliations developed in such fellowships produced changes in the brain neurochemistry of participants. Support groups moderated levels of beta-endorphins, dopamine, and serotonin in the participants. Behavior of the human as well as the infrahuman animal is influenced by changes in brain neurochemistry as a result of social interactions as we noted in the infrahuman animal research described in chapter 3 (Higley et al., 1991; Keverne et al., 1989). Constructions such as self-efficacy and expectancies are primitive and ambiguous indices of the consequences of behavioral changes induced by changes in brain chemistry. Verbal reports of expectancies and self-efficacy are effects not causes of the changes in brain chemistry induced by the "social chemistry" of the group. The close social affiliations that may develop in self-help groups facilitate reversal of the neurochemical imbalances produced by excessive consumption of alcohol and other drugs and predisposing states.

Given the demonstrated superiority of 12-step over CB treatment in the large sample of patients examined in the VA Comparative Outcome Study there is no reason for continued use of CB treatments in VA facilities. It is unethical and cost ineffective to continue providing CB for alcohol and other drug dependency problems in the face of the evidence of greater effectiveness of 12-step treatment programs.

Conclusion

We have completed our selective review of treatment outcome studies. It has been an interesting odyssey. What essentially started in the 1970s with a study by two students, individualized behavioral treatment of gamma alcoholics with the goal of controlled drinking, appeared to hold the promise of a remarkable advance. It was aggressively promoted as a new scientific approach for treating alcoholics. Failures to replicate and allegations of misconduct for a time quieted the enthusiasm for this new form of treatment for alcoholics. Behavioral methods to train alcoholics in controlled drinking were renamed methods for secondary prevention and harm reduction for problem drinkers. Despite the relatively large number of small efficacy studies with questionable results, the hegemony of revisionists grew, helped by the reward of large grants, establishment of research and training centers, and a proliferation of further studies designed to fit the current scene of managed care. Behavioral methods employed in studies with low statistical power, inappropriate measures, and no lasting treatment effects for problem drinkers metamorphosized into abstinence oriented brief interventions for alcoholics. The MATCH Project arrived. Individualized behavioral treatments that failed to have lasting effects with problem drinkers were now used to treat alcoholics as well. Predictably, these methods failed to reach the level of effectiveness of many traditional treatment programs. Hypothesized interactions between patient attributes and specific treatments largely failed to appear or persist. What has been found repeatedly in studies of treatment effectiveness and in the MATCH project is that involvement in 12-step programs such as AA significantly increases the likelihood of maintaining abstinence, is the most effective relapse prevention available.

An enormous effort was invested in the development and refinement of numerous questionnaires, assessment, and motivational tools used in Marlatt and colleagues' harm reduction approach to excessive college drinking (Dimeff et al., l999). The overall endeavor reflects the same problem seen in the MATCH project. Large amounts of research funds financed the two failed projects. Despite the poor outcomes the studies are hailed as successes by spokespersons for the projects and government administrators. Both projects represent the best and the worst in much of clinical psychology. They reflect technical skill in the development of tests and questionnaires and the measurement of outcomes coupled with a lack of creativity in the goals and designs of the projects fostered by wearing ideological blinders. Results are nevertheless promoted with the zeal of snake oil salesmen.

How many times must these "behavior therapy methods" fail before their application to alcoholics extinguish and "harm reduction" for alcoholics and problem drinkers is properly evaluated as a very risky endeavor? They never will, as long as revisionists continue to be reinforced by grant money from NIAAA and they continue their hegemony over relevant review boards of granting agencies and editorial boards of journals. In the meantime the successful treatment of alcoholics in private treatment facilities employing traditional treatments reflected in the CATOR registry and a brief nontraditional behavioral multimodal program used by Schick Shadel have been a well kept secret. Their successful outcomes have been ignored by academic clinical psychologists if not actively suppressed.

A fitting conclusion to this chapter is a slight variation of an ironic declamation: "Clinicians, like scientists, must be willing to test their cherished assumptions against hard data and to relinquish views and practices that do not stand up to the test of evidence." (Miller et al., l995, p. 33).

results contradict the claims by Marlatt et al. concerning the viability of controlled drinking or harm reduction for alcoholics, individuals meeting the criteria for alcohol dependence (see chapters 6 and 7).

Marlatt et al. (1993) further argue: "Opponents of controlled drinking based their opposition on the premise that alcoholism is a physical disease and that the "symptoms" of this biological disorder cannot be voluntarily controlled or regulated" (p.464). It is significant that there are no references to these opponents. My objection to controlled drinking as a treatment goal for alcoholics is based on the research literature not ideology. The assertion that controlled drinking is a viable treatment for alcoholics has been repeatedly contradicted (e.g., Maltzman, 1994; Wallace, 1989a, 1989b, 1990; see chapter 6).

At the turn of the century, in   prebehavioristic times, there were two general kinds of psychopathologies, organic, and functional or mental diseases. Watson (1913, 1916), the founder of behaviorism, accepted psychopathologies as diseases, but suggested that so-called mental diseases are caused by bad habits. A disease need not be "physical", have a known biological etiology and pathophysiology. Supporters of the traditional disease concept of alcoholism (Jellinek, 1960; Keller, 1975) recognized that learning may play an important role in the initiation of heavy drinking. A reasonable hypothesis based on the neuropsychological (Goldman, 1983), necropsy (Harper & Kril, 1990), and neuroimaging research (Cala, 1987) is that a behavioral sign and symptom in that syndrome, loss of control, is peculiar to alcoholics as compared to alcohol misusers or problem drinkers because alcoholics suffer from brain dysfunction which may or may not be reversible. This brain damage differentially affects the frontal lobes which are responsible for self-regulation, "executive functions", the loss of which underly an environmental dependency described as loss of control over drinking (Lemere, 1956; Lhermitte, 1986; Lyvers, 1998, in press; Maltzman, 1991, 1994; Stuss & Benson, 1984).

Marlatt et al. (1993) construct a straw man version of the disease concept and draw the following non sequitur:

Drinkers fall into one of two categories: alcoholic or nonalcoholic. Nonalcoholic drinkers do not suffer from 'loss of control' over their drinking and therefore do not need moderation training. By the same token, alcoholics have only two options: to abstain or to continue drinking in a progressively deteriorating manner. By the standards of the disease model, there is no 'middle ground', no middle way between the two extremes of alcoholic drinking or abstinence. (p.464).

There is no middle ground for Marlatt et al. (1993) because they conflate problem drinking and alcoholism, as does Fingerette (1988a, 1998b). Alcoholics and problem drinkers are explicitly distinguished from one another in the received view as gamma alcoholics vs alpha and beta alcoholics (Jellinek, 1960). The former case involves people classified as suffering from alcohol dependence and the latter, those suffering from alcohol abuse. In principle, problem drinkers, individuals who are not dependent on alcohol according to DSM-IV but who misuse alcohol, could be taught to moderate or control their drinking. However, the problem is not as simple as Marlatt et al. and other revisionists suggest. The difficulty is that there is no reliable established means of determining who is a problem drinker who will remain a problem drinker or improve, and who is classifiable as a problem drinker but if he or she continues to drink will progress into alcoholism. The problem at present is the failure to use assessment tools sensitive enough to predict differential progress, either towards recovery or alcoholism. This is an empirical problem, one which has not been adequately addressed. One of the obstacles to advances in the theory and treatment of alcohol problems is the attitude of many behavior therapists that a treatment is either behavioral or biological and there is a fundamental conflict between the two. They adhere to the ancient mythology of the hair of the dog - the treatment must contain a component of the etiology. If, according to the revisionist straw man caricature of the disease concept, the etiology of alcoholism is biological, then the treatment must be biological. If the etiology is psychosocial, the treatment must be psychosocial. However, an individual may receive a head injury - a physical etiology - and become aphasic, but that individual may be taught to speak again with entirely behavioral techniques. Etiology does not necessarily entail a corresponding treatment.

The continuity principle

A central thesis of Marlatt et al. (1993) is that there is a single dimension or continuity from social drinking to dependence. At different times Marlatt has espoused different forms of a continuity hypothesis. Originally, Marlatt (1979) espoused continuity in terms of the principles of learning:

All drinking behavior, from social drinking to alcohol abuse, is assumed to be governed by similar principles of learning and reinforcement. As such, it is assumed that there is no crucial difference that distinguishes the social drinker and the problem drinker, other than the amount of alcohol consumed. (p.324f).

Now Marlatt espouses continuity in terms of the consequences of drinking. Both conceptions are contradicted by behavioral evidence already at hand. Marlatt originally stressed the notion of continuity in the sense that the same laws of learning hold from social drinking to alcohol dependence. However, no one has ever explicitly delineated what these laws are, how they work, and how it is that most people who consume alcohol do not learn to become dependent.

Examination of the history of medicine indicates that whether or not a disease is observed to be continuous with the normal state such as essential hypertension or qualitatively different as in the case of tuberculosis, is dependent upon knowledge of the etiology of the disease (Reznek, 1987). Phenotypical and genotypical differences must be differentiated. Thus, people with Down's syndrome show a continuum of IQ from severely retarded to normal. But the phenotypical continuum of Down's syndrome in the group is caused by a qualitative difference, a chromosome anomaly in the individual. What appears to be a continuum of alcohol consequences among a group of people can have qualitatively different etiologies in different individuals. However, even at the phenotypical or descriptive behavioral level, notions of continuity and a single dimension are falsified by the evidence at hand. There is striking behavioral evidence that contradicts the notion of continuity, evidence that has been available for many years (see chapter 1 and 3; Hodgson, Rankin, & Stockwell, 1979). Why are such results and their implications ignored?

CONTROLLED DRINKING AS A FORM OF HARM REDUCTION

The fundamental assumption underlying harm reduction according to Marlatt et al. (1993) is the notion of continuity. Why this should be so is not explicated. In any case, there are striking contradictions to the notion of continuity both in presumed underlying principles and in signs and symptoms of misuse and dependence. "Harm reduction" is simply a label for a potpourri of different social and individual problems and approaches to them. Nevertheless, Marlatt et al. (1993) state:

> The purpose of this paper is to integrate controlled drinking into the broader, more inclusive framework of harm reduction. We begin with a review of the controlled drinking controversy as it applies to the treatment of alcohol dependence. The debate over the early behavior therapy research conducted by Mark and Linda Sobell is discussed in some detail, because this study triggered considerable opposition to controlled drinking research and practice over the past decade. Research reporting controlled drinking outcomes in both abstinence-based treatment and moderation training programs is reviewed, followed by a discussion of predictors of moderate drinking outcomes. The choice between treatment goals of abstinence or moderation is discussed for alcohol-dependent clients. (p.466f).

Davies

Marlatt et al. (1993) initiate this controversial area with a discussion of the landmark study by Davies (1962). They state:

> Over three decades ago, Davies sent shock waves through the alcoholism field by publishing the results of a long-term follow-up of patients treated for alcoholism at the Maudsley hospital in London. In a 1962 paper entitled, 'Normal drinking in recovered alcohol addicts'... Davies challenged the traditional emphasis on abstinence as the only acceptable treatment goal for alcoholism by showing that of 93 male alcoholics who were followed up for a period of from 7 to 11 years following treatment, 7 of them reported a pattern of normal or controlled drinking. This outcome occurred despite the fact that the treatment program was geared to the goal of total abstinence. Davies' results sparked a storm of controversy because he challenged the traditional definition of alcoholism ... - that an alcoholic, by definition, is someone who has 'lost control' and is thereby unable to control, regulate, or moderate alcohol use (Marlatt, 1983). The fact that even a single exception (much less 7 exceptions in this case) to this absolute definition existed meant that only one of the two following possibilities could be true: that the patients in Davies' study could not have been true alcoholics to begin with, or that some individuals who have been previously diagnosed as alcoholics do, in fact, engage in moderate 'nonproblem drinking.' (p.467).

Marlatt et al. (1993) overlook a third possibility: the patients misled Davies. They do not consider Edwards' (1985) restudy and follow-up of Davies' 7 subjects purportedly drinking moderately. Edwards (1985) describes the results of his restudy as follows:

The data suggest that two subjects can be confidently described as having "returned to normal drinking," with this pattern maintained from shortly after the original Maudsley discharge up to the present: Case 1 showed evidence of severe dependence before that admission, whereas case 6 was probably never more than slightly dependent. As judged by level of alcohol intake, intoxication, alcohol-related disabilities or dependence symptoms, none of the remaining five cases maintained normal drinking over the total follow-up period; this statement is reinforced by records as well as by information gained at interviews... There is evidence that Cases 2, 4, and 5 were drinking excessively during the original follow-up as well as later. A similar conclusion could be drawn for Case 3 if the uncorroborated memories many years later of the subject's widow are accepted and for case 7 if the unsupported evidence of a previous workmate and drinking companion is accepted. Three subjects manifested at some time a heavy use of psychotropic drugs. (p. 185f).

Edwards (1985) found that five of the seven original patients purportedly drinking moderately and functioning well:

experienced significant drinking problems both during Davies' original follow-up period and subsequently, that three of these five at some time also used psychotropic drugs heavily, and that the two remaining subjects (one of who was never severely dependent on alcohol) engaged in trouble-free drinking over the total period. (p.181).

It is apparent that results for one of 93 patients presumably diagnosed as an alcoholic and engaged in moderate drinking cannot provide the basis for implementing moderate drinking as a viable treatment goal for alcoholics. Davies had been misled by his respondents as Edwards (1985, 1994) clearly demonstrates. It is apparent that Davies' study from the outset supported rather than contradicted the traditional view of alcoholism when the evidence from Edwards' (1985) revealing follow-up is considered.

An interesting insight into how Davies was misled is revealed in an interview Edwards had with Davies. Edwards tells Davies:

'I saw one of these "returned to normal drinking" patients years later... and he confessed that he had been drinking like a fish the whole time, and even during the month when the *QJSA* [*Quarterly Journal of Studies on Alcohol*] published the account of his return to normal drinking, he was... drinking in a very alcoholic way. He told me that when your research follow-up worker came to do an interview with his wife he let her know in advance that he'd bash the living daylights out of her if she told the truth and she gave an account which was entirely false to substantiate his own false account.' (Journal Interview, 1979, p. 240).

Why is there is no mention in Marlatt et al. (1993) of Edwards' reports and his demonstration of the lack of validity of Davies' results, one of the cornerstones of the controlled drinking approach?

The Rand Reports

Marlatt et al. go on to discuss "later replications" and cite the Rand Report (Armor, Polich, & Stambul, 1976, 1978), the second purported cornerstone of controlled drinking for alcoholics:

Davies' findings were replicated by an American group of investigators from the Rand corporation, an independent research contracting firm. The first Rand report, published in 1978... consisted of the results of an 18-month follow-up of male alcoholics treated with a goal of abstinence in 45 alcoholism treatment centers in the U.S. The overall pattern of results showed an improvement rate of 70% for several different treatment outcome indices. Although this is a notable improvement rate, controversy was sparked by the finding that not all of the improved patients were totally abstinent during the follow-up period. (p.468).

A second Rand Report [Polich, Armor, & Braiker, 1981] documented the outcomes over a four-year period following initial treatment for 85% of a cohort of 922 male patients randomly drawn from eight alcoholism treatment centers. The results showed that 18% of the patients were reported to be drinking without problems or symptoms of dependence. (p. 468).

Marlatt et al. (1993) ignore criticisms by Wallace (1989a, 1989b, 1990) exposing the manifest methodological inadequacies in the two Rand Reports. There are several serious shortcomings which make Rand Report I uninterpretable. None of these shortcomings are considered by Marlatt et al. First, the authors of the Rand Reports did not follow Nathan and Skinstad's (1987) recommendation:

When alcoholic patients drop out prematurely from treatment or cannot be found for subsequent follow-up, they must be accounted for. The most defensible explanation for these losses is to consider them treatment failures and to assume that dropouts have likely returned to abusive drinking; most researchers agree that ignoring those who drop out from treatment or who are otherwise lost to follow-up by excluding them from further analyses of outcome unfairly inflates success estimates. (p.332).

Only 21% of the patients in Rand Report I were available for interview at the six month follow-up; 2371 of 11,500 male non-DWI subjects were recovered (Armor et al., 1976, p. 65). Given this unacceptably high attrition rate, a greater effort was made to obtain followup data after 18 months at 8 of the 44 available ATCs. At these latter facilities, 600 male non-DWIs were recovered, 62%, still a serious loss of subjects. In neither case did Armor et al. follow the standard procedure recommended by Nathan and Skinstad (1987): count the people lost to attrition as failures. If this were done, the success rate would have been discouragingly low. As a consequence, the Rand study improvement rate is grossly inflated and the importance of the study is exaggerated.

An additional major shortcoming of the study is that they used "rubberband" criteria for assessing the incidence of controlled drinking versus abstinence at followup. The criterion for judging that someone was "abstinent" was the report that the person had not had a drink for the 6 months prior to the follow-up. But for a person to be judged as engaging in "controlled" or "normal" drinking, they need only to have been drinking "moderately" for the previous 30 days. Why was the criterion for controlled drinking not the same as for abstinence, 6 months, or the criterion for abstinence 30 days? If the former were used, the odds are overwhelming that there would be less evidence of controlled drinking. If the latter criterion, abstinence for 30 days, had been used there would have been a much higher rate of abstinence.

The motivation behind use of these differential criteria is not explained. Its effect is obvious. It makes controlled drinking outcomes appear viable. Marlatt et al. (1993) do not report, much less criticize, this major shortcoming in the methodology of the Rand Report. Still another serious shortcoming of the Rand study ignored by Marlatt et al. (1993) is the criterion for what constitutes "normal" or controlled drinking. Armor et al. (l976) state, "... we... set upper limits for normal drinking at 3 oz/day for daily consumption and 5 ounces for typical quantities" (p.77). That is 3 oz of alcohol not 3 drinks. In other words a six pack a day is normal and 10 beers or shots of whisky a day is typical for a normal or controlled drinker, provided there are not serious side effects. Alcohol consumed in the amounts that Armor et al. consider normal or controlled drinking may lead to physical dependence and serious biomedical consequences, including the increased likelihood of brain damage that may be largely irreversible in many people (Cala,1987, Nicolás et al., 1993) and continued neuropsychological deficits (Eckardt et al., l980).

Armor et al. (1976) assert that of those definitely alcoholic in terms of consumption and behavioral impairment, 12% were drinking "moderately" at 18 months (using the 30 day window). This 12% are 19 people out of 161 (Table 19, p. 87). Thus the evidence that purported alcoholics can return to "moderate" drinking (not more than a six-pack a night on average or 10 drinks on a typical day) for 30 days is based on 19 people. The impression created by revisionists and textbook writers who have failed to study the original sources is that a huge study involving 11,000 - 14,000 people found that alcoholics can return to "moderate" drinking. In fact, this conclusion was based on 19 cases.

According to Wallace (l990):

Even in the so-called four-year study (Polich, Armor & Braiker, l981), the actual window on drinking behavior varied from one to six months, with the bulk of observations on "nonproblem drinking" centering around one to three months.

In general, then, the Rand studies used windows of such short duration that they provided very little evidence in support of stable, sustained moderate or nonproblem drinking among alcoholics. In fact, when estimates of sustained, longer-term controlled drinking are derived from the data for the four-year follow-up, they are quite low. The sustained, stable, long-term nonproblem drinking rate in the Rand studies corrected for the Rand report authors' acknowledged error in their measurement of quantity and frequency of consumption of approximately one-quarter is roughly 3% to 4%. But even this very low, sustained nonproblem drinking rate is probably spuriously high because it was based on those persons who were drinking nonproblematically at three *specific follow-up point* from admission to four-year follow-up. Consequently, it is not known that these patients were drinking in a nonproblem manner *throughout* the four-year follow-up period. (p. 271).

An average of six drinks a day and not more than 10 drinks on a typical day is no longer considered a safe, moderate, level of drinking by proponents of controlled drinking (Sancehz-Craig, 1986; Sanchez-Craig, Wilkinson, & Davila, 1995). It was never considered safe, moderate, normal, drinking by experienced clinicians (Blume, 1977). Additional criticisms of the Rand Reports may be found in chapter 1.

Training In Controlled Drinking

Encouraged by the apparent success of Davies that alcoholics may return to controlled drinking despite a treatment goal of abstinence, behavior therapists set out to train alcoholics to control their drinking. Their reasoning was that such training should increase the success rate of a treatment inherently more attractive to alcoholics than abstinence.

Lovibond and Caddy

Lovibond and Caddy (1970) were apparently the first to report a study explicitly designed to train "alcoholics" to control their drinking, using blood-alcohol level discrimination training and aversive discriminative conditioning, administering electric shocks if participants drank more than a specified amount. We use the term "alcoholic" advisedly since there was no independent assessment of severity of the subjects' drinking problem. Participants in the study were obtained via referrals by general practitioners, psychiatric hospitals or, in most cases, were volunteers who learned of the project through the news media. Most were said to have been hospitalized for alcoholism on "numerous occasions". Absence of obvious psychosis and the willingness to accept electric shocks were the only selection criteria. Marlatt et al. (1993) state:

> The results of this initial study were encouraging: In a follow-up evaluation, Lovibond and Caddy reported that of 31 alcoholics who had received the experimental treatment, 24 had successful outcomes and were able to drink in a 'controlled manner'. Although these preliminary results were promising, the study was limited by the absence of a comparison treatment control group and by the fact that the follow-up period was relatively brief (16-60 weeks posttreatment). (p.469).

Again, we find that Marlatt et al. (1993) are an untrustworthy source. Contrary to Marlatt et al. Lovibond and Caddy employed a control group. It differed from the experimental group in the first three shock sessions: the electric shocks were noncontingent upon alcohol consumption. Thereafter the two groups were treated in the same fashion. After initial improvement comparable to the experimental group, with repeated treatment sessions drinking by control group members increased markedly and a majority dropped out of treatment. Asserting that the 24 successful controlled drinking outcomes were obtained in a follow-up period of "16-60 weeks posttreatment" is a misrepresentation of Lovibond and Caddy's procedure. Twenty-four of 31 subjects reduced their drinking to moderate levels *during* the 10 weeks of outpatient treatment. Posttreatment attrition was marked so that by 50 weeks posttreatment only three participants were found. The purported striking results reported by Lovibond and Caddy were for the period *during* outpatient treatment, not posttreatment as asserted by Marlatt et al. (1993). If we adopt the recommended criterion of counting attrition as failures, obviously, the posttreatment outcome success rate is abysmally low.

THE SOBELL CONTROVERSY

We turn now to the most controversial cornerstone of the controlled drinking treatment goal and the only one that explicitly claimed that they treated gamma alcoholics as distinguished from problem drinkers (Sobell & Sobell, 1978). Marlatt et al. (1993) provide a summary of the procedures employed by the Sobells during the treatment phase of the study and the two-year follow-up period that contain several critical errors of omission and commission. Marlatt et al. (1993) state:

> In addition to regular telephone contacts approximately every other month [sic] with each patient, follow-up procedures also involved obtaining information on the patient's progress from at least three collateral sources, including objective public records. At each follow-up contact, patients were asked a variety of questions about their drinking, including the following: 'How many days since our last contact have you had anything to drink and how much did you drink, on each day?' In a retrospective accounting procedure, each day was classified into one of five categories: abstinent days, controlled drinking days (consumption of less than 6 ounces of distilled spirits or its equivalent), drunk days (consumption over this limit), or days incarcerated in a hospital or prison setting. For overall purposes of comparison, the categories of abstinent and controlled drinking days were combined as 'days functioning well' to be compared with 'days not functioning well' (sum of drunk days and days incarcerated)....
>
> One potential limitation of the study is that most of the follow-up interviews were conducted by Linda Sobell. Because she was aware of the original treatment conditions for each patient, the interviews were not conducted in a 'blind' manner, introducing the possibility that the results may have been biased to some degree by the interviewer's knowledge of the design and hypotheses. The potential for biased self-reports was minimized by the use of standard, objective questions and by the fact that all interviews were tape-recorded [sic] and open to independent verification. As an additional check on the validity of the findings an independent group of investigators under the direction of Glen Caddy... conducted a three-year follow-up of the patients treated by the Sobells (Caddy, Addington, & Perkins,1978)... Caddy and his co-authors reported that the controlled drinking subjects continued their superiority to the abstinence-goal control group on most measures of drinking and adjustment. (pp. 470, 471).

Marlatt et al. (1993) also describe the Pendery et al. (1982) study introducing along the way a remarkable series of errors of commission and omission:

> The authors reported that they had followed up as many as possible of the original patients in the Sobells' study in the late1970's and early 1980's. During this period, Mary Pendery (a graduate student (sic) then working under the supervision of UCLA psychology professor Irving Maltzman) personally interviewed the patients asking each to give a retrospective account of his drinking during the years since the completion of the Patton Hospital program in the early 1970s...

A careful reading of the Pendery study, however, reveals a number of disturbing questions concerning the scientific credibility of the findings reported in the *Science* article. First and foremost is the issue of why the results from the abstinence-goal control group were omitted from the article despite the fact that patients in the control group were included in Pendery's follow-up. A key strength of the Sobells' research design is the fact that patients were randomly assigned to either the experimental controlled drinking treatment or the abstinence control condition... The omission of outcome data for the control group is a crucial flaw...

Another serious problem is that the 'data' reported by Pendery and her colleagues are largely based on retrospective self-reports in which patients were asked to give past accounts of their drinking for periods ranging from five to ten years. The question of biased self-reports is a serious problem, particularly since Mary Pendery was well known for her stand against controlled drinking. In addition, Pendery et al. relied upon interviews in which patients were asked to give retrospective accounts of their drinking behavior that occurred years in the past. In contrast, the Sobells reported their results as part of an ongoing prospective study in which follow-up interviews were scheduled much closer in time to the events they asked patients to report. The Sobells provided quantitative reports of daily drinking dispositions. (pp.471, 472, 473).

Contrary to Marlatt et al. (1993) as indicated in chapter 4, during the period in question Pendery was head of the Alcoholism Treatment Unit in the San Diego VA Hospital. This information was in my article which Marlatt et al. (1993) cite (Maltzman, 1989). Marlatt, not a disinterested reporter, fails to mention that Mark Sobell was a graduate student and Linda was an undergraduate when they started their project. Neither one had formal clinical training. Nevertheless, we are called to seriously consider the results of their abstinence treatment knowing their bias in this regard as well as their inexperience.

Marlatt et al. (1993) turn to the second issue surrounding the Sobell controversy, my allegation of scientific fraud against them. They note that the president of the Sobells' employer at the time, the Addiction Research Foundation, appointed a committee chaired by a professor of law at the nearby University of Toronto to investigate. The Committee found the Sobells innocent of intentional wrong-doing, but careless. Another investigation conducted at ADAMHA, the Alcohol Drug Abuse and Mental Health Administration chaired by Trachtenberg (1984) also issued a report finding no evidence of scientific misconduct. Marlatt et al. (1993) assert:

Unfortunately, the debate about the veracity of the Sobells' findings continues. As recently as 1989, an article by Maltzman appeared in the *Journal of Studies on Alcohol* repeating allegations of scientific fraud against the Sobells (Maltzman, 1989), although several other papers published in the same issue strongly disputed his claims (Sobell & Sobell, 1989; Baker, 1989; Cook, 1989)...

The continuation of this debate, two decades after the original research was published and more than a decade after two independent committees cleared the Sobells, is a testament to the emotional nature of the question of controlled drinking in alcoholics. (p.474).

Issues and diversions in the Sobell controversy

The Sobells (1982) and their supporters (Heather & Robertson, 1983; Marlatt, 1983; Marlatt et al.,1993; Peele, 1983) have adopted a strategy of diverting attention from the two basic issues surrounding the Patton IBTA study. These are the allegations (Boffey, 1982) that, (a) the Sobells (1973a, 1976, 1978) and Caddy et al., (1978) have intentionally misrepresented their procedures and fabricated results, and (b) contrary to their claims, physically dependent alcoholics participating in the studies given a treatment goal of controlled drinking did not engage successfully in nonproblem controlled drinking in sufficient numbers to support controlled drinking as a viable treatment goal for alcoholics.

Attention is diverted from these two issues by attacking our study on the following grounds: (a) we did not compare the experimental and control groups; (b) we depended on patients' verbal reports and memory which are notoriously poor. We must first examine what the Sobells said their treatment outcome measures were, not what Marlatt et al. (1993) say they were. Major discrepancies between the two are apparent. The Sobells state:

> Basically, each subject and as many respective 'collateral information sources' as possible were contacted every 3-4 weeks throughout the entire follow-up interval... While follow-up interviews were regularly conducted every 3-4 weeks, subjects and collaterals were usually unaware of the exact date and time they would be contacted. (Sobell & Sobell, 1973, p. 601).

The Dickens Report lists the data base used in their investigation as those data provided to them by the Sobells (Dickens, 1982, pp. 35-40). This extensive list does not include tape recordings of each of the interviews, contrary to the assertion by Marlatt et al. that these were obtained for each interview. Tape recordings of each of the interviews are not mentioned in the Sobells' procedure section of any of their IBTA reports. In their book (Sobell & Sobell,1978) they state that they tape recorded a final interview (p. 167) which formed the basis of a later article on the interview as brief therapy. According to Sobell and Sobell (1978):

> As part of the IBT follow-up, subjects were asked to consent to a tape-recorded interview at the end of their two-year follow-up interval. The interview was intended to gather information about the subjects' impressions of the study. (p.167).

Marlatt et al. erroneously report tape recordings of all follow-up interviews and incorrectly report the frequency of follow-up interviews as occurring every other month. Research records listed by the Dickens Commission as provided by the Sobells do not include interview sheets containing the information for daily drinking dispositions purportedly obtained from each patient (Dickens et al. 1982, pp. 35-40). Since the patients were purportedly interviewed every 3-4 weeks for two years, there ought to be a minimum of 26-34 follow-up interview sheets completed for each person from which the daily drinking disposition is derived. These are the critical raw data of the study providing the bases, e.g., for the published individual drinking profiles of days functioning well (Sobell & Sobell, 1978, pp.128-132). Published summaries of six month outcomes, are not the raw data, contrary to the Dickens Committee report (p. 32f).

As we discuss in detail in chapter 5, Marlatt et al. (1993) and the numerous other commentators on this controversy note that the Dickens Committee Report found the Sobells innocent of any wrong doing. All of these commentators fail to note what the Dickens Committee Report failed to do - look in the right place. The Dickens Committee nowhere reports that it examined the data obtained at each interview and reconstructed daily drinking dispositions as reported in the Sobells' publications, not even for the four randomly selected subjects.

Marlatt et al. (1993) and other commentators as well as the Dickens Committee declare that the retrospective reports of our participants are subject to fallible memories because of the many years between their interview by Pendery and the original follow-up. The Sobells' study in contrast interviewed relatively frequently and was therefore less subject to errors of memory. Why then did not the Committee interview the patients and determine whether their memories agree with the data on the interview sheets or not, support the Sobells' or our contention concerning the frequency of interviews and the nature of the data? I think the Committee did not take that obvious step for fear of what it might uncover: There were no detailed time-line interview sheets providing the daily drinking disposition for each day of the year for each subject.

Diversionary tactics

Again, Marlatt et al., (1993) attack our paper for failing to compare the two groups, once more an issue considered at length in chapter 5 including evidence that at least one subject was reassigned, and need not be repeated here. As true of the Dickens Committee Marlatt et al. ignore the significant order effect reported in Pendery et al. and additional reasons given for not comparing the two groups, as well as my subsequent replies to critics.

A final question: How can Marlatt et al. (1993) be considered to have provided an objective disinterested review of the controversy, when they make no reference to the evidence presented in my paper (Maltzman, 1989) of reassignment and nonrandom assignment of patients in the Sobells' study? Is this the kind of scholarship that engenders trust and advances the pursuit of the truth?

Validation of Sobells' Research

Marlatt et al. (1993) assert that Caddy et al. (1978) conducted an independent three-year follow-up of the Sobells' patients which validates their results. Marlatt et al. do not discuss the data presented in Pendery et al. (1982) contradicting such an assertion, data which have also been reproduced by Wallace (1990). Additional evidence reported by Maltzman (1989) is also ignored by Marlatt et al. There are sworn affidavits from 10 of 13 living participants in the controlled drinking experimental group who report that they were never interviewed by Caddy et al. or their associates, contrary to the published report (Caddy et al., 1978). Evidence reported by Pendery et al. (1982) contradicting Caddy et al. is reproduced in Table 8.1. Descriptive results are shown for the six highest functioning patients purportedly interviewed by Caddy et al. and are among those whom they report to be among the 50% who were functioning well 100% of the time in their third year follow-up.

Table 8.1 Pendery, et al., (1982), present the following: "findings regarding third-year treatment outcomes of the six subjects ranked highest by Caddy et al., (1976) all of whom they reported as functioning well 100 percent of the days in that year." (p.173).

CD-E 1   Subject and multiple collaterals state he drank heavily throughout year 3, during which he resided in three states. He used an assumed name on his driver's license because of an outstanding alcohol-related felony bench warrant issued in year 2. In February, year 3, police were called by neighbors of subject's mother, when he threatened violence and caused a disturbance while drunk, and in April, he was too drunk to attend his brother's funeral. (This trend continued and in year 4 he was arrested for drunk driving and rehospitalized.)

CD-E 5   Subject states that "the third year included some of my worst drinking experiences. "In August 1972, "after drinking more than a fifth of liquor per day, I went to the San Bernardino Alcoholism Services for help. I was having shakes and other withdrawal symptoms and was very sick physically. By then, a physician had told me I had alcohol cirrhosis of the liver." A record of the subject's application for treatment there, his wife's statement, documentation of subsequent hospitalization for alcoholism treatment, and continued deterioration of his health are consistent with his self-report.

CD-E 11 Subject and collateral state that year 3 was his worst year. His records show he spent time in jail, in a state hospital, and in a Veterans Administration hospital because of actions he committed while intoxicated. Toward the end of year 3, he had additional arrests, including one for drunk driving.

CD-E 13 Subject and multiple collaterals state that he was abstinent throughout year 3. He states, however, that this was in spite of the controlled drinking treatment. He became abstinent only after additional alcohol-related incarcerations in hospitals, jail, and road camp. He then spent 5 months of year 2 at Twelve Step House, an AA-oriented alcoholism recovery home, to which he attributed his abstinence.

CD-E 15 Subject and multiple collaterals state he was drinking excessively (sometimes as much as a fifth per day and some beer) when he was not going to be at work. (His blood alcohol of 0.34 percent on a recent admission to a hospital confirms his high reported tolerance.). He had not yet experienced serious alcohol withdrawal symptoms during year 3 and did not require hospitalization. According to his family, however, his health was already beginning to deteriorate, leading to repeated alcohol-related medical problems and hospitalizations from 1976 to the present.

CD-E 18 Subject and collateral state that he successfully controlled his drinking throughout year 3, although, "it would not be entirely accurate to say I never drank excessively. " We found no evidence of alcohol-related problems in any major life area. In our view this subject, who apparently had not experienced physical withdrawal symptoms, might have been appropriately designated an alpha (psychologically dependent) alcoholic...

Note. From Pendery, et al. (1982). Reprinted by permission from the American Association for the Advancement of Science

---

Four of the six were drinking heavily during the year they were reported by Caddy et al. as functioning well 100% of the time. Note that in all cases the recall of a participant is supported by reports from collateral persons and/or public records. Examination of these descriptive histories contradicts the argument offered by Marlatt et al. (1993) and other critics that the results obtained by Pendery "are largely based on retrospective self-reports" (p. 473). Despite the evidence contradicting the validity of Caddy et al.'s (1978) reported results and the sworn statements of the majority of available participants and collateral persons that they were never interviewed, there has never been an investigation of the Caddy et al. study.

Marlatt et al. (1993) go on to consider the best designed study of controlled drinking training with chronic alcoholic inpatients (Foy et al., 1984; Rychtarik et al., 1987). What is most striking about their treatment of this study is that Marlatt et al. and every other revisionist I have read who has commented on this study has misinterpreted the results. As previously noted (see chapter 1), the study by Rychtarik, Foy, and their colleagues contradicts the notion that controlled drinking is a feasible treatment goal and fails to corroborate the Sobells' results. At six-month follow-up the experimental group that had received controlled drinking training in addition to traditional treatment, was significantly worse than the control group receiving only traditional treatment. A follow-up five to six years later found no significant difference between the two groups (Rychtarik et al., 1987). This means that controlled drinking training had no significant effect. Nevertheless, supporters of controlled drinking have consistently misinterpreted its results as indicating that traditional abstinence and controlled drinking skills training were equally effective.

Marlatt et al. (1993) make the same error in interpretation as other revisionist supporters of controlled drinking. Commentators incorrectly interpret the Rychtarik et al. (1987) study, casting controlled drinking outcomes in a favorable light. I suggest this reflects the powerful biasing effect of their common ideology. The Institute of Medicine (1990) makes the same error in interpreting Rychtarik et al.

Additional controlled drinking outcomes

Treatment outcome studies claimed to demonstrate controlled drinking adopted spontaneously by patients typically do not report assessments of severity of the alcohol dependence or misuse. When studies explicitly distinguish between problem drinkers and alcoholics or obtain independent measures of the severity of dependence, they characteristically find that physically dependent participants do not engage in controlled drinking in appreciable numbers; they abstain or eventually relapse. It is only the problem drinkers who on occasion engage successfully in controlled drinking in appreciable numbers. Edwards et al. (1983) found that 40% of their patients were in the good outcome category 10-12 years after treatment. Of these, approximately 70% were abstaining and 30% were engaged in social drinking. The latter group "had never become severely dependent" as assessed on the Severity of Alcoholism Dependency Questionnaire (Stockwell et al., 1979). Orford, Oppenheimer and Edwards (1976) found that after a two-year follow-up, of those in the good outcome category, participants who were engaged in controlled drinking had all been diagnosed as problem drinkers prior to treatment. Abstainers were physically dependent alcoholics and problem drinkers. None of the alcoholics, independently diagnosed prior to the start of treatment, was engaged in successful social drinking.

Taylor, Helzer, and Robins (1986) reviewed outcome studies of the occurrence of moderate drinking in recovering alcoholics published during the decade since the 1976 Rand Report. They concluded that in large studies with a large evaluation window, the rate of return to moderate drinking is approximately 3%.

Walker (1987) conducted a study of 100 randomly selected cases of inpatients treated in a New Zealand Hospital. Follow-up time varied from 8 - 12.5 years. Forty per cent had recovered clinically and socially with 28% completely abstinent for 2.5 - 12 years. Twelve percent had lapses of less than seven days in any year but had maintained their health and social situation. Some of the patients who were deceased were known to be recovered at the time of death so that the recovery rate actually exceeded 40%. Only 2% had become stable moderate drinkers. Walker concludes, "A return to social drinking for alcoholics is so rarely an achievable goal that it has no place in a normal treatment plan" (p.556).

Marlatt et al. (1993) make no reference to the results of Edwards and his colleagues or to those reported in perhaps the most carefully conducted large-scale multisite inpatient treatment outcome study of all (Feuerlein & Küfner, 1989, Küfner & Feuerlein, 1989) discussed in some detail in chapter 7.

Controlled drinking training for problem drinkers

A difficulty with the controlled-drinking-as-secondary-prevention program is that it presupposes the effectiveness of assessment. Despite Marlatt et al.'s (1993) ideological caricature of the problem of progression from problem drinking to alcoholism, this is a critically important empirical problem. It must be possible to differentiate between individuals who, once learning to reduce their drinking, will continue to drink with moderation, will remain at a moderate level, from those others who may increase their intake and progress into alcoholism. Miller and Joyce (1979) state, "It may be some time before we can a priori empirically discriminate successful candidates for controlled drinking from those with poorer prognosis..." (p. 775). After two decades there is still no progress and even worse, the problem is ignored by Marlatt et al. (1993).

Miller has for years claimed striking success for his variation of behavior therapy, behavioral self-control training (BSCT), in contrast to the purported lack of success for abstinence oriented treatment programs (Hester & Miller, 1995; Miller, 1980; Miller & Hester, 1980). He has reported success rates of from 60% to 80% in his and other studies. Miller and his associates (Miller et al., 1986; Miller et al., 1992) have now reported the results of a long-term follow-up study, 3.5 - 8 years, of the controlled drinking participants in these studies which had been described with enthusiasm. Strikingly different long-term results were obtained from those reported in the original short-term outcome follow-ups (see chapters 1 and 6).

One could not possibly determine from the review by Marlatt et al. (1993) that the long term follow-up results obtained by Miller et al. (1986, 1992) contradict the extravagant claims originally voiced for controlled drinking for problem drinkers. Approximately 10% -14%, depending upon whether or not subjects lost to attrition are treated as failures, were engaged in moderate drinking at follow-up; 23%-31% were abstinent. Even with state-of-the-art training for controlled drinking, more people were abstinent in the long term than were drinking moderately. Neither outcome is impressive, particularly when the base rate of spontaneous remissions after one year is considered: 19% (Miller & Hester, 1980).

In their cursory discussion of these important results, Marlatt et al. (1993) fail to note that Miller and his colleagues explicitly excluded alcoholics from their treatment program, limiting their controlled drinking training to problem drinkers. Alcoholics dependent upon alcohol who had manifested severe withdrawal symptoms including convulsions and delerium tremens were excluded (Graber & Miller, 1988; Harris & Miller, 1990; Miller & Taylor, 1980; Miller, Taylor, & West, 1980). Marlatt et al. do not report that the diagnosis of some of the participants as suffering from gamma alcoholism was made retrospectively with additional information not available at the time the study was initiated. They also fail to note that the detailed interview schedules obtaining self-reports based on long term recall and forming the bases for these classifications were administered 3.5 - 8 years after the initiation of treatment. Marlatt et al. (1993) make a point of observing that at the time of the follow-up an appreciable percentage of the controlled drinkers, 33%, were gamma alcoholics, based upon these retrospective reports. However, they do not point out that the group was only 10% of the sample retrieved, in other words, perhaps three gamma alcoholics engaged in controlled drinking, assuming that one accepts the validity of detailed self-reports 3.5 - 8 years after the fact. Marlatt et al. do not find it necessary to criticize this retrospective assessment of alcohol dependence versus abuse which must rely on detailed recall of events which occurred 3.5 - 8 years earlier, intervals as long and longer than those occurring in the Pendery et al. (1982) study. The latter study is criticized by Marlatt et al. for purportedly having too extreme a time lag between events and their recall.

Marlatt et al. (1993) also fail to observe that Miller et al. (1986) reported that approximately 66% of the subjects were diagnosed as gamma or delta alcoholics at follow-up. These results are in accord with Jellinek's (1996) suggestion that problem drinkers may progress into alcoholism. It must be remembered that at the outset of the treatment program initiated by Miller and his associates participants were all judged to be problem drinkers.

Diagnostic techniques for discriminating between early stage alcoholics or potential alcoholics versus problem drinkers or alcohol abusers, are critically important, especially if controlled drinking is the treatment goal. Controlled drinking as a treatment goal is not necessarily harm reduction. In the long run it may be harm induction, providing an opportunity for individuals to progress in the damage to themselves and to others.

Eckardt et al. (1980) found that there are continued deleterious neuropsychological consequences of post treatment drinking. They comment:

The resumption of drinking following treatment, even at levels of consumption deemed by some as being 'socially acceptable,' was associated with poorer neuropsychological performance than abstinence. Whether the degree of the decrement in neuropsychological function is of clinical significance remains to be determined, especially in light of the assertion that controlled drinking is an appropriate goal for some alcoholic patients .... It is clear, however, that the influence of resumed alcohol consumption on recovery of brain function should be considered by both clinician and the alcoholic patient in determining treatment goals. (p.145f).

Important ethical as well as health issues are raised by Eckardt et al. that proponents of controlled drinking as harm reduction fail to address.

Abstinence treatment outcomes

As discussed in chapters 1 and 7 reasonably high success rates exist for private abstinence treatment programs in the United States and some programs abroad, but they have been a well kept secret by revisionist reviewers who dominate academic publications in the field of alcoholism studies. Abstinence results reported by CATOR (Harrison et al., 1991) are not cited by Marlatt et al. (1993). Despite the supporting evidence abstinence is not considered a successful way of producing harm reduction.

Conclusion: two decades of pettifogging

The basic issue in the past two decades of controversy in the field of alcoholism studies, more important than controlled drinking versus abstinence, is the truth and trust versus mendacity and deceit. Tactics of ideological supporters of controlled drinking have foresaken the former virtues for the latter devices of ambition.

The second issue is whether (a) controlled drinking is a viable treatment goal for alcoholics as distinguished from problem drinkers and whether (b) controlled drinking is a viable treatment and secondary prevention method for problem drinkers.

Research reviewed in chapters 6 and 7 demonstrates that abstinence for alcoholics is a viable treatment goal whereas controlled drinking is not. For problem drinkers, I assume a subgroup of these alcohol misusers may reduce their alcohol consumption to safe limits, i.e., 2 drinks/day for males and 1 drink/day for females and remain at that level without progressing into alcoholism. However, methods for differentiating between such people and those who will progress into alcoholism have not been employed by promoters of controlled drinking. Claims for success of controlled drinking with problem drinkers by Marlatt et al. (1993) and other revisionists far exceed the reach of current research, which at best is preliminary.

Marlatt et al.'s (1993) arguments claiming success of controlled drinking with physically dependent alcoholics are counterfeit. None of the three cornerstone studies of controlled drinking by alcoholics, Davies, Rand, Sobells, withstands scrutiny. Evidence overwhelmingly demonstrates that controlled drinking is not a viable treatment for such individuals. Evidence at hand of effective controlled drinking treatment for problem drinkers is a promissory note at best, since the evidence that appears to support controlled drinking is based on relatively short-term follow-ups and poor methodology, short evaluation windows and inflated measures of "improvement". Long-term follow-up fails to support claims made for controlled drinking and show that an appreciable number of individuals screened as appropriate candidates for controlled drinking because they were problem drinkers, progress over the years into alcoholism (Miller et al., 1986, 1992). Behavior therapists act as though these distressing outcomes do not exist.

Controlled drinking as proposed by Marlatt et al. (1993) has a fatal flaw: It ignores the evidence that alcoholism is a biopsychosocial syndrome. Of critical importance is the evidence that brain dysfunction may develop even in problem drinkers, a dysfunction which may persist with continued drinking (Cala, 1987; Eckardt et al. 1980; Eckardt et al., 1998; Shear et al., 1994). Further evidence for the critical role of biobehavioral factors is the finding that neuropsychological and electrocortical measures of brain function can predict the occurrence of relapse with some success (Bauer, 1994; Parsons, 1994). Assessments required to differentiate those who may benefit from controlled drinking from those who will be harmed must include measures of brain structure and function to ensure that brain disease is absent. It must be remembered that, in contrast to controlled drinking, abstinence as a treatment goal does not carry the danger of inducing further brain damage (Eckardt et al., 1980) and progression into alcoholism.

When all of the outcome evidence for abstinence as a treatment goal is considered, it is apparent that some of these programs have attained higher success rates than any controlled drinking program. Effectiveness and harm reduction with controlled drinking depends on effective assessment. Such assessment, it appears, must involve measures of brain structure and function.

The above documentation of the numerous errors of omission and commission in Marlatt et al.'s (1993) review of one segment of the harm reduction literature, that concerned with controlled drinking, suggests that it fails to provide an appropriate guide through the complex of issues for which harm reduction is offered as a solution. The article under consideration has been adapted by Marlatt et al. and is now part of a chapter on harm reduction with some additional material (Larimer et al., 1998). Errors of omission and commission noted in the present chapter remain.

When a community is directed to a single objective, its code of conduct becomes simpler and more severe than the easy-going code of compromises which does duty for most people. In daily life few of us are entirely rigid about white lies and tax-deductible expenses and other small evasions. We accept, even if we do not condone, such venial sins. But the professional morality of scientists allows no compromises. It tells each man that he must report what he believes to be true, exactly and without suppression or editing. Nowhere in a research journal is a scientist allowed to minimize an awkward discrepancy or to stress a comforting confirmation. Nowhere is he allowed to put what seems expedient in place of an unpalatable truth. A scientist takes it for granted that when another scientist reports a finding, he can be believed absolutely - by which we mean, that we can be certain that what the man reported is exactly what he thought he saw or heard, no less and no more.

This absolute trust of each man in the word of every other man is remarkable in the society of scientists. Yet it is not by itself the whole of scientific morality. For a morality embraces not only the individual and his trust, but a whole community, and it therefore has to provide for all the subtle relations between the members of the community. The morality of science is subtle in this way, but it has grown from a simple principle - the principle that the community of scientists shall be so organized that nothing shall stand in the way of the emergence of the truth. (Bronowski, 1977, pp.199-200).

9

LITTLE ALBERT REDUX:
OR WHATEVER
HAPPENED TO SCHOLARSHIP

> Whoever controls the present controls the past as well as the future.
>
> -Orwell (1984)

Many students of psychology probably know the story of Little Albert. He was the subject in the first study of human classical conditioning of fear, a study by Watson and Rayner (1920). They initially demonstrated that nine-month old Albert displayed no fear when shown live animals such as a rat, rabbit, dog and monkey as well as inanimate objects, cotton, a human mask, burning newspaper, etc. Albert showed fear when a loud noise was suddenly produced by striking a steel bar with a hammer. Two months later fear was conditioned to a rat by pairing the loud noise with occasions where Albert touched the rat. After two sessions involving a total of seven trials, a test trial, presentation of the rat alone without the noise, resulted in the occurrence of fear responses defined as crying and attempts to avoid the rat. Five days later generalization test trials were introduced by presenting familiar wooden blocks, a rabbit, dog, sealskin coat, cotton, etc. Albert displayed generalized fear to the rabbit, dog, and seal skin coat, but not many other objects. Circumstances prevented Watson from determining the persistence of the fear and from attempting to extinguish the crying and avoidance elicited by the rat and generalization stimuli. A number of writers (Cornwell & Hobbs, 1976; Harris, 1979; Prytula, Oster, & Davis, 1977) have observed that with the passage of time, accounts of this classic experiment on fear conditioning drifted from the original in a variety of details, some quite important.

Cornwell and Hobbs (1976) and Harris (1979) report that the deviations from the original encountered in secondary sources in several instances modified the details to make the original appear better, more acceptable, and more in keeping with present ethical standards. Very often the errors were trivial. Various textbooks examined by Harris (1979) misrepresented Albert's age, his name, whether the CS was a rat or a rabbit, and the list of stimuli purporting to elicit generalization. Some secondary sources added a cat, a man's beard, a fur muff, and a teddy bear, etc. An extinction session was invented in later accounts where Watson eliminated the fear in little Albert, thus bringing closure and a happy ending to the experiment. Extinction of fear was studied by Jones (1924) several years later in a different child with guidance from Watson (Jones,1974).

Samelson (1980) notes the inconsistencies and contradictions found in various reports of the Little Albert experiment that Watson himself published. The paper originally published is a preliminary pilot study at best. Samelson observes that in the original report of the study, but subsequently ignored by commentators:

> Whenever Albert was emotionally upset, he would 'continually thrust his thumb into his mouth... [thus becoming] impervious to the stimuli producing fear'....

The extraordinary appeal of the Albert story must have come from the fact that it was.... a beautiful illustration of an idea already congenial to its audience. (Samelson, 1980, p. 621).

Samelson's observation is particularly pertinent to the case we will consider, the saga of the Sobells' controlled drinking study (Sobell & Sobell, 1972, 1973, 1978, 1984a, 1984b, 1989). Results purporting to show that behavior modification/therapy may be applied with striking success to a new area of problem behavior, alcoholism, would be most congenial to clinical psychologists of a behavior modification/therapy persuasion. It fit the Zeitgeist. It was compatible with the apperceptive mass of the new clinical psychologist and was accepted as another demonstration of the superiority of behavior modification based upon laboratory principles of conditioning over psychodynamic and folk psychology. It opened a new area of research for which funds were becoming available in the recently formed National Institute on Alcohol Abuse and Alcoholism (NIAAA). It also provided access to a new practice domain for behavior therapy, the lucrative alcoholism treatment field, currently estimated to cost more than five billion dollars a year, dominated by Alcoholics Anonymous and the "medical model".

The controlled drinking saga we will consider involves more significant consequences than Little Albert. Its consequences may affect public policy, civil and criminal justice proceedings, treatment and mistreatment of an unsuspecting public, misuse of public funds, and the promotion of cynicism and moral laxity in professionals and students. These may be some of the consequences when there is uncritical and zealous acceptance of myths having direct impact upon the well-being of the public.

Compounding the difficulty in ascertaining the truth about the Sobell study and its aftermath is that several sources of pertinent information are not readily accessible. For example, a report for which one must contact an institute and pay for a copy (Dickens et al., 1982), or request from a government agency (Trachtenberg, 1984). In such cases free and open access to the information permitting verification of events is hindered. Difficulties are compounded when the information sought concerns an alleged ethical violation where the proceedings are confidential, or a lawsuit and its outcome. Disinterested authors of review articles or textbooks and handbooks are unlikely to make the extra effort needed to obtain a report or confirm an assertion under the above conditions. Potential authors would be even less likely to pursue independent confirmation of assertions if they received a summary of the report that purports to provide its principal conclusions or when there is available an apparent authoritative account (Marlatt, 1983, 1985; Marlatt, Lorimer, Baer, & Quigley, 1993) or readily accessible reviews (Brownell,1984; Foreyt,1987,1990) by like-thinking pundits. Under these conditions the reader will most likely rely on secondary sources that are readily available. This is evident in textbook accounts (Barlow & Durand, 1995; Goldstein, Baker, & Jamison, 1986; Logue, 1988; Thombs, 1994; Wortman, Loftus, & Marshall, 1988). It is even evident in monographs purporting to report upon fraud or controversies in science (Hunt, 1999; Kohn, 1986).

Some may wonder, "why dredge up the Sobell's alleged misconduct when they have been exonerated by five different investigations" (Baumeister, Heatherton, & Tice, 1994; Nathan, 1989; Sobell & Sobell, 1989)? I "dredge up" the story because: (a) there have not been five different investigations; (b) the ones that have been conducted are fundamentally flawed as seen in chapter 5; and (c) the system that permits perpetuation of this sort of myth has serious inadequacies that can only be corrected if there is a free and open airing of the factors that perpetuate myths such as those surrounding the controlled drinking controversy.

The focus of the first section of the present chapter is the by now familiar Sobell IBTA study (1972,1973a, 1976, 1978), designed to train physiologically dependent alcoholics to take up controlled drinking. It is the Little Albert of alcoholism treatment. Our net will be spread further in the second section of the chapter, catching the errors of omission and commission in treatments of alcoholism found in undergraduate elementary and advanced textbooks and handbooks on alcoholism designed for graduate students and professionals (Hester & Miller, 1995; Thombs, 1994). Implications of this catch are that generations of students are being fed ideologically driven constructions of the alcoholism field that are contradicted by the research literature that is ignored or misrepresented by textbook writers especially those of a behavior therapy persuasion. Potential harm to the unsuspecting public that may read or be advised and treated by students reading this material cannot be estimated and may be considerable.

At the time of its publication the IBTA study appeared to be the most rigorously designed and executed treatment experiment ever conducted in the field of alcoholism studies. It purported to have had random assignment of patients to an experimental and control group and a two-year post-treatment follow-up with interviews every 3-4 weeks. Each interview obtained a daily drinking disposition and determined for each day for two full years whether the subject: abstained, drank less than 6 oz of spirits or the equivalent, drank more than 6 oz of spirits or the equivalent (drunk day), was incarcerated in jail or was in a hospital for alcohol related reasons. Information concerning drinking behavior was also obtained from each participant's collaterals.

Papers reporting the follow-up after one year (Sobell & Sobell, 1973a), two years (Sobell & Sobell, 1976), and the description of the study in book chapters were widely read and cited (Franks & Wilson, 1975, 1978), as was the book reporting the entire study (Sobell & Sobell, 1978). Based upon a review of *Current Contents* I estimate more than 350 journal citations of IBTA study reports for the 10 year period 1976-1985.

Our concern is not over drift in the Sobells' original accounts of their procedures. Relatively little occurred, in part because they were repeated so frequently. However, following my allegation of fraud (Boffey, 1982) apparent misinformation by the Sobells appeared and was disseminated by others. For example, it was said (Dickens et al., 1982) that the Sobells' law suit attempting to prevent our follow-up of the patients in the IBTA study terminated because of their lack of funds (Heather & Robertson, 1983; Hunt, 1999). In fact, the lawsuit was decided in our favor on the merits of the case. The number of investigations of their alleged fraud ballooned into five. These purportedly include a congressional investigation (Baumeister, Heatherton, & Tice, 1994; Hunt, 1999; Marlatt, 1983, 1984; Marlatt et al., 1993; Nathan, 1989; Peele, 1984; Sobell & Sobell, 1984b) and a medical malpractice lawsuit which dragged on for 4 years. All five purportedly exonerated the Sobells (Baumeister et al., 1994; Nathan, 1989; Sobell & Sobell, 1989). These "investigations", as we have seen, are not what they have been made out to be.

Errors of commission and omission in secondary sources tend to cluster around specific issues and occurrences. We shall consider some of the most frequent and significant errors found in secondary sources and then turn to misinformation that has been widely circulated and cited.

THE SOBELLS' PROCEDURE

Frequency of interviews

All of the Sobells' descriptions of the research procedure employed in their study stated that the patients and their collaterals were interviewed every 3-4 weeks. A time-line follow-back procedure was said to have been employed (Sobell & Sobell, 1989) in which subjects' drinking disposition for every day of the previous 3-4 weeks interval was accounted for in terms of days abstinent, drunk, drinking in a controlled fashion, or incarcerated in jail or hospital for alcohol related reasons.

As we saw in chapter 5 the Dickens Committee found that the Sobells interviewed their subjects less frequently than reported in their publications. Nevertheless, Marlatt et al. (1993) state that there were regular telephone contacts, "approximately every other month" (p.470). Thombs (1994) on the other hand asserts that the Sobells contacted "their subjects every 2 weeks" (p.99) as does Peele (1983). Further variation is contributed by Nathan and Lipscomb (1979) who state that, "patients were contacted every 2 or 3 weeks to enable the follow-up worker to keep track of their whereabouts for the formal follow-up interviews scheduled at 6-month intervals." (p.338). When the data were collected is unclear from this erroneous description, implying that data were collected at 6-month intervals. Two kinds of interviews, frequent informal and semi-annual formal interviews are not described in any of the Sobell reports or in the Dickens Committee Report. For example, the Sobells (1973a) state: "Each time that a subject or a collateral information source called or was contacted, various information was obtained concerning the subjects' functioning since the last followup contact". (p. 602).

Taped daily drinking disposition interviews

Another type of error in the description of the Sobells' procedure is the claim that they tape recorded each of the interviews in which they obtained reports of the daily drinking disposition. Marlatt et al., (1993) are explicit, "The potential for biased self-reports was minimized by the use of standard, objective questions and by the fact that all interviews were tape-recorded and open to independent verification" (p.471). Other writers are somewhat ambiguous. For example, Cozby (1985), states,..."a 'blue-ribbon panel' ... investigated the Sobells' original work. Fortunately, the Sobells had kept extensive records of their research activities, including audiotapes of interviews of the patients in a follow-up study" (pp.206-207). Nathan and Niaura (1985) also report that the Sobells had tape-recorded interviews, but do not specify the nature of the interviews. A similar ambiguous assertion is made by Heather and Robertson (1983, p. 268).

Time-line follow-back interviews that provided the follow-up data for the Sobells' study were not audiotaped. Taping of an interview was done at the end of the second year follow-up. These latter tapes did not provide the daily drinking disposition data that constitute the primary dependent variable used in the Sobells' IBTA study. "As part of the IBT follow-up, subjects were asked to consent to a tape-recorded interview at the end of their two-year follow-up interval... to gather information about the subjects' impression of the study" (Sobell & Sobell, 1978, p. 167). Contrary to Marlatt et al., (1993), the Sobells (1984b) state quite clearly, "The taped interview was not used for the purpose of routine data collection or to provide evidence of our contact with subjects." (p.165).

Despite the above errors in his description of the procedures and data obtained in the IBTA study, Nathan (1985) asserts, "I know the Sobells, I know their data. They did not commit fraud." (p.172).

Random assignment of patients

According to Marlatt et al. (1993), "A key strength of the Sobells' research design is the fact that patients were randomly assigned to either the experimental controlled drinking treatment or the abstinence control condition" (p.472) (see also Marlatt, 1983, 1985). Marlatt et al. (1993) assert: "A careful reading of the Pendery study, however, reveals a number of disturbing questions concerning the scientific credibility of... the *Science* article. First and foremost is the issue of why the results from the abstinence-goal control group were omitted..." (p.472).

"The Sobells did have a control group consisting of patients who had been treated with the goal of abstinence. However, Pendery and her coworkers did not report follow-up data on the members of this group. " (Logue, 1986, p. 213).

Thombs (1994) in a textbook for alcoholism counselors uses a secondary source and sarcasm to observe: "As Peele (1985) and others have subsequently pointed out, Pendery et al. (1982) in their investigation of the Sobells' research, conveniently ignored the outcomes among the abstinence treatment group." (p. 98).

Nathan and Niaura (1985) state, "It is unfortunate that Pendery and Maltzman failed to report on a parallel follow-up of control subjects; the absence of data on control subjects makes valid conclusions from their data on experimental subjects impossible." (p.433).

All of these comments asserting that the two groups in Pendery et al., (1982) were not compared diverts attention from the issue the Dickens Committee (Dickens et al., 1982) was appointed to address: The validity of the Sobells' research report. Did they do what they said they did and did they find what they said they found? Whether or not the control and experimental groups differed in treatment outcome in the Pendery et al. study would neither prove nor disprove the allegation of the Sobells' misconduct. It would only indicate whether controlled drinking and abstinent treatment effects were the same or different, were reliable or not. This latter question presupposes the trustworthiness of the reported data and procedures. Examination of Patton State Hospital records (Pendery et al., 1982) revealed a significant difference between the two groups in the order in which they entered the hospital (p < .002). Most of the experimental subjects entered the hospital before the control group patients. Since we found this significant order difference which violates the assumption of random assignment of any statistic we might use to compare the two groups, we could not compare the groups further. Our significant difference in order is also the Sobells' significant order effect. Their two groups cannot meaningfully be compared. Pendery et al. (1982) explicitly state that the two groups were not compared further for three reasons:

(1) There is a difficulty in interpretation of differences between groups because the control patients volunteered, were selected as appropriate for controlled drinking, and controlled drinking was considered an attainable goal yet these patients were given the abstinence treatment goal instead.

(2) Patients in the control group were exposed to laudatory reports concerning successful controlled drinking while some were still in treatment for abstinence, and when all were still being interviewed during the follow-up period. Television programs such as CBS News reported on the Patton successes with controlled drinking in the winter of 1971; the Sobells and two patients were on the Ralph Story TV program extolling the success of controlled drinking in February 1971; in March 1971 *Time* published an article on the Patton study extolling the advantage of controlled drinking. Half the control group had not yet been run when this story appeared. A story appeared on the front page of the metro section of the *San Diego Union* in March, 1973 describing the remarkable success of controlled drinking reported by Linda Sobell during a talk she gave at Sharp Hospital in San Diego.

(3) Pendery et al. (1982) wished to address the question of whether or not controlled drinking itself is a desirable treatment goal. Were 85% of the participants in the controlled drinking group functioning well 85% of the time as claimed by the Sobells (1978)?

What the Dickens Committee meant by their finding, "no evidence of departure from randomization" is that they found no evidence of intentional deviation from random assignment. Reports by members of the research staff that a coin toss determined membership in the experimental or control group was taken as evidence that the patients were randomly assigned. The Dickens Committee never demonstrated why our statistical finding of nonrandomness and its implication should be ignored. Neither did Marlatt et al. (1993), Thombs (1994), nor the numerous other critics who castigate Pendery et al. for failing to compare the two groups with one exception, Heather and Robertson (1983). The latter simply consider our reasons for not comparing the groups unimportant. However, they were unaware of the extensive media coverage received by the Sobells' experimental subjects almost from the outset of the study continuing through the follow-up period.

INVESTIGATIONS, REAL AND ALLEGED

Misinformation has enveloped the Sobell affair, including the legal actions that they have taken and the number and kind of investigations of their alleged fraud. For example, Nathan (1989) asserts that Maltzman (1989), "repeats a series of allegations that have been considered and rejected by five separate and competent investigative groups." (p. 465).

Dickens Report exonerates Sobells

The first and most extensive investigation of the Sobells alleged fraud was conducted by the Dickens Committee appointed by the Sobells' employer at the time allegations of misconduct appeared (Boffey, 1982). Discussion of the fundamental flaws in the Dickens Report are presented in chapter 5 and need not be repeated here.

Premature termination of legal action

According to Heather and Robertson (1983):
> The Sobells became aware of this (Pendery et al.) projected investigation and there then followed a long and protracted legal battle over access to the list of names and details of subjects. The Sobells argued that they were prevented by the ethics of confidentiality from handing over this list to any unauthorized person... Eventually in 1976 lack of funds forced the Sobells to retire from the legal dispute and access to their patients was granted by the courts to Pendery and Maltzman. (p. 262).

The apparent source of this misinformation is the Dickens Report, and therefore ultimately the Sobells. A similar reason for the termination of the lawsuit is given by Hunt (1999) who also invents the legal parties representing me.

A congressional inquiry exonerates Sobells

Chapter 5 presents the evidence contradicting the Sobells' claim that a congressional investigation exonerated them of wrong doing. Nevertheless the Sobells as well as a number of commentators have asserted that they have been exonerated by a congressional investigation (Baumeister et al., 1994; Brownell, 1984; Hunt, 1999; Marlatt, 1983,1984; Peele, 1984; Roizen, 1987; Sobell & Sobell, 1984a,1984b). For example, Roizen (1987) states, "The Sobells' research was also reviewed by the Subcommittee on Investigations and Oversight, Committee on Science and Technology of the United States House of Representatives, which conveyed its conclusions by letter to the Sobells in March 1983..." (pp. 269-270).

A further lack of scholarship is evident on the part of some commentators (Brownell, 1984; Hunt, 1999). They quote portions of Jensen's letter to the Sobells as though it were the original source but use a sanitized version correcting the typographical and grammatical errors.

Trachtenberg Committee Report exonerates Sobells

The Sobells (1989) and others (Baumeister et al., 1994; Foreyt,1987; Hunt, 1999; Marlatt et al., 1993; Nathan, 1989) have stated that the Trachtenberg Committee (Trachtenberg, 1984) under the aegis of the Alcohol Drugs and Mental Health Administration (ADAMHA) investigated the Sobells and exonerated them of wrongdoing. A description of the enforced incompleteness and superficiality of the investigation is provided in chapter 5. Commentators have uniformly ignored the admitted shortcomings of the investigation by the Trachtenberg committee (Trachtenberg, 1984), assuming that they read it.

APA Ethics Committee exonerates Sobells

The Sobells (1989) assert that an investigation by the Committee on Scientific and Professional Ethics and Conduct (CSPEC) of the American Psychological Association has exonerated them. Baumeister et al. (1994) and Nathan (1989) reiterate this claim. Actually, over the years there were at least two complaints against the Sobells brought to the CSPEC. Both were brought by me and the two are in a sense related. Shortly after the injunction and lawsuit filed against us, the Sobells also brought an ethics complaint against Pendery and me for lack of consideration of patient welfare, a major complaint in the lawsuit. Following the court decision in our favor I brought an ethics complaint against the Sobells, October 13, 1976, alleging that they committed fraud. After charges and counter charges, correspondence and several meetings of CSPEC, I received the letters from Brenda Gurel, Secretary of CSPEC at the time which are quoted in chapter 4. There was no investigation.

In October 1983, I again brought a series of ethics complaints to CSPEC against the Sobells. I alleged that:

the Sobells: (1) did not follow the procedures they said they employed; (2) did not accurately report the condition of their patients; (3) intentionally fabricated results; (4) made public statements misrepresenting the nature of the outcome of their study; (5) never corrected the misconceptions of the outcome of their study; (6) never corrected the misconceptions patients had of the treatment they received or provided alternatives to them when it must have been apparent that the treatment had failed; (7) did not protect the confidentiality of their patients by obtaining written consent from all of the patients prior to giving the names of the patients to Glenn Caddy and David Perkins; (8) have not corrected the misrepresentations cited and others since their confirmation in the inquiry known as the Dickens Committee Report (Dickens et al., 1982). Furthermore, the Sobells continue to commit acts of ethical misconduct in an effort to discredit me and Dr. Pendery in our efforts to report what actually happened in the Patton study. (Maltzman, October 13, 1983).

The committee replied that they could consider alleged misconduct which "could only have been discovered as a result of the Dickens Commission Report" (Mills, June 13, 1984). There was no CSPEC investigation of the data obtained by the Sobells; there was no investigation of fraud.

Failure to retract previous statements does not adequately constitute a *current* violation of ethical principles, even if those statements are based on prior unethical conduct. Our position on this complex procedural issue does not reflect a judgment by the committee regarding the substance of your complaints, since the Rules and Procedures prevent us from considering further their merits. (Mills, February 13, 1984).

There was no suggestion that the CSPEC had, or ever would, conduct an investigation of the validity of the Sobells' data. There was no exoneration from allegations of fraud with respect to fabrication of results or misrepresentation of procedures. The CSPEC found that the Sobells' public statements were not self-contradictory and there was no need to retract or clarify earlier published statements. The CSPEC concurred with the Dickens Committee that there was no evidence that the failure to accurately report the frequency of their contacts with patients affected their results. This conclusion by both committees is gratuitous, since they never determined whether or not there are time-line follow-back interviews obtained at each contact and that these data generate the published results. We already know from the meager results described in the Trachtenberg Report that the interview data cannot reproduce the published results in all cases. To find intent to misrepresent by examining published reports alone is an impossibility and this essentially is what the CSPEC found.

Patients' malpractice lawsuit exonerates Sobells

Finally, the Sobells have claimed that they were investigated and exonerated in the course of a $96,000,000 medical malpractice lawsuit brought against them by patients or their estates. Nathan (1989) and Baumeister et al. (1994) echo these claims. We saw in chapter 5 that this is one more blatant form of misinformation floated by the Sobells and promoted by their sympathizers.

Martyrs for science

Revisionists have engaged in a brilliant strategy. They have reinterpreted an allegation of fraud as an attack by an outdated ideology threatened by their scientific approach to problems of alcoholism. The Sobells paint themselves as martyrs in this ideological attack upon them as suggested by the title as well as the content of their reply to Pendery et al. (1982), "The aftermath of heresy... " (Sobell & Sobell, 1984a). Barlow (1993) editor of the book series containing a book by the Sobells' (1993), states in a prefatory note: "Few individuals have made more substantial contributions or have had to endure more controversy along the way than Mark and Linda Sobell" (p. xiii). Segal (1987), editor of a series including a book edited by the Sobells (1987a) states:

Although this new approach, labeled as 'controlled drinking,' was yet to be fully evaluated, its inception evoked a significant reaction from traditionalists in the field of alcoholism. Rather than exploring the utility of the new model it was summarily rejected. Peele, writing in 1984, noted then that not only was controlled drinking rejected, 'no clinician in the United States publicly speaks about the option of controlled drinking for the alcoholic' (p. 1342). This rejection resulted in large part from criticisms of the Rand Study (Polich et al., 1981), and the insinuation by Pendery et al. (1982) that the pioneering controlled drinking research by Mark and Linda Sobell was fraudulent (Sobell & Sobell, 1973, 1976, 1984). As a result of the Pendery-Sobell controversy little progress was made in examining the utility of behavioral methods to help persons with alcohol-related problems. Behavioral scientists and clinical practitioners in the United States had to invest their energy to repel the onslaught brought only (sic) Pendery et al., and could not move ahead until the controversy was settled. (p. xi).

To think that Pendery et al.(1982) and my one statement to the *NY Times* (Boffey, 1982) required hundreds of scientists and practitioners to divert their energies from behavioral research in order to respond and thereby retard progress in helping people with alcohol related problems is an extraordinary claim that is beyond all bounds of reason and evidence.

A similar and ironic lack of self-regulation is apparent in the comments by the authors of a book on self-regulation, Baumeister et al. (1994), who state:

A study by Davies (1962) provided an initial challenge to the notion that alcoholism is a progressive disease that can only be treated with abstinence... The debate that followed has been heated and occasionally vicious. For instance, Mark and Linda Sobell conducted a controlled drinking study in the early 1970s in which operant techniques were used to teach alcoholics to control their drinking behavior. The Sobells concluded that, at least for some individuals, a return to moderate drinking was a viable outcome (Sobell & Sobell, 1973). An article in *Science* by Pendery, Maltzman, and West (1982) criticized the Sobells' research on a number of grounds, including charges that the Sobells misrepresented their findings. These charges of scientific misconduct were evaluated by no less than five international panels of inquiry, including the United States Congress and the American Psychological Association. In a nutshell, the Sobells received some criticisms for minor experimental sloppiness, but there were no indications that any fraud or misrepresentation had occurred (Sobell & Sobell, 1989). Marlatt has summed up the controversy in this way: 'Anyone who suggests controlled drinking is branded as an agent of the devil, tempting the naive alcoholic back into the sin of drinking. If drinking is a sin, the only solution is salvation, a surrendering of personal control to a higher power' (1983, p.1107) (Baumeister et al., 1994, p.167).

A confabulation in the above passages by Baumeister et al. (1994) and Segal (1987) is that Pendery et al. (1982) made allegations, insinuations, or suggestions that the Sobells had committed fraud. This assertion is false. Philip Abelson (1983), editor of *Science* at the time, is explicit in characterizing the editors' care to avoid any such attribution. The source of the allegation of scientific misconduct is my belief that the Sobells committed fraud reported in the *NY Times* by Boffey (1982) after he informed me that Mark Sobell asserted that the paper by Pendery et al. is nothing but an ideological attack.

A series of commentaries on the controlled drinking saga found in a behavior therapy handbook series also suggests the role of martyr adopted by the Sobells and the biasing influence of ideology. Foreyt (1990) states:

there is an article written by the Sobells (Sobell & Sobell, 1989) entitled 'Moratorium on Maltzman: An Appeal to Reason.' in which they carefully review once again the allegations raised by Maltzman and colleagues, and they summarize the findings of each of the inquiries into the conduct of their study. Reading the article by the Sobells again reminded me of the agony and suffering they must have gone through during the past several years. Reviewing the entire controversy one more time, I was again impressed with how thoughtfully and impressively the Sobells handled each of the attacks on them and their work. Although minor errors in the reporting of their data were found, none of these errors appeared to have affected the study's outcome. Only because the Sobells kept such detailed records of their study, including original tapes and notes,

'disease model' or the 'learned behavior' perspective. The data showed that the 'controlled drinking' approach achieved significantly better results than did abstinence training (Rand, l980). (McConnell, l989, p.258).

The above is pure invention. An experiment was not designed and conducted by investigators at the Rand Corporation. A subgroup of subjects, from a select number of facilities described in the first Rand report were followed up for four years and the outcome reported in the second Rand report (Polich et al., l980).

The study [the second Rand report] is based on a random sample of 922 males who made contact in l973 with any one of eight Alcoholism Treatment Centers (ATCs) funded by the National Institute on Alcohol Abuse and Alcoholism. The same cohort was interviewed in previous followups at 6 months and 18 months, and has been the subject of other research, including an earlier Rand study.... The 4-year followup study was not designed as an experimental study of alternative treatments, but its detailed history of treatment over 4 years did permit some analyses of treatment relationships. (Polich et al., l980, pp. v-vii).

McConnell invents an experimental study and results which never existed. His treatment of alcoholism reflects the powerful influence of bias combined with a reliance on secondary sources, primarily Marlatt and William Miller. A distorted and inaccurate review of the field is the consequence, including inventions that complete the, "gestalt": the whole picture of a successful approach to the problem of alcoholism by cognitive behavior therapy. It is a pity, because there is so much in the learning and behavioral neuroscience area that is exciting and relevant to alcohol use and the etiology of alcoholism and its characteristics permitting its classification as a disease. Set and setting are among these variables once we go beyond the simple description of an effect which is a function of the specific situation in which the organism, human or infrahuman is stimulated or receives a drug. A response is always a function of the state of the organism at the moment - how it is "set" and the situation which influences that state (Gauvin, Briscoe, Goulden, & Holloway, 1994; Maltzman, 1990; Rusinov, 1973; Stewart, & Grupp, 1985). Worst of all, McConnell's book provides a misleading, and inaccurate depiction of a major social problem, one that may directly influence the lives of students reading the book.

A second introductory text came to my attention by "accident", Wortman, Loftus, and Marshall (1988). Wortman is a well-known social psychologist; Loftus a well-known experimental psychologist, an expert in human learning and memory and eyewitness testimony; Marshall is a professional writer.

My daughter, Sara, was a graduate student in the Department of Psychology at the Univesity of Minnesota. It has a tradition of teaching the entire introductory course in one large section where the lectures are given by a master lecturer and the class is divided into small discussion sections which meet with graduate student teaching assistants. The head teaching assistant selects the textbook that will be used in any given year. Since the University of Minnesota is one of the largest state universities in the country, approximately 2,000 students a year will take the course given once in each of two semesters/year. Given an estimated price of $50/book at the time, textbook sales for an adoption results in the tidy sum of approximately $100,000/year. Sara happened to be the head teaching assistant one year, busily going through textbooks in the fall trying to decide on one to use for the introductory course in psychology. As I recall, she called one evening rather disturbed, and informed me that she had read a text that had been given to her by a field representative for its publisher. Scanning it, she came to the section on alcoholism where she noticed that my name was mentioned. She exclaimed that the book is libeling me within earshot of the field representative. She photocopied the relevant section of the book and mailed it to me. It did not libel me, but it was an inaccurate and biased presentation of the problem of alcoholism, its characteristics, and treatment. An editor with the publisher called me a few days later. She was coming to the west coast and asked to see me to discuss the material in the book. I agreed. A few days later we met and had a cordial conversation. I said I would write to Wortman and describe my concerns. I sent her an eight page single-spaced letter including references presenting my critical comments. Wortman called and we had an amiable conversation. She thanked me for the information I provided. It was apparent, and she readily admitted, that neither she nor Loftus were knowledgeable in the field of alcoholism and that the section was written by one of the consultants who contributed to the book. I then realized that McConnell's text was an exception. He had written the entire book himself. Most introductory texts have become encyclopedic in length and detail and specialized sections are subcontracted out and written by "experts" in the particular fields. That is what happened in the Wortman et al. book.

Some of the inaccuracies and errors found in the text are as follows: Davies' (1963) classic study is described as a landmark showing, "a small percentage of alcoholics were able to resume drinking in moderate amounts.... How was this possible, psychologists wondered, if alcoholism is a disease whose major symptom is a total breakdown of control if *any* alcohol enters the body?" (p.460). Edwards' (1985) study indicating that patients had misled Davies was not acknowledged.

Jellinek (1960) distinguished among alcoholics and different varieties of what we call problem drinkers, in DSM-IV terms, alcohol dependence and alcohol abuse. That the textbook never makes explicit the distinction between the two diagnostic categories is misleading and poor pedagogy.

The following is a real blooper: "Less than 10 percent of alcoholics in traditional abstinence programs actually manage to give up drinking entirely (Miller, 1985)." This statement is false and is based on an erroneous reading of Miller. He reported that less than 10% spontaneously adopt controlled drinking and suggests that if a treatment program had controlled drinking as its goal it would have a higher percentage of people engaged in successful controlled drinking - greater than 10%. An error of the above sort stating that only 10% of patients in traditional treatment programs gain abstinence in a text read by students who may have a relative with a drinking problem or who themselves are in need of help is unfortunate. It most likely would discourage seeking professional help.

Wortman et al. (1988) describe the Sobells' study and report what the Sobells described as their procedure; subjects were interviewed every three to four weeks, etc. I pointed out to Wortman that this is what the Sobells said they did at the time, not what they actually did, as reported by the Dickens Committee and which the Sobells admitted was the case. A lack of familiarity with the Dickens Report is obvious. One of the cruelest cuts of all occurs when the text turns to the criticisms of the Sobells and describes the critics (Pendery et al., 1982) as "therapists", a term used by Cook (1985), the probable source of this erroneous attribution. It is designed to contrast the Sobells, scientists, with their adversaries, "therapists", who are ignorant of the scientific method.

These therapists reexamined the outcomes for the experimental subjects who had participated in the Sobells' research. Their findings showed a change from the earlier studies. Most of the men had serious alcoholic relapses... Some critics went so far as to suggest that the Sobells may have misrepresented their data (Boffey, 1982)... The Sobells and like-minded psychologists answered that the data from this study must be viewed in comparative perspective... the Pendery critique never compared the outcomes for those in the controlled-drinking group with the outcomes for those in the group that received conventional hospital treatment.... The controlled-drinking subjects may not have turned out to be models of reform, but the men given traditional abstinence-oriented therapies fared even worse (Sobell and Sobell, 1984). (Wortman et al., 1988, pp.461-462).

The standard revisionist interpretation of the Sobell controversy is given. Fraud was not committed, because if one examines the control group it did even more poorly than the experimental group. "Thus, in comparison with the conventional treatment the controlled-drinking program did seem to have advantages." (Wortman et al., 1988, p.462). Another blooper follows:

Subsequent data have tended to support the Sobells' conclusion that it is possible for some alcoholics to become controlled drinkers. One major study of alcoholics across the country found that four years after treatment, 18 percent of the controlled-drinking group had reduced their alcohol consumption to nonproblem levels. In contrast, less than 10 percent of the conventionally treated group were totally abstaining (Polich, Armor, and Braiker, 1981).

As was true of McConnell, Wortman et al. are implying that an experiment was conducted comparing two groups, one receiving treatment for abstinence and the other receiving treatment for controlled drinking. That is not true. Figures offered for the two kinds of outcome are also incorrect. Polich et al., (1980) state: "46 percent of the sample were found to be in remisssion: 28 percent were abstaining throughout the 6-month period before the followup interview, and 18 percent were classified as 'drinking without problems' " (p. vi).

Advocates of abstinence are not convinced by the findings and are not likely to be in the near future. They continue to see controlled drinking as a threat to successful long-term treatment. Behaviorally oriented therapists disagree, however. Some see the goals of abstinence and controlled drinking as compatible. According to Alan Marlatt, learning not to drink (how to say no) is an important part of controlled drinking (Marlatt, 1983). The two goals, in his view, can work together for the benefit of patients.

Although there is still widespread and heated debate over controlled-drinking programs, their use for some problem drinkers is gradually growing. The best candidates for this form of treatment seem to be those who are younger (under forty), with shorter histories of excessive drinking (less than ten years), no strong physical addiction to the drug...

As controlled-drinking programs spread, so does awareness that it is often counterproductive to be tied to a single form of treatment for all people with a certain disorder (Cook, 1985). Since the sources of people's problems differ in the first place, it makes sense that they would benefit from more individualized treatments. Such treatments can include a variety of biological, psychological, and social therapies. This is the direction in which the treatment of alcoholism is currently moving. (Wortman et al., 1988, p.462).

There is no recognition of the evidence that alcoholism treatment is not moving in the desired direction. It has been there for years in the form of the Minnesota Model. Their presentation of alcoholism treatment distorts the present scene, fails to recognize the existence of private treatment facilities and their high rate of success in treatment outcomes at least as represented by the CATOR results discussed in chapter 7. Wortman was very gracious in receiving my comments and references and was determined to eliminate errors and misconceptions in her textbook. I took her at her word.

Roediger, Capaldi, Paris, and Polivy (1991) have produced another well-received encyclopedic introductory textbook, more than 700 pages of text plus another approximately 150 pages of indices and glossaries. Each of the authors is well-known in their specialties, fields of human learning and memory, animal learning and behavior, developmental psychology, and eating disorders. Sections on clinical psychology and personality, including alcoholism were written by Polivy, a professor at the University of Toronto and therefore a former colleague of the Sobells. Each chapter in this well organized book contains a section labeled "Controversy". "One of the compelling aspects of contemporary psychology is its intellectual ferment. Many issues are unsettled, many controversies exist. In each section we take one such controversy, present its opposing viewpoints, and, if possible, draw tentative conclusions." (p. xix). Unfortunately, they do not meet these conditions in the controversy section related to substance abuse. An entire page is devoted to the Sobells and controlled drinking all based on secondary sources, primarily Marlatt (1983) and Cook (1989). These are hardly opposing points of view. "Controlled Drinking or Abstinence for Alcoholics: One Treatment for All Patients?" (p. 595) is the title of the controversy in question.

Marlatt (1983) is the source for the description of Davies' (1962) study that purportedly sent shock waves through the alcoholism treatment field. The Sobells' study is briefly described as comparing traditional abstinence treatment with behavioral training designed to enable alcoholics to become moderate drinkers, which is not defined.

To therapists who were dedicated to treating the miseries of alcoholism and had been trained to believe that 'once an alcoholic, always an alcoholic,' this study bordered on the sacrilegious-trying to teach an alcoholic to keep drinking sounded harmful rather than helpful.

In 1982, the fears of the abstinence-treatment establishment seemed confirmed. A study, in *Science*, by Pendery, Maltzman, and West, 1982) *alleged* that the Sobell and Sobell (1973) patients had been recontacted, reinterviewed, and were no longer successful social drinkers- the treatment had actually failed. This allegation touched off a controversy so heated that Maltzman actually accused the Sobells of scientific fraud (Marlatt, 1983). (Roediger et al., 1991, p.595) (italics added).

This is a new twist. The question is raised as to whether there actually was a follow-up of the patients in the Sobells' study. By using the term "alleged" it is suggested that perhaps we invented the entire story. The author(s) is unaware, of course, of the letter in *Science* written by Abelson (1983) stating that every assertion in our paper was supported by an objective source reviewed by the editorial board of *Science*. Certainly, the students could not know that there is no basis for the insinuation. They trust the authors of their text, especially since the authors state that the opposing sides are represented in the controversy.

The text states that the results were as the Sobells reported them (Sobell & Sobell, 1984) because the Sobells say they are. Furthermore, the memories of the patients 10 years or more after they participated in the study is at fault, an argument we have encountered before.

Cook (1989) has suggested that the attack may have been motivated more by a desire to discredit research on controlled drinking than by concerns about scientific rigor. Indeed, the persistence of these attacks despite five separate investigations by independent commissions, funding agencies, and even Congress vindicating the original investigation suggests that more is at stake than the validity of one study (Sobell & Sobell, 1989). (Roediger et al., 1991, p. 595).

It is significant that both Cook's (1989) and the Sobell and Sobell (1989) reply to my (Maltzman, 1989) article are cited, but my article to which they are responding is not cited, much less discussed.

While this controversy has raised questions about the ability of science to protect itself against both fraud and false accusations, for the most part it has tended to ignore the bulk of the evidence about the actual issue at hand, treating alcoholism. The study by the Sobells was merely one of the first published investigations of controlled drinking (an Australian study appeared in 1970, [Marlatt, 1983]). Since then, there have been many more, and more sophisticated experiments demonstrating the effectiveness of controlled drinking at least for some patients, some of the time (Cook, 1989). (Roediger et al., 1991, p. 595).

Polivy goes on to cite Marlatt (1983) as the source for the information that some alcoholics even those treated for abstinence go on to moderate their alcoholism. She then provides Marlatt's (1983) bromide based on Rand Report II that those under 40 who are less severely addicted, with fewer life problems do best with controlled drinking whereas those over 40 who are more severely addicted and lack social support would do better with abstinence training. "Thus, while neither treatment can be said to be a real 'cure' for alcoholism, the evidence seems to indicate that treatment should be matched to the patient who will receive it...." (Roediger et al., 1991, p.595).

It will be interesting to see how a later edition of this text, as well as others, will deal with the results of project MATCH which failed to support the matching notion. Little will probably appear in the textbooks until one of the gurus such as Marlatt or William Miller publishes an article about MATCH in a popular psychology journal and it will become the secondary source for the texbook writer after passing through the ideological filter.

Abnormal psychology textbooks

Davison and Neale (1996) two well-known behavior therapists have written a popular abnormal psychology textbook which is in its sixth edition. It emphasizes expectancies and cognitions:

For example, alcohol is commonly thought to stimulate aggression and increase sexual responsiveness. Research has shown, however, that these reactions may not be caused by alcohol itself but by the drinker's belief about alcohol's effects. In experiments demonstrating these points, subjects are told that they are consuming a quantity of alcohol but, in fact, are given an alcohol-free beverage with its taste disguised. (Davison & Neale, 1996, p. 289).

As usual, no alternative interpretations are suggested. Contrary results are not mentioned, and the problem of ecological validity, generalizing from a laboratory experiment with college student as participants to life outside the laboratory is not raised.

Jellinek's phases in the development of alcoholism are described with an emphasis upon purported contrary results such as the unpredictability of blackouts and the variability in the course of alcoholism as reflected by the research reported by Cahalan and his colleagues and more recently in detail by Schuckit, Tipp, Smith, & Bucholz (1997). Descriptions of major fluctuations in the amounts consumed by alcoholics ranging from abstinence to heavy drinking for periods of time are ascribed to Cahalan's research. Again, there is a lack of familiarity with the literature, including the recognition that alcoholism defined by Cahalan is a much broader category than gamma alcoholism as defined Jellinek and alcohol dependence as defined by DSM-IV. Extensive research supports Jellinek's general formulation of a progression in severity of symptoms in alcoholics, including the course of alcoholism in women, and has been described in chapters 1 and 2. None of this literature is cited. Periods of abstinence as well as controlled drinking in alcoholics have been described by clinicians for years (Mann, 1950). What characterizes their alcoholism is that they cannot consistently regulate their drinking or refrain from drinking. Schuckit et al. (1997) have provided quantitative data on the extended periods of abstinence experienced by many alcoholics. Such evidence does not contradict Jellinek's conception of progressive worsening of dependence syndromes. It simply is not a smooth progression, which is true of the symptoms of many other diseases as well.

Etiology of alcoholism and drug misuse in general is discussed in terms of sociocultural, psychological and biological factors. Consideration of psychological variables has expectancy emerging as a major factor. In contrast to McConnell's treatment, it is not tension-reduction that promotes alcohol use but the expectation that alcohol reduces tension. Davison and Neale do not ask what causes the expectancy. They do recognize the problem of individual differences and in this regard turn to personality characteristics as a solution to the puzzle of individual differences in the risk for alcoholism. Longitudinal studies spanning early childhood to young adulthood are cited in support of the hypothesis that personality dispositions are risk factors for alcoholism.

Alcoholism treatment is presented in a biased and incomplete manner. Miller and Hester are cited as providing evidence that the more expensive inpatient treatment is not more effective than outpatient treatment. "Higher costs of inpatient treatment are not matched by higher degrees of effectiveness" (p.315). Chapter 7 provides evidence indicating that the above generalization is meaningless unless individual differences among patients are controlled. Inpatient and outpatient treatment cannot be directly compared because more people with a poorer prognosis, severely dependent people lacking social support, as well as people with comorbidity and polydrug use, tend to self-select or be placed in inpatient rather than outpatient facilities. Individual patient variables must be equated before the two treatment modalities can be compared. Here is an opportunity to educate the student in research methodology and critical thinking. Instead, the text blindly follows the party line and provides the reader with potentially harmful misinformation. Davison and Neale assert:

> Because inpatient treatment is much more expensive than outpatient treatment, its cost effectiveness should be questioned. From the available data, Miller and Hester found that the higher costs of inpatient treatment are not matched by higher degrees of effectiveness... in general, the therapeutic results of hospital treatment are not superior to those of outpatient treatment. (p.315).

Davison and Neale describe AA and present the 12 steps. They state:

> Unfortunately, the claims made by AA about the effectiveness of its treatment have rarely been subjected to scientific scrutiny. [I have never seen such claims; they would be out of character; AA does not claim to be a treatment.] Findings from uncontrolled studies must be viewed with caution: AA has high drop-out rates, and the dropouts are not factored into the results... In addition, there is a lack of long-term follow-up of AA clients. Results from the best controlled study to date are mixed (Walsh et al., 1991).

> Alcohol-abusing workers at a General Electric manufacturing plant were randomly assigned to one of three treatments: three weeks of hospitalization followed by AA; AA alone; or a choice of treatment. Of the seventy-one people in the choice group, twenty-seven elected hospitalization, thirty-three AA, and six no treatment [sic]. At a two-year follow-up of the entire group, 23 percent of the hospitalization group had required rehospitalization for alcoholism, compared to 63 percent of the AA group and 38 percent of the choice group. On the other hand, it is important to note that those who *chose* AA did well in the study; it is when alcoholics were randomly assigned to AA that they did not fare at all well. (p. 316).

There are several errors of omission and commission in the above passage. The number of subjects in the choice group do not add up to 71, the total in the group. Davison and Neale neglected to mention a subgroup that chose outpatient treatment; the total choosing hospitalizaiton is incorrect. Results are reported in a confusing manner. Walsh et al. (1991) do not report specific results for the subgroups within the choice group, only the overall results for the choice group as compared to the participants in the AA group and the hospitalization group. Davison and Neale fail to mention that all three groups improved significantly over their pretreatment condition as reflected by a variety of measures. Hospitalization was significantly superior to AA and the choice group where the latter two groups generally did not differ significantly from each other. Walsh et al. did not compare outcomes of AA patients randomly assigned to AA as compared to those who chose AA voluntarily.

The statement, ".... it is important to note that those who chose AA did well in the study; it is when alcoholics were randomly assigned to AA that they did not fare at all well ...." (p.316), is a confabulation. Davison and Neale fail to comment on the fact that hospitalization was significantly better than choice despite the insistence by cognitively oriented clinical psychologists that choice of treatment is an important variable in determining recovery because it builds self-efficacy and the latter is a critical determiner of recovery. Self-efficacy produced by choice as a determiner of recovery is contradicted by Walsh et al., (1991). They also fail to note the demonstration by Walsh et al. that inpatient hospitalization treatment is cost effective in the long run.

Concerning controlled drinking, Davison and Neale state:

Until recently it was generally agreed that alcoholics had to abstain completely if they were to be cured... for they were said to have no control over their imbibing once they had taken that first drink. Although this continues to be the abiding belief of Alcoholics Anonymous, the research mentioned earlier called this assumption into question: drinkers' *beliefs* about themselves and alcohol may be as important as the physiological addiction to the drug itself. Indeed, considering the difficulty in our society of avoiding alcohol altogether, it may even be *preferable* to teach the problem drinker to imbibe with moderation. A drinker's self-esteem will certainly benefit from being able to control a problem and from feeling in charge of his or her life. (p. 318).

Note the substitution of vague mentalistic notions for established principle. Poorly conceived balanced-placebo experiments contradicted by experimental evidence are the basis for the myth promulgated by two cognitive behavior therapists who rely on selected and biased sources from fellow revisionists. Also note the sleight of hand, shifting from alcoholics to problem drinkers as though these are equivalent diagnostic categories.

Controlled drinking refers to a pattern of alcohol consumption that is moderate and avoids the extremes of total abstinence and inebriation. During early controlled drinking programs, [sic] outpatients were allowed to drink to a moderate level of intoxication and blood alcohol. They were then informed if the level of blood alcohol rose above a certain percent (Lovibond & Caddy, 1970). Thereafter when they drank, they were supposedly able to keep the blood level of alcohol low. (p. 318).

The study in question was examined in chapter 8 where we saw how it was misinterpreted by Marlatt et al. (1993). Participants were not simply verbally informed when their blood alcohol level was too high. They received a strong electric shock. Davison and Neale do not define "moderate", leaving it to the student to decide what is "moderate" - which usually becomes whatever they and their friends are doing. Note also that Davison and Neale dignify a small and poorly conducted efficacy experiment with the attribution of a "program", a gambit they also use in describing the Sobells' IBTA study.

Findings of one well-known treatment program suggests that at least some alcoholics can learn to control their drinking and improve other aspects of their lives as well (Sobell & Sobell, 1976, 1978). Alcoholics attempting to control their drinking were given shocks when they chose straight liquor rather than mixed drinks, gulped their drinks.... Their improvement was greater than that of alcoholics who tried for total abstinence and who were given shocks for any drinking at all.

In contemporary controlled drinking treatment programs, patients are taught other ways of responding to situations that might lead to excessive drinking. Learning to resist social pressures to drink: assertiveness, relaxation, and stress management training, sometimes including biofeedback and meditation... They are also taught that a lapse will not inevitably precipitate a total relapse and should be regarded as a learning experience (Marlatt & Gordon, 1985)...

The trend toward controlled drinking, however, has not gone unchallenged. An attack against the early work of the Sobells was launched by Pendery, Maltzman, and West (1982), who argued that some of the patients believed to have been drinking moderately had in fact reverted to uncontrolled and self-destructive drinking. Groups like AA also object to moderation in drinking as a sensible treatment goal. A Rand Corporation study (Armor, Polich, and Stambul, 1976, 1978) [sic] offered a way to resolve the controversy by suggesting that abstinence is a better goal for older, more addicted drinkers, while moderation is viable for younger, less dependent drinkers. [This is the wrong reference. They mean Polich, et al., (1981). This generalization is contradicted by Welte, et al., (1983) and by Küfner and Feuerlein (1989) as discussed in chapter 7.] ... Success at controlled drinking is especially associated with younger age and lighter drinking, as suggested by the Rand study (see reviews by Miller & Hester, 1986a, and by Sobell, Tonneato, & Sobell, 1990, of studies other than their own). The patient's ability to choose his or her own goals may also improve outcome (Sanchez-Craig & Wilkinson, 1987).

The abstinence versus controlled drinking issue is controversial, for it pits influential forces, such as AA, who uphold abstinence as the *only* proper goal for problem drinkers, against more recent workers such as the Sobells and those adopting their general approach, who have shown that moderation can work for many alcoholics, even those with serious drinking problems. If the therapeutic means of achieving the goal of moderate drinking are available-and research strongly suggests that they are-then controlled drinking may be a more realistic goal even for an addicted alcoholic. As of this writing, controlled drinking is much more widely accepted in Canada and Europe than it is in the United States. (p. 318).

Ideologically driven assertions best described as propaganda and numerous errors of omission and commission as well as a superficial acquaintance with the pertinent literature characterize the passages quoted above. Davison and Neale cite Sanchez-Craig and Wilkinson for the advantages of choice, yet the Walsh et al. (1991) study which they cited earlier demonstrated that choice of treatment was significantly worse then assigned hospitalization, although the study has difficulties because the treatments assigned as chosen were not identical. However, our discussion of Sanchez-Craig's study in chapter 6 indicates that it also has serious methodological problems, for example excluding individuals who accepted the disease concept of alcoholism.

Barlow and Durand (1995) have also written a current abnormal psychology text. Barlow is a well-known behavior therapist in the field of anxiety and panic and a supporter of the Sobells (Barlow, 1983, 1993). Alcoholism in Barlow and Durand's textbook, as was true in the Davison and Neale (1996) text, is discussed within the context of a chapter devoted to "substance-related disorders". In contrast to Davison and Neale's textbook, Barlow and Durand devote considerable space to a definition of terms such as "intoxication", "abuse", and "dependence", and reproduce the DSM-IV criteria for substance abuse. Unfortunately, during the course of the chapter they do not adhere to the distinction between abuse and dependence, problem drinking and alcoholism. Ideology takes over once the discussion turns to characteristics of alcoholics and problem drinkers. Jellinek is the straw man:

An early notion of alcohol use and dependence was that, once problems arose with drinking, these problems would continue to become worse and follow a predictable downward pattern if the person kept drinking (Sobell & Sobell, 1993). In other words, like a *disease* that isn't treated properly, alcoholism will get progressively worse if left unchecked. First championed by Jellinek several decades ago, this view of alcohol abuse (sic) and dependence continues to influence the way people view and treat this disorder... Unfortunately Jellinek based his model of the progression of alcohol use on a now famous, but faulty study (Jellinek, 1946) which we will briefly review.

In 1945, the newly formed self-help organization Alcoholics Anonymous (AA) sent out some 1,600 surveys to its members asking them about symptoms related to drinking... they were given a list of problems and asked to think back and report if and when they had happened. Only 98 of the almost 1,600 surveys were returned, however. As you know, such a small response could cause serious problems in interpreting the data. Obviously, this group of 98 may be very different from the group as a whole... A number of attempts by other research to confirm this progression of stages has not been successful (Schuckit, Smith, Anthenelli, & Irwin, 1993).

It appears instead that the course of alcohol *dependence* may be progressive for most people, although the course of alcohol *abuse* may be more variable... This study [Schuckit et al., 1993] suggests, that, among people with chronic alcohol abuse and dependence, a pattern of increasingly severe consequences of drinking is common. This progressive pattern is not inevitable for everyone who abuses alcohol. (p. 479).

Of course, this is precisely what Jellinek said. A progression characterizes gamma alcoholics, people who develop alcohol dependence, as distinguished from alpha and beta alcoholics, problem drinkers or people who abuse alcohol. Schuckit et al. (1993) studied people who were all alcohol dependent, not alcohol dependent and alcohol abusers. Barlow and Durand (1995) conclude: "...we do not as yet understand what distinguishes those who do and those who do not display this negative progression (Sobell & Sobell, 1993). " (Barlow & Durand, 1995, p. 479).

Faulty scholarship, errors of commission and omission, plague the above passage. Once more, "the big lie" promulgated by Mendelson and Mello (1985) and by Fingarette (1988b) that Jellinek based his progression generalization on a biased sample of 98 members of AA is offered by Barlow and Durand (1995).

Relevant studies, discussed in chapter 1 have repeatedly demonstrated a progression in symptoms reported by alcoholics.

The purpose of examining the progression of a disease is to obtain knowledge useful to the clinician and research investigator. While knowledge about the usual clinical course of most medical disorders, such as diabetes mellitus, and psychiatric syndromes, such as schizophrenia, has been extremely useful, it is important to remember that these are general descriptions that rarely apply perfectly to an individual. This heterogeneity in the clinical course of a problem is the result of subgroups within populations, differences in the severity of the disorder in individuals at the time of first identification, additional aspects of the life situation including available social and financial support systems, levels of stress, and genetic differences inherent in each individual. Despite this diversity of influences, it is still possible to describe a usual clinical course for diagnostic entities. (Schuckit et al., 1993, p. 786).

Using a structured interview Schuckit et al. (1993) interviewed more than 600 male inpatients receiving treatment for alcoholism. A collateral was also interviewed. Verifiable objective questions were used to assess the occurrence of symptoms and the age at which they first appeared. They were not the questions used by Jellinek. Data obtained from the participants showed, "that the progression of problems can be simplistically divided" (p. 788) into five phases. Schuckit et al. then categorized the participants into a number of subgroups to determine whether or not the progression held for subgroups categorized as a function of age of onset of alcohol dependence, whether or not a family history of alcoholism was present, and primary alcoholics with and without psychiatric diagnoses of other disorders such as depression, drug dependence, etc. Progressions of symptoms in a subgroup were all highly correlated.

The evidence of a *general* progression of alcohol related life problems is consistent with the prior research by Jellinek as well as the several additional attempts to replicate his earlier findings... On the other hand, as has been reported by other investigators, the *specific* items Jellinek cited are not identical to those reported here. This probably reflects changes in social mores and legal sanctions over the years as well as different study groups...

The demonstration of a roughly predictable rank ordering of events in the lives of primary alcoholics has several implications. First, it is possible to teach physicians, counselors, and other deliverers of health care about a logical progression of problems among persons with severe alcohol-related problems. Second, the data will help clinicians predict the probability of future problems. This can be important information to share with alcohol-dependent individuals..(Schuckit et al., 1993, pp. 789, 790f).

Finally, I believe it may be possible to predict who progresses and who does not progress in severity of dependence with continued drinking, if examinations of brain structure and function became part of the routine intake assessment of people entering treatment for drinking problems.

Miller and Hester (1986) and Hester and Miller (1995) are the major sources of information on alcoholism treatment outcomes and therefore the usual source of ideologically contrived myths. Barlow and Durand (1995) assert:

Research on the comparative effectiveness of treatments for alcohol abuse suggests that there may be no difference in the outcomes for alcoholic patients between intensive residential setting programs and quality outpatient care (Miller & Hester, 1986). Although some people with alcohol dependency problems do improve in these inpatient settings, they may not need this expensive in-hospital care.

In the alcoholism treatment field, the notion of teaching people controlled drinking is extremely controversial, in part because of a study showing partial success in teaching severe abusers to continue to drink in a limited way (Sobell & Sobell, 1978). In this study the subjects were 40 male alcoholics who were at the time in the alcoholism treatment program at a state hospital and were thought to have a good prognosis. The men were assigned either to a program that taught them how to drink in moderation (experimental group) or to a group that was abstinence oriented (control group). The researchers, Mark and Linda Sobell, followed this group of men for 2 years... during the second year after treatment, those who participated in the controlled drinking group were functioning well for 85% of the days while the abstinence group were reported to be doing well for only 42% of the days... The results of this study suggested that controlled drinking may be a viable alternative to abstinence for some alcohol abusers, although it clearly wasn't a 'cure'.

The controversy over this study began with a paper published in the prestigious journal *Science* (Pendery, Maltzman, & West, 1982). The authors reported that they had contacted the men in the Sobell study after 10 years [sic]... and found that only one of the men in the controlled drinking group continued to maintain a pattern of controlled drinking. Although this reevaluation made headlines and was the subject of a segment on the 60 Minutes television show, it had a number of flaws (Marlatt, Larimer, Baer, & Quigley, 1993). Most serious of the problems with this study was the lack of data on the abstinence group over the same 10-year follow-up period...

Despite these problems, the controversy over the Sobell study had a chilling effect on the treatment of alcohol abuse with controlled drinking in the United States ... Among the research that has looked at controlled drinking as an option, the results seem to show that this treatment is at least as effective as abstinence approaches, but that neither treatment is successful for 70%-80% of patients over the long term-a rather bleak outlook for people with alcohol dependence problems. (pp. 507, 509).

There is no reference for the study(s) reporting this bleak outlook. Only 20%-30% are successfully treated? Among others discussed in chapter 7 CATOR shows that the average abstinence rate is far better than 20% to 30%. Where is the evidence that controlled drinking is at least as effective? What is the impact upon students who read that alcoholism treatment is effective for only 20% to 30% of patients? It seems likely that such information in a textbook written by well-known clinical psychologists would discourage friends or family, or they themselves, from seeking help with such a dismal success rate presented as fact. Misinformation which may discourage people from seeking treatment that may help them is inexcusable and unethical. Unfortunately, this textbook which has numerous errors of omission and commission in its treatment of alcoholism will probably be widely adopted because of the reputation of the authors in clinical areas other than alcoholism.

Conclusion

Lack of scholarship, the failure to critically study original sources, is an essential aspect of the "Little Albert phenomenon", including the present saga. Casual observers and unsophisticated students who limit their knowledge of the saga to secondary sources or superficial readings of primary sources, may be victimized by ideology. Casual scholarship, citing primary sources that are not read, reliance on unreliable secondary sources, and confabulations driven by ideology cannot advance knowledge, and is unethical. It may cause harm to the public. Concern for the truth and the trust necessarily dependent upon the truth, entails an even greater responsibility in areas where there are relatively direct consequences for the public well-being. Scholarship is not limited to original papers and chapters in handbooks. It is essential in textbooks where the student and the public have a need to know and their well-being is at risk.

Rosenthal (1994, 1995) suggests that poor quality research is ethically indefensible. Conduct of research, data analysis and reporting of results all have valuative components, ethical implications. One more dimension must be added to the research enterprise: quality of scholarship. Literature reviews are also valuative. The first principle of the Helsinki accord of the World Medical Association guiding biomedical research asserts that research must be based upon, "a thorough knowledge of the scientific literature" (Levine, 1986, p. 428). Violation of this ethical principle has repeatedly occurred in lecture halls and textbooks as well as in the professional literature. It is time professors and publishers assume responsibility for their products.

10 SITTING PRETTY

What have the principals in our drama been doing lately? In the present chapter we shall review some of the more recent activities of leading revisionists in the field of alcohol studies and what we may anticipate in the future.

When Mark Sobell is invited to address the Research Society on Alcoholism on methodology, a society founded by the National Council on Alcoholism and dominated by MDs and neuroscientists you know that he has been rehabilitated. When Linda Sobell is elected president of the Association for the Advancement of Behavior Therapy, the largest speciality organization of clinical psychologists in the United States, you know that she has been rehabilitated. When they are both invited by the journal *Addiction* to write an editorial with experts from around the world invited to comment, you certainly know they have been rehabilitated (Sobell & Sobell, 1995a). *Addiction*, formerly the *British Journal of Addiction*, is the oldest journal in the English language devoted to the study of alcoholism and other addictions. As I indicated in chapter 4, it is the journal which was threatened by a lawsuit from the Sobells if they published my manuscript examining the Dickens Committee Report. Eventually, the editor, Griffith Edwards, after some three years, bowed to the fear of a lawsuit and returned the manuscript to me. Those same Sobells are now invited by that same editor to write an editorial with invited commentaries reviewing 25 years of controlled drinking controversy and their role in shaping current alcoholism studies and treatment policy. I was not invited to comment. It's interesting how controversy is defined by politics - and the fear of controversy. How true Tey's insight was - and Orwell's. The Sobells' editorial and some of the comments it elicited are examples of the basic principles of Orwell's (1949/1950) Ministry of Truth (Propaganda) - IGNORANCE IS STRENGTH, DOUBLE THINK, and WHOEVER CONTROLS THE PRESENT CONTROLS THE PAST AS WELL AS THE FUTURE.

From the outset the Sobells (Sobell & Sobell, 1978) adopted the position that they are the advance guard of a new and, for the first time, a scientific approach to problems of alcohol misuse and their treatment. They were attacked by Pendery et al. (1982) and others because controlled drinking, "threatened an entire culture based on the philosophy of Alcoholics Anonymous (AA)" (Sobell & Sobell, 1995a, p. 1149). They go on to write:

We believe that the major reason why debate about controlled drinking has waned is because the old battles have little relevance to today's leading issues in the alcohol field. Many things have contributed to the change, three of which are discussed below: (1) epidemiological studies that have identified a large population of people with low severity alcohol problems; (2) introduction of the alcohol dependence syndrome concept; and (3) consideration of alcohol as a public health concern. (p.1149).

We would add two important variables contributing to the apparent waning of the old battles: (a) politics and, (b) pusillanimous editors. One dimension to the "battle" continues to be ignored: the truth and the trust essential in science and society as a whole which must rest upon the truth. The truth is still the basic issue in the alcohol studies field and the battle goes on.

Whether or not the Sobells' research threatened the culture of AA is irrelevant to the truth or falsity of their critics' assertions. Criticisms of the Sobells' work (Pendery et al., 1982; Maltzman, 1989) the Rand studies (Blume, 1977; Wallace, 1989a) and Davies (Edwards, 1985, 1994) were issue oriented, concerned with the methodology and validity of the research in question. The Sobells need to explain how they could have interviewed a subject only twice in an entire year, provide daily drinking dispositions for 365 days, and insist that they thought they were interviewing patients every three-four weeks. They never have. This is not a question of culture, ideology, or philosophy. It is a question of scientific integrity. Not only is the integrity of the Sobells involved, but of an entire community of behavior therapists and others claiming the mantle of "scientists" who rallied around the Sobells. By framing the issue from the outset as a clash of cultures, their scientific approach versus lay superstition, the Sobells could rationalize the attacks on their work and adopt their role as martyrs for the new science.

The Sobells' stance elicited energetic support over the years from other social scientists and especially behavior therapists because their work represented the conquest of a new area, opening up new job and research opportunities for behavior therapists. Their fallacious line of reasoning confusing the truth status of assertions with motivations and attacking the messenger because they cannot refute the message continues in the Sobells' editorial. As the Sobells (Sobell & Sobell, 1995a) put it: "Central to the battle, however, was the legitimacy of taking a scientific approach to test basic assumptions about the nature of alcohol problems, and the practical implications of such an approach (Cook, 1985)." (p.1149). In other words, they are denying, among many other research accomplishments, the existence of the Yale Center on Alcohol Studies and the voluminous amount of work it produced, and especially the scholarly research of Jellinek (1960) prior to their appearance on the research scene in the early 1970's.

The Sobells (1995a) suggest that controlled drinking research shifted direction from treatment of alcoholics to secondary prevention with problem drinkers because the epidemiological work of Cahalan and colleagues showed that, [a] "chronic alcoholics represented a minority of those with alcohol problems, and [b] by introduction of the dependence syndrome [Edwards & Gross, (1976)] which conceptualized individuals as varying in levels of dependence severity." (p.1149). The Sobells continue, "Consequently, individuals with less serious alcohol problems (i.e., problem drinkers) became the main target of research examining moderation goals (Miller & Caddy, 1977; Sobell & Sobell, 1978)." (p. 1149).

Note above that the Sobells cite the book describing their IBTA research (Sobell & Sobell, 1978) as a study of problem drinkers with "less serious alcohol problems". Talk about revisionism! The IBTA study at Patton State Hospital that launched their meteoric careers states under the heading of "Experimental Design" and "Subjects": "A group of 70 male gamma (Jellinek, 1960) alcoholic patients who had voluntarily admitted themselves to Patton State Hospital for treatment of alcoholism served as subjects in the IBT study. All subjects had experienced physical dependence on alcohol and had several previous alcohol-related arrests and hospitalizations..." (Sobell & Sobell, 1978, p. 82).

Cahalan and his colleagues did not show that problem drinkers far exceeded the number of alcoholics, implying that a much larger group of problem drinkers than alcoholics exist and are underserved, a lucrative market for behavior therapists providing brief outpatient interventions. Cahalan and Room (1974) did not provide a basis for this fallacious argument because they did not employ dependent variables that differentiate between individuals diagnosable as alcohol abusers as distinguished from those suffering from alcohol dependence. We discussed this issue in chapter 1 in our review of the study by Hasin et al. (1990). A study of a community sample by Hasin, Rossem, McCloud, & Endicott (1997) using DSM-IV criteria indicate a greater incidence of people with alcohol dependence than alcohol abuse. Grant et al. (1994) report the results of a National Longitudinal Alcohol Epidemiologic Survey involving face-to-face interviews with more than 42,000 people 18 years or older. Using DSM-IV criteria 4.38% were classified as suffering from alcohol dependence whereas 3.03% were abusing alcohol. Corresponding results were obtained by Schuckit (1988) in his longitudinal study of young men differing in their level of responsiveness to an alcohol challenge. As noted in chapter 3 Schuckit found a higher percentage of men developing alcohol dependence than alcohol abuse within both the FH+ and FH- subgroups. These studies using current diagnostic criteria show that there is not a large unserved class of problem drinkers who cause most of the problems as compared to a small class of alcoholics receiving most of the current treatment resources.

Revising revisionism

It may seem self-serving, but I believe that there is a more reasonable interpretation than the one offered by the Sobells for the shift in emphasis from controlled drinking treatment studies of alcoholics to controlled drinking studies of problem drinkers, to secondary prevention. The study by Pendery et al. (1982) raised grave concerns about the reliability and validity of the Sobells' study although the faithful defended the Sobells to the best of their ability. They also buried the study by Caddy et al. (1978) because of its obvious lack of validity when compared with the results reported by Pendery et al. for Caddy et al.'s most successful controlled drinkers (see chapter 5). Although the results reported by Pendery et al. could be rationalized as occurring 10 years later, lacked a control group, and my allegations of fraud were inappropriate, they nevertheless raised doubts. However, the death knell of controlled drinking as a treatment for alcoholics came from within the fold.

Foy (Foy et al., 1984), Rychtarik (Rychtarik et al., 1987) and their colleagues are behavior therapists and had published previously in the alcoholism field. They began their study of controlled drinking believing their results would support the successful outcome reported by the Sobells. Theirs was the best designed study of controlled drinking training for chronic alcoholics in the treatment field. Participants were randomly assigned to treatment conditions and interviewers were blind to the treatment assignment of the participants. When their study found that after six months participants in the group that received controlled drinking as well as abstinence training were significantly worse than the participants receiving only abstinence training and 5-6 years later there was no effect due to controlled drinking, grounds for supporting controlled drinking for alcoholics vanished. Even Nathan (1985), a champion of the Sobells, made his famous pronouncement that the Sobells' work was an anomaly. It turns out that the unwashed luddites of AA and their camp followers were right about controlled drinking for alcoholics. It does not work. The Sobells could never admit this outright of course. They do now after they and their fellow revisionists found a new and more lucrative research field: study the large numbers of heavy drinkers who have occasional problems, or even many of the alcohol abusers, who still may be distinguished from alcoholics. They now open this field to research and label it secondary prevention, a public health problem.

The Sobells attribute the current lack of controversy over controlled drinking treatment for problem drinkers to: (a) the public health approach which considers controlled drinking a secondary prevention approach to forestalling alcoholism by preventing people with minor problems from progressing, and (b) the recognition that there are degrees of severity of dependence. Optimal efficiency and success requires a matching of treatment goal with severity. Severely dependent alcoholics are best served by an abstinence treatment goal whereas moderately dependent problem drinkers are best served by a controlled drinking goal. The latter assertion is not supported by evidence we reviewed in chapters 6 and 7.

There are multiple reasons for the apparent acceptance of controlled drinking for problem drinkers and lack of controversy among academics, the people who write about clinical treatments. Acceptance of controlled drinking is lacking among alcoholism counselors, although a concerted public relations effort is being made to convert them. There are now continuing education programs for alcoholism counselors offered by Nova University, the Sobells' new home base, and articles in the counselors' magazine promoting the revisionist view (Phillips, 1995; Rotgers, 1996a). Lack of controversy over controlled drinking may be found among behavior therapists in academic psychology but not within the community of credentialed alcoholism counselors treating people with alcohol problems or research psychologists, neuroscientists, pharmacologists, and MD's.

A major reason for the growth in influence of the controlled drinking movement within clinical psychology and its current noncontroversial standing in large part is fortuitous. It is a matter of timing, a matter of chance. What made it possible was a receptive audience tuned to accept certain results and their interpretations, and leaders, or more appropriately, sales people, to promote the revolution. Controlled drinking as a treatment modality and as a goal found a receptive audience among academic clinical psychologists of the behavior therapy persuasion. As Samelson (1980) observed, a receptive audience tuned towards the message provided the fertile field for the growth of behaviorism in the 1920's. A similar situation was present in the 1970's in the form of behavior therapy as the dominant approach to clinical research and treatment. The Sobells' research fit with the behavior therapy movement and the two embraced. Masterful salesmanship promoted their rise to the top of academia and concomitant financial success and influence. A major new movement in clinical psychology in the 1960s toppled the hegemony of the psychodynamic, primarily Freudian, position in academic clinical psychology and practice. The victorious movement grew out of the conjoint influences stemming from Wolpe's (1958) influential book inspired by Hullian and Pavlovian research and theory and the application of Skinner's form of behaviorism to applied problems. There are still distinctive differences between the offshoots of behavior therapy and applied behavior analysis. Today the former has evolved into cognitive behavior therapy which is probably the most popular variety of current psychotherapy, whereas applied behavior analysis is still largely true to Skinnerian behaviorism and has its greatest successes in application to severe behavior problems such as autism (Lovaas, 1993).

Behavior therapy adopted by the younger clinical psychologists with training in some experimental as well as clinical techniques and influenced by the dominant position in experimental psychology at the time, learning theory, replaced psychodynamics as the most influential ideology in clinical psychology. Like any successful new movement, behavior therapists proselytized adherents, and started their own journals and handbook series. It came to be the major force within clinical psychology in the United States.

From the outset the Sobells and their research were adopted by the aggressive new clinical movement. They were hailed as champions of the new wave of enlightment and their research and interpretations were quickly incorporated in handbooks and textbooks. The IBTA study was an apparent successful application of a new approach to an entirely new problem area. It opened up new possibilities for research with funding from the new, at the time, National Institute on Alcohol Abuse and Alcoholism (NIAAA). The Sobells' research represented another triumph for the new kid on the block in opposition to the outmoded psychodynamic position which never was particularly successful in treating alcoholics or obtaining research funding. By the 1970s academic clinical psychology was dominated by behavior therapists. Clinical psychologists most likely to conduct research on alcoholism and write about it were therefore in allegiance ideologically with the Sobells who were treated as champions of the new behavior therapy approach to alcoholism fighting the evil darkness of ignorance represented by AA and their followers.

Clinical psychologists who actually worked with alcoholics in treatment facilities and the alcoholism counselors who were the largest group of people working with alcoholics on a day-to-day basis did not publish in academic journals. For one thing, they were too busy. For another, counselors do not have the training or the interest to conduct treatment evaluations and other kinds of clinical research. Psychiatrists and internists who were working full time in the alcoholism treatment field, like the clinical psychologists in the field, do not usually write for professional journals. Publishing and reviewing in academic journals and books concerned with alcoholism treatment are now dominated by academically based behavior therapists. Outsiders who wish to write in opposition have a difficult time publishing their work because of the hegemony of the dominant ideological group, the behavior therapists.

There are several reasons for the purported success of controlled drinking for problem drinkers, its acceptance and lack of controversy among academics, the people who write about clinical treatments. Revisionists work at obtaining and publicizing some apparent evidence of success as would manufacturers of a new cereal or cigarette brand. They sold themselves and a product. With the aid of money from NIAAA they received lucrative grants over the years and promoted each other at every opportunity. Nathan as associate editor for the *American Psychologist* made sure that Marlatt's paper and others supporting their views would be published. They had a built-in support group: other behavior therapists.

The *Annual Review of Behavior Therapy* was a staunch supporter regardless of who wrote the chapter on addictions in a given year. Section writers were usually not experts in the alcoholism or drug addiction field. Two successive editors who wrote the chapters on addictions were in the field of obesity (Brownell,1984; Foreyt, 1987). They were careful to toe the party line, praised controlled drinking and vigorously defended the Sobells once they came under attack. After all, their own scientific view was being attacked by the know-nothing luddites, camp followers of AA who knew nothing about research. An attack on one behavior therapist is an attack on all. All for one and one for all - a nice rallying call for a political party but not for scientists. These influences made controlled drinking noncontroversial within academic psychology and related disciplines. Orwell and Tey anticipated such events in their fiction. Unfortunately, what happened in the field of alcoholism studies is not fiction. It is a true social tragedy.

More recently Nathan became an associate editor for *Contemporary Psychology*, the journal of the American Psychological Association that reviews books in psychology and related disciplines. It was fortuitous. He accepted a high level administrative position at the University of Iowa, my alma mater. Harvey, the editor of *Contemporary Psychology* is in the University of Iowa Psychology department. He appointed his distinguished new colleague, Nathan, to the editorial board. As a result Nathan would choose reviewers of books on alcoholism. It is no accident that books within the revisionist fold were given favorable reviews. However, the high academic position Nathan held suggests that he will gradually disappear from the alcoholism scene. His sights are set on higher goals. He was acting president of the University of Iowa, but could not retain the job. A permanent president was selected from off campus. Nathan has returned to a chaired professorship in the Psychology department. His most recent attempt for higher office was running for president of the American Psychological Association. He lost the election. He is probably searching for a high level administrative position worthy of his many apparent administrative successes. Nathan continues to wield influence within the American Psychological Association. For example, he participated in five different events at the 1998 American Psychological Association Convention in San Francisco, including a discussion session called: "Distinguished Scientists meet with students to discuss critical issues in psychological science" and one of greater irony: a discussion session on "Ethics code revision". Nathan apparently is on the task force revising the ethics code of the American Psychological Association. His influence within the alcoholism field will continue to wane, especially with the change in editorship of *Contemporary Psychology*. His political influence within the profession remains high as illustrated by his 1999 award by the American Psychological Association's Board of Professioanl Affairs for his Distinguished Contribution to Knowledge.

Marlatt for years was the editor for psychological studies in the *Journal of Studies on Alcohol*. Nathan as head of the Alcoholism Research Center at Rutgers University was executive editor of the *Journal* which is published by Rutgers University. They controlled what would be published in the area of human psychology. The *Journal* has improved with both of them gone, but not in the field of psychology or the book review section of the *Journal*. The editor for psychology, Blane, is biased and superficial as seen in his personal publication efforts (Leonard & Blane, 1987). The editor, for a time, of the book review section, Rotgers (1996b), is biased - witness his glowing review of

Hester and Miller (l995). Entire journals are under the wing of revisionists - *Addictive Behaviors*, and for years *SPAB*, the *Bulletin of the Society of Psychologists in Addictive Behaviors*. The latter has undergone a name change since the Society has become a division of the American Psychological Association.

Every psychology journal that publishes clinical articles that may include studies of alcoholism contain Marlatt, Miller, the Sobells, or some of their former students on the editorial board. Journals of the behavior therapy movement such as *Behavior Therapy* and *Behaviour Research and Therapy* are controlled by revisionists. I have had the distinction of having manuscripts rejected by both of the above journals.

The chilling effect of the threat of legal action hangs over all journal editors, even without action on the part of the Sobells, as was true of the *Ethics and Behavior* journal and before them, the book publisher, Wiley. Is it surprising that controlled drinking is no longer a controversial subject within academic psychology? Behavior therapists at present control the major avenues of academic professional communication that carry research concerned with alcoholism treatment. They and their fellow ideologues also control much of the sources of government funding for research on alcoholism treatment.

Another source of power and influence of academic behavior therapists which has lead to the noncontroversial current status of controlled drinking in academia is that they train graduate students in clinical psychology in the behavior therapy mold. Their former Ph.D students following graduation or a postdoctoral position obtain positions in the clinical and/or academic field and continue to write, spread the word, and assume positions of influence aided by the influence of their mentors and the "old boy" network.

Clinical psychologists working in the alcoholism treatment field who are not members of a university faculty do not create followers since they do not teach in graduate schools and direct doctoral dissertations. When they retire or die there is no one to replace them. Someone like myself is an outsider on all counts. I am not a clinical psychologist. I do not treat alcoholics and I am not a recovering alcoholic. I am an experimental psychologist who entered the field of alcohol studies late in my career, coming from a completely unrelated field of research. I was too old to start a new career and training program in alcoholism research. Besides, I would not receive funding from NIAAA since their review boards contain former students of Marlatt and the Sobells or their sympathizers. It takes only one low rating by a member of a review board to sink a grant proposal competing for limited federal funds.

There is another simple but basic reason for the current noncontroversial nature of controlled drinking within academia: Wait long enough and the opposition will die or retire. Since they do not train people to succeed themselves in the field, the opposition dies with them. Clinical psychologists today who dare disagree with the behavior therapists would have a difficult time advancing in many clinical specialities within the academic field. I do not have that problem since my career did not depend upon publications in the field of alcoholism. My publications in the alcoholism field are limited by the fear of editors, the fear of threats of litigation by the Sobells or imagined threats, as well as the ideological biases of behavior therapy reviewers. If I was starting out now as an assistant professor with a speciality in alcoholism research, I probably would not attain tenure because it would be too difficult to publish my work on alcoholism.

Public health approaches had nothing to do with the Sobells' influence and the apparent noncontroversial nature of controlled drinking as secondary prevention. Their promoting a public health approach is a relatively recent development. It is a marketing device that fits with the development of managed care and the related view that less treatment is better because it costs less. Managed care in the alcoholism treatment field is being translated into minimal care. A critical issue ignored by behavior therapists and managed care administrators is that in the long run their relatively brief behavioral self-control and coping skills, motivational enhancement, etc., methods will cost more in human suffering and dollars than more intensive traditional treatment because the former are not as effective in the long term. The Sobells' editorial and reply contain no references to any studies, much less well-controlled studies, showing that stepped-care is successful, cost effective, and causes more good than harm to the individual patient, their significant others, and society at large, in the long run.

Autonomy versus paternalism

In her commentary in support of the Sobells, Duckert (1995) states:
In my opinion the real paradigm shift is not so much the choice of different treatment methods as in the choice of model for understanding human nature. Is the problem drinker to be met as an ally or as an untrustful adversary? Shall we trust the person's ability to evaluate his/her own situation and needs and his/her capacity to make adequate choices about future relationship to alcohol - or shall we as therapists be the ones who decide what is the best alternative for him/her? (p. 1169).

Duckert in the above passage raises a fundamental ethical issue, one about which the Sobells (1995a, 1995b) are quite definite: choice of treatment should be left to the patient. To do otherwise is paternalistic. Duckert, the Sobells, and many other revisionists fail to recognize the complexity of the ethical problem at hand. They also fail to recognize the existence of a large body of scholarship related to issues of autonomy and informed consent (Beauchamp & Walters, 1992; Beauchamp, Faden, Wallace, & Walters, 1982; Grisso & Appelbaum, 1998). Behavior therapists engaged in delivering controlled drinking treatments deal with the problem of autonomy and informed consent as though the patient is an equal in understanding and rationality and therefore a true partner in the decision making process leading to choice of treatment. There is no consideration on the part of these treatment providers of the possibility that someone who has been drinking excessively for years and probably using other drugs as well, engaging in irrational, impulsive, and at times dangerous behavior, can now calmly and thoughtfully reach a decision concerning their treatment goal.

Ethical treatment which involves respect for autonomy and self-determination requires that pertinent information be provided the decision maker, the patient, concerning the possible alternative treatments, and the possible positive and negative consequences of these treatments. Patients must understand the information provided and be capable of weighing the possible positive and negative consequences of controlled drinking described to them to reach a truly informed consent. If such information is not provided or participants do not understand the information or cannot comprehend its implications, the treatment is unethical and fails to meet federal regulations governing informed consent in the United States (Fadin & Beauchamp, 1986). Does Duckert present the evidence to her patients that heightened irreversible brain damage may occur with continued alcohol consumption whereas with abstinence there would be no further brain damage due to alcohol? Does Miller, Hester, the Sobells, Marlatt, etc. provide such information? Does Duckert and the other behavior therapists promoting harm reduction obtain an adequate assessment of brain structure and function from their patients before offering them the opportunity to make this important decision? From the nature of Duckert's and the Sobells' discussion and the description of their research and that of other behavior therapists, I doubt it.

Before offering controlled drinking as an alternative to abstinence an essential first step must be taken: obtain a thorough neuropsychological and neurological assessment. A great advantage of abstinence is that such an assessment is unnecessary before proceeding with treatment. A basic ethical principle is to do no harm. Advocacy of controlled drinking without prior assessments of brain structure and function violates this fundamental principle. When there is diminished capacity, as is the case in the majority of problem drinkers and alcoholics, paternalism overrides autonomy, is required, contrary to Duckert (1995), the Sobells (1995a), Hester and Miller (1995), and other controlled drinking advocates. At stake is the fundamental ethical principle to do no harm which in many cases is violated by the so-called harm reduction procedure of training for controlled drinking.

Miller promotes motivational enhancement as a technique facilitating patients' active involvement in treatment. Imagine the motivational enhancement for abstinence if alcoholics entering treatment were given neuroimaging scans of their brains and the brains of abstinent people of the same age. They have an opportunity, literally, to see the consequences of drinking and abstinence.

Another important but neglected issue is raised by Glatt (1995): the family of the patient should be party to the informed consent since they are also influenced by the consequences of treatment decisions. Glatt is an experienced and wise physician who has been in the treatment field for many years. He does not accept the judgment of the Sobells that their controlled drinking study had a revolutionary impact upon the treatment of alcohol misuse problems. Glatt observes from his personal experience that Davies (1962) had a great impact upon the thinking of physicians treating alcoholics in the 1960s, a decade before the Sobells' work. Abstinence versus controlled drinking was vigorously debated among physicians treating alcoholics. Physicians arrived at an abstinence position because of careful observation of their patients not because they blindly adopted an AA ideology.

In their reply the Sobells (1995b) derogate the role of careful and thoughtful clinical observation and emphasize the importance of trained observation necessary to avoid bias and the influence of ideology, the type of training they received as scientists. Sounds reasonable to the innocent reader. However, the book you are reading is a refutation of the self-aggrandizing argument that behavioral scientists are cloaked with armor protecting them against their expression of bias, ideology, self-aggrandizement, mendacity, sloppy scholarship, and other venal and crass motives.

Interest in controlled drinking and the attempt to train alcoholics to engage in controlled drinking was not initiated by the Sobells. As Glatt (1995) describes the 1960s, Davies' study in 1962 caused the big furor. Other behavior therapists (Lovibond & Caddy, 1970) employed aversive conditioning and blood alcohol concentration discrimination training in an attempt to train moderate drinking, work reported before the Sobells' conducted their research at Patton State Hospital. Operant conditioning studies by Mendelson and Mello (1966) and others had considerable impact upon behavior therapists, because they showed that alcohol consumption by alcoholics could be brought under control of environmental contingencies. Such results purportedly refuted the notion that alcoholics suffer a loss of control over their alcohol consumption, the linchpin for the insistence that abstinence is the only feasible treatment goal for alcoholics. Operant conditioning studies provided a tremendous lift to behaviorally oriented psychologists, especally those of a Skinnerian bent, including the Sobells at the time who assumed that alcoholism is nothing but a discriminated operant (Sobell & Sobell, 1975).

Stepped-care

Stepped-care is the term the Sobells use to describe their public health approach to controlled drinking. It corresponds to Marlatt's harm reduction. Not long ago I experienced stepped-care in physical medicine. How it differs from the Sobells' recommendation for alcohol misuse is revealing. I have had difficulties with my left foot for some time and I don't mean because I keep putting it in my mouth. Severe attacks of acute pain occur unpredictably. At times it feels as though I stepped on hot coals, or a sharp nail punched into my heal or toes. My internist at my HMO sent me to a specialist in physical medicine. After examining my reflexes and vascular system, pushing, pulling, jabbing, and getting my verbal reports of the kind, frequency, and location of pain he suggested a stepped-care plan. His diagnosis was deterioration of the metatarsal arch in my foot, a peripheral skeletal disorder not related to a previous problem I had of a pinched spinal nerve. I should try a Dr. Scholl insole insert in my shoes, an orthotic device that costs about ten dollars. Make an appointment in two months from now so that he can check on my progress. If the insert does not work he would write a prescription for a custom made orthotic device that would cost about $100. He was sorry but the HMO does not cover the costs of such items. If neither of these alternatives works, we will have to consider more radical alternatives. Injections of steroids would be tried next. If that failed, the last resort could be taken, surgery.

This is a stepped-care approach to my painful and distracting but not fatal problem. It differs in certain fundamental ways from the stepped-care recommended by the Sobells. Most importantly, the origin of my problem is in my peripheral skeletal system. My brain function is presumably normal for a person of my advanced age, i.e., compared to my age cohort. I can give an informed consent to a treatment based upon adequate understanding of the information offered. Presumably I have the capability of weighing the positive and negative consequences of choosing a particular treatment which by no stretch of the imagination is potentially harmful to me except in the later steps and certainly not harmful to others.

Stepped-care for people misusing alcohol or other drugs is a different story. Nowhere do the Sobells suggest an assessment of brain structure and function before people in need of treatment for alcohol related problems undertake controlled drinking. If the patients' brief intervention with moderate drinking does not work, they put themselves and others at risk for serious injury, accidents, and rending emotional experiences for themselves, their family and friends and monetary costs born by themselves and to varying degree society at large. Has anyone conducted a study of what happens to people with this moderation training in the case of those few for whom it works in the long term and the majority of those for whom it does not - as in the long-term follow-up by Miller et al. (1992)? For the majority of people who relapsed in the study by Miller et al., how many accidents occurred, what injuries took place, what was the cost in lost working hours, job performance, and inpatient and outpatient medical treatment as compared to those who attained abstinence? What was the accident rate, general medical expenses, etc., of those few who attained long term controlled drinking? Why are not ratings and family climate scales administered to significant others including the family that the patient interacts with during the time when they are engaged in controlled drinking and when they relapse completely? What kind of damage occurs to the patient and to others if the first step fails? Why are not the consequences of excessive drinking, the failures in social adjustment, job performance, etc., detailed by the very people who insist that presence or absence of drinking is an insufficient measure of recovery? Why is such poor research as the BSCT brief intervention studies by Miller and his colleagues, poor in their failure to obtain social adjustment and medical cost measures, as well as in long term drinking outcomes, so praised and promoted by revisionists? I think the answer is rather obvious.

The Sobells, Duckert, and other revisionists write as though the stepped-care approach to alcohol problems is dealing with as inoffensive a problem as my deteriorating metatarsal arch. It is not. It is dealing with potential permanent brain damage that affects every aspect of the individual's emotional life, performance, and intellectual capabilities. The Sobells and other revisionists cannot get it through their heads that alcohol is a powerful drug and that excessive drinking affects brain function and structure with striking individual differences in the degree of dysfunction and in the degree of reversibility. Problem drinkers in large numbers as well as alcoholics may suffer irreversible brain damage with continued drinking, even drinking in small amounts. The evidence is in Cala's (1987) CT scans and a host of other studies using neuroimaging, electrocortical and neuropsychological test batteries to assess brain function (Eckardt et al., 1980, 1998; Muuronen et al., 1989; Nicolás et al., 1993; Wilkinson & Sanchez-Craig, 1981). None of these asssessments are recommended, much less required prior to the initiation of stepped-care. Why not? Information obtained from such tests are essential for a truly informed consent. Anything less is unethical and opens the door to litigation when relapse occurs. Failure to obtain a proper informed consent in controlled drinking studies with problem drinkers is apparent from the discussions of the Sobells (1995a,1995 b); Duckert (1995) and from moderation treatments described in Miller and Hester (1986).

Among the additional ethical issues overlooked in the   Sobells' public health approach are the negative public health consequences. Mixed messages are sent to providers, the public, and patients. Uncertainty of goals, the myth promoted by Hester, Miller, the Sobells, Marlatt, and other revisionists, that there is no good evidence that abstinence works and there are no differences among treatment modalities or goals, reduces the ability to attain abstinence (Hall et al., 1990, 1991; O'Malley et al., 1992). People who might have been helped with abstinence oriented treatment would be delayed in their recovery by trying controlled drinking under the encouragement of providers who consider the short rather than the long term outcome. If patients attempt abstinence, their motivation and the mixed messages sent by their stepped-care oriented health provider reduces the probability of success.

Current public health interest in secondary prevention for heavy social drinkers and problem drinkers prior to their reaching the stage of alcohol dependence would have occurred regardless of the Sobells' IBTA controlled drinking study. More important for the development of secondary prevention than controlled drinking efficacy studies is the involvement of primary care physicians. Many knew of the dangers of excessive alcohol consumption from their clinical experience and epidemiological surveys on alcohol consumption and morbidity and mortality and some used brief interventions - advice - on the basis of such epidemiological information before controlled drinking experiments attained notoriety. Given their assumption that alcoholism is a disease, it is unlikely that physicians would be impressed by the notion that problem drinking is nothing but a bad habit.

I remember in the 1960s and 1970s my primary care physician at Kaiser Permanente, one of the pioneer health maintenance organizations, at my yearly visit would tell me to stop smoking and cut down on my alcohol and coffee consumption. He did not provide this advice as the result of research on controlled drinking by behavior therapists but as the result of his extensive clinical experience and epidemiological information. Only in the case of coffee may he have been mistaken. My HMO had adopted a public health view of prevention as cost effective as well as in the best interests of its patients from the time of its creation in the early 1950s. Advice and especially brief counseling given by a primary care physician or nurse may make a difference in reducing problems of some heavy social drinkers reached before brain dysfunction has occurred. (Fleming et al., 1997; Israel et al., 1996; Paton, 1996; Wallace, Cutter, & Haines, 1988). It may help some, and is essentially cost free. That is not the same sort of program promoted by the Sobells and other behavior therapists which is controlled drinking by more serious problem drinkers treated by clinical psychologists such as themselves in their own private clinics.

What if....?

Several things would have been different if the Sobells had never conducted their controlled drinking research. First, many alcoholics would not have suffered staggering down the blind alley of controlled drinking. No one considers, much less has assessed the cost of following the Pied Pipers in terms of human suffering as well as in monetary terms.

The mind-boggling $27,000,000 spent on project MATCH could have been put to better use elsewhere. After decades of support from NIAAA for the poorly conceived and conducted efficacy studies by Miller, Marlatt's continuous financial support and those of their students and others, the political influence of the behavior therapists led to their control of social science research funding at NIAAA. Enhanced support could have been provided instead for studies of treatment effectiveness and biobehavioral research that would lead to basic understanding of the biology of alcoholism and its interactions with the social environment as well as the area suffering most from inadequate support, prevention research, by which I do not mean interdiction.

What if the Sobells, Marlatt, and others had not made Jellinek into a bogeyman and fellow-traveler of AA? Novices in the field of alcohol studies might have delved into his work and have been much the wiser for the effort. What follows are a few quotations from Jellinek's (1960) classic work, *The disease concept of alcoholism*, correcting some of the misrepresentations by behavior therapists (Marlatt et al., 1973).

If it should be conceded that morphine, heroin and bariturate addiction involve grave physiopathologic processes which result in 'craving,' then they may be designated as diseases. (and they are included in the American Medical Association's nomenclature of diseases)... The current majority opinion to which the present writer subscribes, and subscribed before it was a majority opinion, is that anomalous forms of the ingestion of narcotics and alcohol, such as drinking with loss of control and physical dependence, are caused by physiopathological processes and constitute diseases...

Recovered alcoholics in Alcoholics Anonymous speak of 'loss of control' to denote that stage in the development of their drinking history when the ingestion of one alcoholic drink sets up a chain reaction so that they are unable to adhere to their intention to 'have one or two drinks only' but continue to ingest more and more - often with quite some difficulty and disgust - contrary to their volition.

It should be mentioned at this time, however, that the loss of control does not emerge suddenly but rather progressively *and that it does not occur inevitably as often as the gamma alcoholic takes a drink...* (italics added) (Jellinek, pp. 40, 41, 42)

It seems that some species of alcoholism show a progression which strongly suggests a true disease process, but apparently as yet no one has given proof that a specific disease condition gives rise to the heavy drinking at the beginning of the alcoholic career. For the initiating phase, the postulation of psychological and cultural factors seems adequate, but not beyond that. (p.66).

The learning theory, as Conger readily admits, does not exclude any other etiological theories; it can be complementary to any of them. Neither would it conflict with a disease conception of one or the other species of alcoholism.

What has been said here of the importance of the learning process as bringing about necessary conditions for the emergence of addiction holds true for many of the symbolic (psychological) mechanisms which have been suggested as etiological factors in alcohol addiction. The most inveterate pharmacologists would not deny that symbolic factors are at work in creating the terrain for the development of addiction in the strict pharmacological sense; as a matter of fact, they insist on the psychological factors for the initiating process... The psychological hypotheses are of greater relevance to alpha alcoholism than to alcohol addiction with its stringent criteria. (p. 77).

Alcoholism as a public health view is not new, is not a product of the inventive thinking of Marlatt and the Sobells with their harm reduction and stepped-care approaches. Jellinek discusses the public health view of alcoholism decades before revisionists hit upon this marketing approach for controlled drinking. If a public health position had been adopted following Jellinek's interpretation in the 1960's and earlier, an approach that corresponds to the one adopted by public health officials would have been embraced. It would not train underage heavy drinking freshman college students to engage in controlled drinking and to continue breaking the law in the manner practiced by Marlatt and his colleagues (Marlatt et al., 1998; Larimer et al., 1998). A community approach would be adopted, one that changes the normative behavior of college students.

Jellinek (1960) reviews all of the theories concerning the etiology of alcoholism and the pertinent research available at the time. He considers the notion that alcoholism is an allergy, the notion adopted by Alcoholics Anonymous. He cites experimental research by Robinson and Voegtlin... which "in a definitive experimental study entirely refuted the allergy hypothesis." (p.87). Jellinek concludes:

> This discussion of the allergy view has not been presented here in order to persuade Alcoholics Anonymous to abandon their conception. The figurative use of the term 'alcoholism is an allergy' is as good as or better than anything else for their purposes, as long as they do not wish to foist it upon students of alcoholism. (p. 87).

Jellinek (1960) also examines the evidence for theories that assume a nutritional deficiency provides an etiological basis for alcoholism. He concludes, "Neither Willaims nor anybody else has ever shown that a craving or need for alcohol exists in the pre-alcoholic state of alcoholics." (p.95). With respect to etiology in terms of brain pathology, he states:

> Recently... an hypothesis has been presented which assumes that brain damage acquired in the course of initial heavy alcohol intake may produce in the course of time those characteristic behaviors which distinguish 'alcoholism' from ordinary drunkenness... More recently Lemere (1956), apparently on the basis of some of these reports has favored this sort of explanation of the etiology of alcoholism... the higher cerebral areas and thus their functions are most subjected to the effects of alcohol and that the cells constituting those areas are also the first to be anesthetized by alcohol. Thus Lemere feels it is justified to assume that, with progressive destruction of the frontal cortex, less alcohol will be required to produce that stage of anesthesia where control is lost... (pp. 88, 89).

While Lemere's hypothesis is limited to lesions subsequent to heavy alcohol intake, there is a hypothesis which postulates a cerebral anomaly preexistent to alcoholism... Little and McAvoy (1952). (p.91).

Jellinek astutely notes that the presence of low levels of EEG alpha activity could be a preexisting condition, a consequence, of heavy alcohol consumption, or a

doing. It questions their training and the adequacy of their treatment. Miller provides a grossly inappropriate parallel of resistance to novel ideas from the history of medicine gleaned from an historical event described by Broad and Wade (1982). It is the story of Semmelweis' heroic battle for the public health. He is the 19th century physician who tried to reform hospital sanitary procedures to stem an epidemic of childbed fever responsible for the deaths of up to 30% of the mothers and their newborn infants in Europe. Physicians rejected his recommendations for improved sanitary procedures, primarily washing their hands in chlorine before attending a pregnant woman or her infant, because it would be an admission of their responsibility in the unnecessary deaths. They drove Semmelweiss from his profession and he eventually died in a mental hospital. Aside from this distasteful and inappropriate analogy to the present state in the alcoholism treatment field in relation to behavior therapy research, Miller neglects several crucially important ingredients in the treatment of Semmelweis by the physicians in control of hospitals in Europe.

Broad and Wade (1982) use the illustration of Semmelweiss to emphasize the point that an isolated fact, failure to wash hands properly, is unpersuasive in the absence of satisfactory theory. Simmelweiss' observations of the fact that clean hands was followed by a decline in cases of childbed fever needed the germ theory of Lister and Pasteur to provide the necessary impact to persuade physicians to change their practice. A second critical ingredient that makes Miller's analogy inappropriate is the virulent role antisemitism played in the ostracism of Semmelweis and his recommendation for improved sanitation. Failure to adapt practice to the empirical results reported by Miller, Marlatt, and the Sobells, does not have a parallel in the outrageous treatment received by Semmelweiss. Failure to adopt the behavior therapy goal of controlled drinking is based on the wisdom of counselors derived from extensive clinical experience with alcoholics.

Following a variety of explanations accounting for the failure to penetrate the unyielding traditional treatment industry, Miller turns instructor in marketing and sales and suggests that the solution is to be proactive. Do not passively wait for the opposition to see the light. Intentionally plan strategies for shaping the treatment industry. Guide their decisions and meet their needs in a more direct fashion:

A first step... is to set clear goals. To whom should the results be disseminated?... What audiences would have a natural interest in the findings?... Some of the possible audiences to reach with the findings of alcoholism treatment research include: alcoholism counselors, psychologists working with addictive behaviors, primary health care professionals, pastoral counselors, authors of major textbooks, insurance company executives, congressional and legislative representatives, employee assistance program counselors, family practitioners, judges who handle alcohol-related offenses, state planners for health and human services, alcoholism information centers, other alcoholism treatment researchers, administrators of alcoholism treatment centers, and university professors training new professionals in psychology, medicine, social work, nursing, counseling, public administration, law, etc... Each of these potential audiences is served by a few major information sources. Many of these are 'trade' journals, for which researchers are typically neither readers nor contributors... To reach a specific audience, it is sensible to publish in their most-read trade periodicals.

Other possible dissemination routes include the annual meetings or mailing lists of organizations such as the Association of Labor-Management Administrators and Consultants on Alcoholism, the National Council on Alcoholism, and the American Personnel and Guidance Association. Specific selected mailings may be planned to reach key textbook authors, legislators, federal officials, judges, or state and local decision-makers. (p.158).

Miller also suggests providing therapist handbooks, video and audio tapes, workshops, and consulting. All are nice incoming generating devices while educating the ignorant insecure alcoholism counselors. Miller concludes:

It is habitual to end with a statement that more research is needed on the topic being addressed... Those of us who do research in the modification of addictive behaviors may be particularly well-suited to conduct such studies. We are accustomed to dealing with seemingly intransigent behaviors, overcoming resistance, instilling motivation for change, and replacing overpracticed habits with novel alternative responses... Perhaps it is time we focussed our expertise on a genuinely challenging problem: how to motivate, evoke, and maintain the behaviors that constitute research utilization. (p. 159).

In other words, "how do we best sell our snake oil". After reading Miller I wondered, as I have often in the past, "do they really believe what they say"? Are the Sobells, Miller, Marlatt, etc., deceiving themselves as well as their audience or are they aware, can they verbalize, their intent to deceive their audience? Is their goal to succeed, conquer, win, so overpowering that it inhibits rational, critical thought, and provides the cloak of self-deception, or are they engaging in a completely calculated strategy? How, after reading it, can any serious scientist believe that their research is impeccable? I have asked myself these questions since 1972. I still cannot decide on an answer.

Unfortunately, revisionists are succeeding in their penetration strategy, at least in coopting government granting agencies and professional societies. Evidence is the fact that Marlatt and Miller have well-funded alcoholism and addiction research centers at their respective universities. They have large grants for research, provide graduate and postdoctoral training, and hire additional faculty to conduct research and provide training. They are past and present officers in various professional societies and serve as consultants to federal granting agencies. They and their former students sit on review boards of granting agencies and journals.

How has all this been possible? Their success rests not so much on the brilliance of their research, but on their ability to suppress the successful research of their opposition or prevent such research from occurring. Suppression is simple. Keep opposing views out of the major journals and handbooks. Never invite the authors to conferences and subsequent edited books in mainline psychology and clinical psychology; never cite their studies. This is obvious in relation to the CATOR registry and publications describing these results, and to Küfner and Feuerlein. Repeated failure has also been my personal experience in attempting to publish articles critical of revisionists, organize symposia on abstinence treatments at meetings of the American Psychological Association, and attempts to obtain research funding from federal agencies. How many research projects from a competing point of view never were funded because they could not muster support for funding from review boards containing revisionists? We will never know. One thing is for certain: Revisionists are sitting pretty.

11 THE PLACE OF FACTS IN A WORLD OF VALUES: WHAT IS TO BE DONE?

MISCONDUCT IN SCIENCE

Personal note

Am I confusing fraud, the intent to misrepresent, with error, the inadvertent mistake which may occur during the normal practice of science? Doob (1984) suggests as much. As one anonymous reviewer for the *Psychological Reports* put it:

> There are many scientists who adhere strongly to a particular theoretical position and simply ignore counter evidence. (How many times are unsuccessful experiments placed in 'File 13' but the one successful one submitted?). I am not condoning such a practice, but in some instances they are eventually proven right and in other instances proven wrong. In that sense, it is not a deliberate effort to deceive, it is the result of strongly held beliefs.

The above conclusion is a non sequitur. Intentionality is not dependent on the presence or absence of strong beliefs. I do not think there is a necessary difference between withholding negative results and fabricating, inventing results, inventing investigations that never occurred, including congressional investigations and court actions. Intent to deceive differentiates fraud from an unintentional error. Strongly held beliefs may lead to intentional deception such as the fabrication of results, the suppression of undesired results, or to an unintentional error. Intentional withholding of results can be devastating, as is evident in the case of tobacco companies withholding evidence that cigarette smoking is addictive (Kluger,1997). If there is intent to deceive, there is little difference between fabricating evidence and withholding evidence. In one case, serious harm can result in the treatment of alcoholics; in the other, harm can occur to the smoker. In both cases potentially serious harm may occur to consumers as well as violations of the fundamental values of truth and trust. The fact that many investigators withhold negative results - even if the majority of scientists indulge in such practice - and I am not convinced that this is the case - it is not to be condoned. It is unethical practice and its consequences may cause serious damage to the health and well-being of the public. That suppression of evidence or invention of evidence is due to strongly held beliefs is no justification for the practice and is to be condemned. That a reviewer of a manuscript and therefore an established professional could reach a different conclusion is a disheartening illustration of the fate of facts in a world of values - or their lack.

In case there is remaining doubt, I believe the following is a fabrication that cannot be taken as an unintentional error. Sobell and Sobell (1978) assert that limiting evaluations of remission or recovery from alcoholism to drinking behavior does not suffice. To illustrate their point the Sobells use a vignette concerning a "sober sociopath". Subject JL is described as functioning well in terms of controlled drinking and abstinence, 96.4% of the days in the second year of the follow-up. However, other measures of JL's interpersonal behavior reveal a different picture:

(a) repeatedly moved from city to city leaving a trail of unpaid bills, (b) obtained welfare and funds for the indigent while working full-time, and (c) fraudulently staged a marriage in order to obtain funds and material goods from his friends and relatives.... This example points out that while the subject's drinking behavior had improved to the point where drinking interfered very little with the rest of his life, his total adjustment can be described in terms of his having become a 'sober sociopath.' (Sobell & Sobell, 1978, p.160).

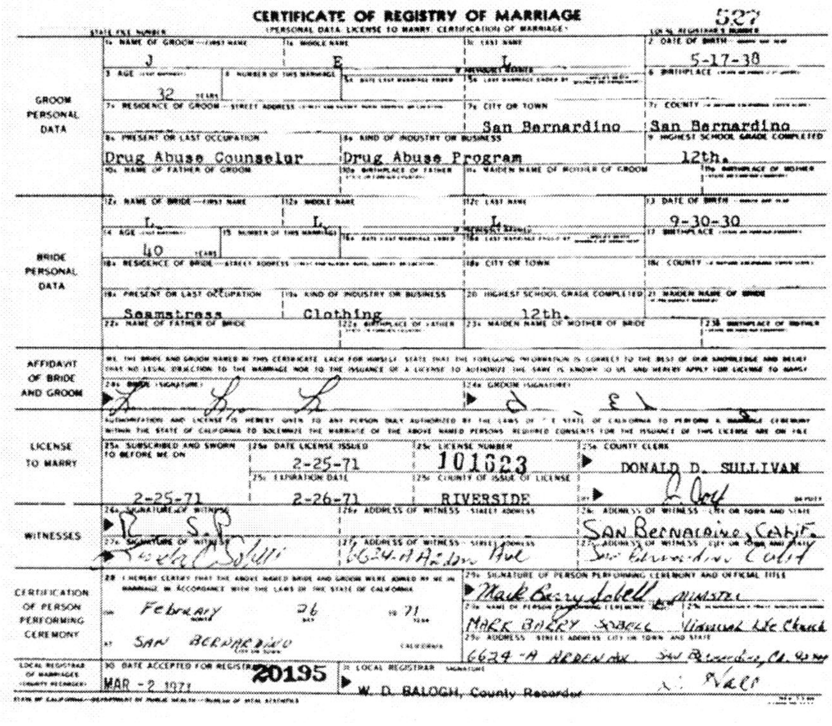
CERTIFICATE OF REGISTRY OF MARRIAGE

527

GROOM PERSONAL DATA

J | E | L | 5-17-38

32 YEARS

7b CITY OR TOWN: San Bernardino | 7c COUNTY: San Bernardino

8a PRESENT OR LAST OCCUPATION: Drug Abuse Counselur | 8b KIND OF INDUSTRY OR BUSINESS: Drug Abuse Program | 9 HIGHEST SCHOOL GRADE COMPLETED: 12th.

BRIDE PERSONAL DATA

L | L | L | 9-30-30

40 YEARS

19a PRESENT OR LAST OCCUPATION: Seamstress | 19b KIND OF INDUSTRY OR BUSINESS: Clothing | 20 HIGHEST SCHOOL GRADE COMPLETED: 12th.

AFFIDAVIT OF BRIDE AND GROOM

LICENSE TO MARRY

25a SUBSCRIBED AND SWORN TO BEFORE ME ON: 2-25-71 | 25b DATE LICENSE ISSUED: 2-25-71 | 25c LICENSE NUMBER: 101623 | 25e COUNTY CLERK: DONALD D. SULLIVAN

25d EXPIRATION DATE: 2-26-71 | COUNTY OF ISSUE OF LICENSE: RIVERSIDE

WITNESSES

San Bernardino, Calif.

6624-A Arden Ave | San Bernardino Calif

CERTIFICATION OF PERSON PERFORMING CEREMONY

February 26 71

SAN BERNARDINO CALIFORNIA

Mark Barry Sobell, Minister

MARK BARRY SOBELL | Universal Life Church

6624-A ARDEN AVE. San Bernardino, Ca.

LOCAL REGISTRAR OF MARRIAGES

MAR - 2 1971 | 20195 | W. D. BALOGH, County Recorder

Figure 11.1 Copy of JL's marriage license.

Notice the signatures at the bottom. Mark Sobell is the officiating minister and Linda is a witness. Figure 11.2 is a copy of an affidavit by JL. Could the Sobells have written the vignette of the sober sociopath because they inadvertently forgot to mention that Mark was the minister officiating at the wedding ceremony and Linda the witness? The wedding, by the way, is legal. Mark was ordained as a minister through a correspondence course. There were some advantages to ordination in addition to officiating at weddings. His house could be considered a church since he held "church meetings" in it and as a church the house would be tax exempt.

(1)

I the undersigned was very shocked and hurt when Dr. Sobell used my case history in his publication

I am JL who to whom he referred. At no time did I give my permission for Dr. Sobell or anyone else connected with the research program to use my initials or any part of my case history for publication.

Both Dr. Sobell & his wife advised me that I was a Gamma Alcoholic and that if I participated in their research program I could drink again socially with no adverse effects either socially or physically ever again upon completion of their program

I was so convinced by them that upon completion of the program I and another former patient appeared on the Ralph Story AM Los Angeles T.V. Show and proclaimed to the world that the Sobell's had found a way to let Alcoholics return to " Normal

Figure 11.2 JL's statement Page 1 of 3.

334

Social Drinking." __ That evening
After Appearing on the show
Dr. Sobell performed a marriage
ceremony in his home, with Mrs.
Sobell as maid of honor + Mr. R.
P   , Research Assistant, As
best man. He married me + my
girlfriend, h   h   . He had
A mail-order Ministers license
From the Universal Life Church in
Modesto, Calif. and Assured us
both that the marriage was
legal. He gave us $200.00 + loaned
us his car for a weekend
honeymoon. When we returned
From our weekend he asked me
To give an interview to Time
Magazine which I did.

For years I have lived with
the hope that Dr Sobell was
correct. However I have lost
many jobs, lost (2) wives +
my self Respect while trying to
control my drinking. I had a
card issued by Dr. Sobell showing
me how to drink socially but
I lost it on one of my drunks.
(over)

Figure 11.2 JL's statement Page 2 of 3.

As For Follow-up Interviews by
the Sobell's I was only interviewed
once by Linda Sobell Approx 2 yrs
after completion of their program.
At the time of the interview
I was once again an inpatient
at Patton for Alcohol Treatment.

Since completion of the Research
Program I have been in Detox
Centers 7 times, ~~Be~~ Hospitalized
5 Times and am now presently
living in A Recovery Home for
Alcoholics in

I do hereby authorize you
to use my full name and any
information I have written here
for publication at any time.
I am doing this in hopes that
I may help other Alcoholics
Realize that there is no Turning
back. We either must Totally
Abstain or ~~die~~ we shall
surely die.

Figure 11.2 JL's statement Page 3 of 3.

We must have ideals such as truth to strive for, goals beyond our reach, but "our reach must exceed our grasp" if we are to be a civilized society, including a science that we wish young people to pursue. We all make mistakes, unintentional errors, but I believe that the incidents concerning us are not mistakes and are not trivial deceptions lacking consequences for the well-being of science and society.

Ideology and the truth

A criticism of the traditional, received, view of alcoholism is that its objections to controlled drinking were motivated by politics. Of course. They were also motivated by a concern for the truth and the well-being of alcoholics. Methodologically, the RAND report was a poor study. Davies was wrong, misled by alcoholics because he failed to obtain independent corroboration of their self-reports. The Sobells I believe invented much of their interview data and misrepresented their procedure and results. I believe that the RAND report authors and the Sobells were motivated by ambition. Davies was simply naive.

Now that motivations are settled, what is the truth status of each side's assertions? That is the issue. Professional behavior nowadays is motivated to a great extent by ambition, greed and power. Yet such motives are irrelevant to the truth status of an assertion. We must distinguish between the motivation for an assertion and its truth or falsity, its correspondence with the facts. Evidence that we have reviewed in previous chapters indicate that much of what behavior therapists promote in the field of alcoholism does not work. Whether the research was motivated purely by a search for the truth or a means of supplementing the investigators' income is beside the point. Examination of much of their research reveals that it is poorly conducted and/or improperly interpreted and does not merit the claims made for it. Evaluations of the treatment effectiveness of abstinence programs reported by Küfner and Feuerlein and by Harrison and Hoffmann for the CATOR registry, Smith and his colleagues for aversion conditioning, have a higher success rate than controlled drinking efficacy studies, even those using problem drinkers. All this is aside from the problems that these controlled drinking efficacy studies have when one attempts to generalize their results to clinical practice.

Revisionists have had a double standard in their treatment of the first RAND Report. They did not criticize it for using an unacceptably high criterion for controlled drinking, for having an extraordinarily high attrition rate, or for not having independent corroboration of self-reports. Neither the first nor the second Rand reports were published in peer reviewed journals. They were introduced by press conferences, appearing first as in-house monograph publications accompanied by extensive media coverage, and then in commercially published books. Questionable practices of this sort were greated by silence on the part of the revisionists. In contrast, they resorted to ad hominem attacks when the reports were criticized by Pendery and others because of the inadequacies apparent in the Rand Reports and their misleading message.

A question of character

There is an apparent disdain for boundaries, truth and accuracy, among revisionists. It is not merely a question of carelessly counting the number of interviews. The Sobells initially stated that they were subjected to a Congressional inquiry, further implying that such an inquiry had subpoena powers at their disposal and they were exonerated following such an inquiry. Marlatt (1983) repeated this sensational report as did Brownell (1984) who quotes a sanitized version of Jensen's letter as though it were the original as does Hunt (1999). By 1984 the Sobells knew they could not continue to report the congressional inquiry story in this manner. At our colloquium talk at the University of Washington with Marlatt in the audience I stated that we had a letter from Congressman Gore stating that there had been no congressional investigation. However, the Sobells, Marlatt, and others continue to report some variation of the story that a congressional inquiry exonerated the Sobells and they and others continue to state that there have been five investigations exonerating them.

As we learned from Trachtenberg's report and from the patients' lawsuit, subpoena powers do not cross the border. Residing in Canada provided the Sobells with immunity from subpoena. Since this information is not well-known, they and others continue to report that they were investigated in the course of a major medical malpractice lawsuit brought against them by the patients and once again they were exonerated. They were never served with a subpoena in the case. They were never exonerated because they never came to trial. There could be no mistake.

Stories by the Sobells and other revisionists appear to change with the circumstances. There is a corresponding principle in administration, Parkinson's law (Parkinson, 1957): Activities will expand to fill the available space; work expands to fill the available time. In like manner, here is Maltzman's law, the rubber band theory of truth: the truth will be stretched to meet the available boundaries.

Why?

The major objection to the study by Pendery et al. (1982) expressed by Marlatt, the Dickens Committee and a host of others (Heather & Robertson, 1983; Nathan & Niaura, 1995; Peele, 1985; Thombs, 1994) was that we failed to compare the experimental and control groups. What if we compared the two groups and the experimental group was significantly better than the control group, would that mean that the Sobells did not commit fraud? What if we compared the two groups, controlled drinking versus abstinence, and they were not significantly different or the control group was significantly better? Would this mean that the Sobells committed fraud? It could be argued in the first case that the controlled drinking training really did work 10 years later and in the latter case it could be argued that 10 years later the controlled drinking effects had worn off. In neither case could the comparison prove or disprove fraud.

Emphasis on our not comparing the two groups is a diversion from what has been my concern for almost three decades: the Sobells alleged fabrication of their results. Marlatt's letter and the Dickens Committee report which built upon it emphasized our failure to compare the two groups. It was not the issue for which the Dickens Committee was charged: determine whether or not the Sobells committed fraud. The Dickens Committee failed to fulfil their responsibility because they never obtained and studied the raw data that constituted the basic dependent variable that I alleged the Sobells fabricated, the daily drinking dispositions recorded on time-line follow-back interview forms. Instead, they introduced a red herring: Pendery et al. conducted an inadequate study because they failed to compare the experimental group with the control group.

It would have been quite simple to determine whether fraud was committed or not. Obtain all of the time-line follow-back interview forms of the kind shown in Figure 5.1 and determine whether the information contained therein can reproduce the results published for individual subjects such as JPr. He was reported as having had 282 days abstinent, 27 days drunk and 57 days of controlled drinking (Sobell & Sobell, 1978, p.134) all derived from two interviews using the time-line follow-back method during the course of Year 2 of the follow-up.

Simple. That's it. Why didn't the Dickens Committee do it? Why didn't the Trachtenberg Committee attempt to do it? Why has not a single critic pointed out this crucial first step is missing? I suggest that these committees did not because they could not - and then whitewashed the affair. Why? Who is James Jensen? Why did he write the letter he did? Why could not the APA Ethics Committee (CSPEC) simply say they do not have the subpoena and judicial powers to conduct an effective investigation? Instead, they provided another whitewash of the affair. Why did not Rutgers University write a correction in the *Journal of Alcohol Studies* or give an interview to the *Chronicle of Higher Education* denouncing the misuse of their professional journal? Why did they not fire Nathan for costing Rutgers University and the taxpayers of New Jersey a fortune in the effort to thwart publication of my paper?

Why do dozens of academic authors blindly accept whatever is written as the truth without consulting the original sources or critically evaluating the issues? Why do textbook writers and instructors who use these textbooks disregard their responsibility for the intellectual development of their students and the health and well-being of some of these students, their families and friends and the public at large? Why do these authors ignore their responsiblity to determine the truth status of assertions they make, especially those that may have significant impact upon the readers?

Providing a single answer to all of these complex questions is impossible. Complex kinds of behavior of the sort in question are multidetermined and in different people there may be different determiners - as is true of alcoholism. Some speculation seems warranted if nothing else to try to bring some closure to these vexing questions and to stimulate further inquiry and judicious discussion. First, let us examine what answers traditional sociology of science offers.

Traditional sociology of science

Merton (1968), the preeminent sociologist of science of our time, asserted that science is self-correcting. Fraud is uncovered and punished and cannot ordinarily escape exposure because science replicates its results, especially important results. Self-correction functions through general norms for appropriate scientific conduct which are internalized by students and aspiring scientists during the course of their education and training.

Perhaps Merton's interpretation was correct at one time and still is under certain, unspecified, circumstances. It is an ideal which we should strive to attain. I suspect that it does not hold true to the degree we would like to think it does in broad areas of biobehavioral science and its institutions. It does not hold true, because of the impact of two important factors, one old and the other new: (a) power and politics in science and its institutions, energized by ideology, is as old as science itself (Gillispie, 1960), and (b) the rise of litigation and threats of litigation. Jointly as well as separately these factors have a chilling effect upon truth and the process of self-correction in science. I believe these forces worked to suppress evidence supporting my allegation of fraud in the field of alcoholism treatment by Mark and Linda Sobell (1972, 1973, 1976, 1978) and by Caddy et al. (1978).

Ideology, value judgments in the guise of statements of fact (Bergmann, 1954), and explicit value judgments may determine what is published, the nature of the research conducted, and the very facts that are collected. But there is another, aberrant, way in which values determine facts or the appearance of facts, theories and their social significance. Fraud accomplished under the protective umbrella of ideology, power and politics, is a serious threat to self-correction in science and the public well-being. By fraud we mean the intentional misrepresentation of methods, research results or their import, or the fabrication of data.

How common is fraud in science? Is it an issue to be concerned about?

It may be argued that fraud in science is rare and the chilling effect of libel litigation on the processes of self-correction even rarer. Spokespersons for the science establishment make such arguments concerning the frequency of occurrence of fraud. They also argue that when fraud occurs it is an aberration. These assessments, as well as opposing judgments, that fraud is common or that it is on the increase, are oversimplifications without firm empirical support. However, this question may be less important than it appears because it is not addressing the important issues centering around fraud in science. We must consider the kinds of fraud now being committed, who is committing the fraud, and the circumstances fostering its occurrence.

Fraud may be the consequence of a momentary impulse due to pressure to publish, frustration, or emotional unbalance. Fraud under such circumstances is presumably a temporary aberration due to a disturbed person working under pressure. A classic example is that of Summerlin at Sloan-Kettering who painted his mice, had a nervous breakdown when the fraud was discovered by a technician, and confessed what he had done (Broad & Wade, 1982). However, the more striking cases of alleged fraud that have been described in some detail in recent years, such as those by Darsee and by Soman (Broad & Wade, 1982), the case of Bruening (Holden, 1987), and the Sobell affair that has engaged my efforts since 1972, are different in nature. They have extended over several years or more and I believe involve ongoing misrepresentations and scientific misconduct. In such cases, scientists engaging in fraud characteristically do not confess. Instead, they attempt to brazen it out and may continue to misrepresent events in order to defend themselves. They may take the initiative and attack the accuser. These kinds of cases produce extensive contamination of the database of science, far greater than the case where the scientist is guilty of a temporary aberration. They are also more serious than the latter type incident.

It has been argued by leaders of the science establishment that there is no relative increase in fraud (Koshland, 1987). There may be an absolute increase in fraud, but this should not be misinterpreted. It is due merely to the vast increase in the number of scientists. This line of reasoning overlooks an important change in science, especially bio-behavioral science. When I was a graduate student in experimental psychology in the late 1940s we argued about and investigated latent learning: Does learning and conditioning occur on the basis of drive reduction or mere contiguity of cue and reward? My doctoral dissertation was on the arcane topic of simultaneous vs. successive discrimination learning in the hooded rat. Today, among many other problems, psychologists conduct research on training alcoholics and purported problem drinkers to adopt controlled social drinking in contrast to the traditional treatment goal of abstinence, and report research on the administration of amphetamines to the severely retarded. I conducted research on the determinants of chemical dependence in adolescents - as well as on the esoteric problem of the orienting reflex. Psychology has expanded into areas of research that directly affect the public. Such research was rare in the 1940s and 1950s. As a consequence, there are issues concerning fraud in science including psychology related to the public interest and safety and the public need to know which did not exist in past generations.

What is true of psychology is true of biomedical science in general. Many more scientists work in areas directly related to the health and well being of the public than in the past, in relative as well as absolute numbers. If the same percentage of cases of fraud occurred today as in earlier generations, there is a greatly increased threat to the safety of the public. The numbers game played by spokespersons for establishment science misses the point because fraud in science now may directly affect the health and well-being of the public. Whether increased in absolute or relative numbers over the past, it is a problem of major concern. The Sobells' alleged fraud has potentially enormous impact because it has influenced treatment and public policy that in turn may affect the estimated 8% of the adult population that have a serious drinking problem, their immediate family, and many segments of society at large, as the result of drunk driving and industrial accidents, etc. Its purported results also emboldened other behavior therapists to employ controlled drinking and related methods and induced the NIAAA to fund similar studies and support the research and careers of behavior therapists culminating in the 27 million dollar MATCH project.

Determinants of fraud

We need to examine some of the factors that may influence the occurrence of fraud, factors not considered in the idealized image of science conceived of as a community of scholars engaged in the disinterested objective search for the truth. Fraud may be a function of an approach-avoidance conflict or decision process influenced by costs/benefits as noted by Broad and Wade (1982). A similar analysis has been made by Wilson and Herrnstein (1985) in their examination of the roots of criminality.

Factors operating to deter fraud include a high probability that, (a) fraud will be discovered, (b) it will be reported, and (c) there will be negative sanctions. It will be swiftly and severely punished. A low probability of discovery, reporting it, and punishment, increases the likelihood of fraud, other things being equal. Furthermore, the more attractive the fruits of fraud the greater the likelihood of its occurrence. Given that there is no established mechanism in science and scholarship generally for detecting, reporting, and dealing with fraud and its sanctions, the deterrent threat of the possible apprehension and punishment for fraud is not great.

What has kept fraud in check in the past are the norms for scientific conduct discussed by Merton and the variables that influence these norms, including the character of individual scientists. Resolution of the conflicting tendencies whose outcome determines fraudulent behavior, is moderated in important ways by individual differences in personality. These include such factors as the impulsivity and emotional imbalance of the individual, but more importantly, the scientist's character and normative code of conduct. If these norms are changing in the direction of greater permissiveness, and I believe they are, then the relative and absolute incidence of fraud, and especially fraud in areas that directly affect the well being of the public will be on the rise. National representative studies (Rokeach & Ball-Rokeach, 1989) indicate that there has been a shift in values over the past several decades. If scientists are no different than other people, and I do not believe that they are basically different, then there should be a change in the values of scientists as well. However, the one factor generally assumed to inhibit fraud is the practice that makes science uniquely different from all other activities: controlled experimentation and observation and their replication. I shall argue that this characteristic does not invariably have the assumed self-correcting effect.

ASSUMED PROCESS OF SELF-CORRECTION

As suggested earlier, there are at least three critical decision points which determine whether or not self-correction will occur: (a) If it occurs, is fraud readily detected? (b) If detected is it readily reported? (c) If reported, is anything done about it? There are serious obstacles to self-correction at each of these decision-points.

Reasons for breakdown at each of the decision points

Among the obstacles is the potential selective filter of ideology and   politics which may interfere with self-correction at all decision points. Detection of fraud and its reporting is most likely to occur from an adversarial quarter not from friends or fellow ideologues. If one ideology dominates an area, there are few critical adversaries serving as watchdogs; fraud is less likely to be detected. If detected, it is less likely to be reported by a fellow ideologue, and if reported, less likely to be acted upon. Diversity and pluralism, in science as well as in other institutions and in society at large, help safeguard against fraud. Dampening effects of ideology on self-correction may be present to a far greater degree than the casual observer imagines. Interference with the process of self-correction occurs because adherents to a common ideology react to an attack upon or criticism of one of their members as an attack upon themselves. They will therefore attempt to avoid, defend against, or suppress such an attack. Ideologues are more forgiving of each other than of their common foe. It may all be rationalized as serving a greater good. In practice it promotes the common good. If controlled drinking is purported to be a successful new treatment goal, federal research funds become available, behavior therapists can offer new treatment modalities, employment opportunities multipy, clinical practices increase in size, invitations for lectures, conferences, and workshops multiply, and graduate students are attracted to a new area, all of which facilitates promotions and salary increases for the new ideologues.

Another obstacle to self-correction at the second and third decision points is an imbalance in power and status between the accused and accuser. A graduate research assistant or a technician may be in the best position to detect fraud if it occurs in a laboratory. They conducted the experiment, ran the subjects, analyzed the data, etc. But because of their lack of power and status, their careers depend upon the goodwill and positive recommendations of their supervisors, mentors, and professors. They risk their graduate and professional careers by bringing a complaint against their relatively powerful supervising professor. Furthermore, administrators are unlikely to act on the basis of a complaint by a graduate student against an influential professor, one who brings grant money into the institution, enhances its reputation by their presence, may actually sit on the academic review board of the administrator, or is a personal friend of the administrator, etc. Few protections exist to guarantee normal progress in the career of the relatively powerless accuser and freedom from retribution from the accused, their friends and fellow ideologues. There is thus considerable pressure against reporting and acting upon an allegation of fraud when the accuser is relatively powerless and the accused is relatively powerful. Instances of alleged fraud that are reported, investigated, and dealt with in an even-handed manner usually involve scientists relatively low in the academic power hierarchy, postdoctoral fellows, or investigators on soft money (Broad & Wade, 1982). Powerful people accused of fraud have the resources to fight back, a deterrent against reporting and acting upon fraud, especially for potential accusers with relatively little power.

Fraud is not revealed by failure to replicate

(1) Most observers would probably agree that fraud is not readily detected. If detected, it is often the result of a chance observation by a co-worker, or the curiosity or suspicions of a reviewer. Detection of fraud is not ordinarily a consequence of a failure to replicate an experiment. Most, or certainly many, reported cases of fraud do not seem to be the consequence of failure to replicate, but the whistle blowing of a co-worker, technician, or a knowledgeable scientist (Broad & Wade, 1982). An example of the latter is Sprague's exposure of the alleged fraud committed by Breuning (Holden, 1987). It must be further noted that even after failure to replicate, the intent to misrepresent the findings must be established. Failure to replicate by itself does not establish fraud.

However, it may be argued that in physical science replication readily occurs and therefore its database will not be contaminated as readily as in biobehavioral science. If nothing else, there is a loss of status due to the failure to replicate one's experiments. Fraud is therefore less common in physical science than biobehavioral science. However, there is no evidence that such replications generally occur with their potential for deterrence. Results obtained by Tangney (1987) from a questionnaire study of physical and behavioral scientists suggest that there is little difference in the reported detection of fraud in the physical and behavioral sciences. It may also be wrong to assume that overall, replication is more common in the physical than the social sciences (Hedges, 1987). Perhaps replication is more common for important experiments, but not for all experiments.

Failure to replicate is important in cleansing the database of science from unreliable and invalid data. But there remains the fundamental issue of cleansing the field of unreliable scientists, of recognizing their fraud, meting out sanctions, and setting an example for future generations of scientists. Replication by itself accomplishes none of these important aims. My experience suggests that failure to replicate an allegedly fraudulent study does not entail negative sanctions when influential figures in the field defend the alleged perpetrators of fraud. Nathan, a major figure in the field of alcoholism, then Director of the Center of Alcohol Studies, Rutgers University, states:

> When you look carefully at the series of studies on which the presumed efficacy of controlled drinking treatment was based, you quickly come to realize that only one study, the very well-known study by Mark and Linda Sobell... yielded positive data... basically only the Sobell study yielded data that strongly encouraged the view that controlled drinking treatment could work. That study, I think, was an anomaly. While there are a variety of reasons to question the data, none of them involves fraud. I know the Sobells. I know their data. They did not commit fraud, as has been claimed. However, these data are an anomaly. No one else has reported data of this kind. (Nathan, 1985, p. 172).

Rychtarik et al. (1987) failed to replicate the results of the Sobells but the results obtained by Rychtarik et al. are consistently reinterpreted to support the Sobells' outcome and controlled drinking treatments. This is ideologically driven revisionism, poor scholarship, and lack of curiosity at work. My count is that at least nine different publications have failed to properly interpret Rychtarik et al.'s (1987) study.

(2) If detected, is fraud reported? Sigma Xi (1988) published results of a survey of their active membership which included a question concerning direct knowledge of fraud on the part of a professional scientist. Nine percent agreed emphatically they had such knowledge, 10% agreed in substance, and 9% neither agreed nor disagreed. In response to the question concerning the responsibility of the scientist to expose such fraud on the part of another, 43% agreed emphatically they had such responsibility, 43% agreed in substance, and 9% neither agreed nor disagreed that they had a clear responsibility to expose fraud. Membership of Sigma Xi was listed as 115,000. We do not know the rate of return for the questionnaire or the percentage return by science field. Nevertheless, this is a rather considerable number of scientists who have knowledge of fraud. It could be in the neighborhood of 20,000 cases. Apparently there were no questions on the number of cases of fraud known by the respondent or their actions in response to their knowledge.

Tangney (1987) found that fraud is no more frequently reported by behavioral than by physical scientists. Thirty-two percent of scientists responding to her survey on a large state university campus had suspected a colleague of falsifying data and 54% of these scientists took no action. Of those who reported responding in some manner to their belief that fraud had occurred, we have no information as to the outcome of their actions. A possible sampling bias may be present, however, since a response rate of only 22% was obtained following distribution of 1100 questionnaires.

I believe that there are a number of reasons for the failure to report the occurrence of fraud: (a) The selective effects of ideology; (b) fear of retaliation and litigation; (c) the politicalization of the field promoted by balkanization. It is easier for pressure, fear of retaliation, and loss of perquisites, etc., to operate successfully in a small area of specialization where many investigators know each other personally and where the individual's professional progress and status is largely determined than in the larger discipline as a whole; (d) a drift towards permissiveness in the norms of scientific conduct is reflected in the reasons for not reporting fraud. This increased permissiveness is pervasive within academic life from lowered standards for promotion to the review of manuscripts for professional journals. It is due to many things, expanded size, rapid growth, a great deal of money, and the attraction of individuals to the field with no intrinsic or prior interest in the goals and values of science, among others. Changes in norms of conduct are intimately related to the growth of politics and ideology in biobehavioral science. It must be recognized, however, that these changes are not universal. There are still many journals that maintain rigorous criteria, and I assume that there may be departments of psychology and other disciplines that rigorously but fairly review their members, although I do not, and cannot know, this personally because of reasons of confidentiality.

(3) Finally, if fraud is detected and reported, is effective action taken? My experience is especially relevant to this last decision point. As I have tried to show in the preceding pages the forces of politics, networking of scientists energized by ideology and the threat of libel actions, real or imagined, may prevent the appropriate action at this last critical point in the idealized process of self-correction.

Presence of conflicts of interest that would interfere with the free play of self-correction also limit the ease with which fraud is uncovered and action is taken. When an institution investigates possible fraud by one of its members, it runs the risk of reporting that the alleged fraud did occur and the consequent implication that the institution is at least partially at fault. If nothing else, the institution may suffer a loss of credibility. It displayed poor judgment in hiring such a person in the first place and for being so careless as to permit the fraud to occur. Opposing institutions or professions competing for fees or funding by its members will gain an advantage by its loss of credibility. Philanthropic gifts may decline as a result of the "bad image". These are all reasons for reluctance on part of a university to report statistics of crimes occurring on its campus - or vigorously pursue alleged fraud by a member of its faculty. Pressures are therefore operating against an institution finding or reporting that one of its members or grantees committed fraud. If there are injured patients, the institution may be party to a lawsuit. An attractive solution from the point of view of an institution caught in this difficult conflict is to manifest the style but not the substance of an investigation. Conduct an investigation but omit the important first step, examination of all of the raw data in the alleged fraudulent study. Do the raw data exist, and do they permit reconstruction of the published results in the alleged fraudulent study? To accomplish these ends it may be essential to possess judicial powers, the power to subpoena the raw data, witnesses who testify under oath, and the power to grant immunity to witnesses.

Lack of judicial power by investigating committees has important implications for who will or will not be subject to a searching investigation. Instances of alleged fraud where self-correction has operated successfully characteristically involve junior research investigators or individuals on "soft money". Senior professors, individuals with a network of friends and colleagues, especially when they share a common ideology, are not as easily subject to self-correction. Senior investigators, especially those with an ideological network, have the personal and group resources to intimidate and influence the decisions of journals and professional societies, their university, institute or hospital, the institutions through which self-correction might occur or be induced to occur. If senior investigators refuse to give up their records for investigation, there is no authority other than judicial that can force them.

Appropriate action may be thwarted because there is no effective established mechanism for dealing with fraud. Government agencies will not investigate alleged fraud if government funds were not used. Not all universities have codes of conduct for faculty or procedures for providing an investigation with due process. Ironically, universities and colleges may have a code of conduct with sanctions for plagiarism committed by their students, but not for faculty who commit plagiarism or fraud. When it was pointed out to the administration of the home universities of Caddy and Perkins that allegations had been made that they committed fraud, their administrations essentially did nothing. The president of one university said it was none of her business. A regulation has since been introduced requiring institutions administering federal research grants to provide assurance of the existence of established procedures for investigating fraud. This requirement involves an inherent conflict of interest, as previously noted. Courses in ethics in science are also being introduced in universities as the result of requirements for receiving and administering research training grants. Effects of such requirements remain to be determined, not an easy matter.

Background factors contributing to a change in normative values

A self-fulfilling prophecy may operate to promote fraud in science. A scientist's implicit understanding that difficulties exist in the self-correction process will tend to promote fraud, because such an understanding tends to vitiate the inhibitory potential of punishment. If the potential perpetrator believes that fraud is unlikely to be detected, if detected nothing will be said about it, if brought to the attention of some official body there will be little if any punishment, then the likelihood of fraud is increased. Misconduct will cost nothing but may reap great benefits in academic advances, grant awards, and enhanced status within the profession, university or research facility.

I am in basic agreement with Merton (1968) that the internalized norms of science, an implicit ethical code of conduct, influences the occurrence of fraud in psychology and science in general. However, these norms have drifted from what Merton believed them to be when he wrote on self-correction in science. This has happened, in part, because the social mores and norms of acceptable behavior in large segments of middle class society have drifted and scientists are part of that society. Some evidence for shifts in values stems from studies of national representative samples using the Rokeach Value Survey (Rokeach & Ball-Rokeach, 1989). Samples obtained between 1968 - 1981 indicate that there has been a shift away from social values towards personal values. There has been a decline in the importance of equality accompanied by the continued high priority of personal freedom. There is a relative increased emphasis upon the pursuit of self-centered goals rather than goals of equality and justice. Shifts in goals and attendant standards of conduct of the above sort are the kind that would promote the changes in standards of conduct in research and academic pursuits that are under consideration here. Why societal norms generally have shifted is a difficult multidetermined problem. One important factor I believe is the breakdown of the influence of the extended family with the great increase in mobility that followed Word War II. The villain is not the loss of religion but the airplane and automobile. Ease of travel has meant the dispersing of the extended family and the norms for conduct that the extended family can more readily reinforce and maintain than the single parent family or the isolated couple. Declining norms, accepted and reinforced standards of behavior, are responsible for the decay in morality in our society including the society of scientists.

Alcoholics Anonymous and other self-help groups provide a kind of extended family and concomitant norms, the new way of life, that Fingarette (1988b) emphasizes as necesssary for improvement in the heavy drinker's existence. Alcoholics have to substitute one way of life for another. It is remarkable that Fingarette never recognizes that the very sort of thing that he asserts is necessary for changing a problem drinker or alcoholic is the sort of program implemented by the AA fellowship.

Increase in perquisites

Some of the developments within the bio-behavioral sciences conducive to promoting a decline in normative standards and therefore fraud need to be noted. One such development is the enormous increase in funding and perquisites in science and the consequent increase in temptation and the opportunity for corruption. To a great extent scientists are now business people with the same interests, needs, attitudes, and temptations as the market place. There are many and relatively handsome direct and indirect rewards in bio-behavioral science. Payoffs for fraud which produces seemingly important research results are many. Not the least important is the successful funding of research grants, attendant summer salaries and facilitation of progress up the academic ladder. Rewards may also take the form of invitations to conferences, symposia, and workshops worldwide. These kinds of meetings have proliferated in part as the result of laws requiring continuing education to maintain professional licensure. Such workshops offered for clinical psychologists are dominated by behavior therapists. A recent law in California requiring a course in alcoholism and other drug use for licensure as a psychologist has further increased the number of workshops given by behavior therapists emphasizing "harm reduction" approaches to treatment. Government and industry funding are also available for conferences which often result in edited books that are not carefully refereed. Contributors have free rein for the expression of personal bias, unsubstantiated claims and careless scholarship. They add to the size of one's vita. Minor variations in the same material can be published repeatedly as the consequence of nondiscriminating edited books.

There are also more modest invitations for colloquia presentations and workshops, many for a fee. Even in the absence of fees, they are pleasant experiences, build social and professional networks, and enhance one's vita, thereby facilitating merit increases and promotions. Mutual invitations and networking help every one involved and provide a source of mutual references when institutions require outside evaluations for promotions, or references are needed when a new job is in the offing. Networking is facilitated by the balkanization of psychology. Increasing specialization spawns large numbers of discrete areas of specialization where all prominent investigators know each other. Each speciality wishes to establish its own journal and editorial board, society, or division, with its own officials, within the parent body such as the American Psychological Association and its more than 50 divisions. Or, because of disenchantment with the constituency and goals of the parent body, a group of scientists or practitioners with a common interest form their own independent society.

There is a decrease in the likelihood of critically reviewing or alleging fraud against a member of your own ingroup for several obvious reasons. One is the role of ideology. It protects ingroup members from criticism, since criticism of another member is a criticism of oneself. Furthermore, a criticism or attack upon a member of a small group with a common ideology may lead to retaliation by that person or their colleagues and friends. Your grant or manuscript will be reviewed by them some day. It is a small step from hesitating to criticize a colleague's poor experimental design to ignoring their fabrication of results. In either case, the movement as a whole is hurt if you publically blow the whistle. Since the whistle blower, not the perpetrator, is often accused of damaging the image of the group as a whole, there is the real possibility of being ostracized from the group with the consequent loss of perquisites. There will be no more invitations to international symposia. It will be more difficult to obtain grants and to publish articles in the inner circle of journals. Promotion will become more difficult. These are powerful forces inhibiting the detection or reporting of fraud in a specialized research area.

Some of the force promoting the ill-effects of networking, the fear of whistle blowing, and the blunting of critical evaluation in general, stems from the centralized source of research funding in the federal government. Concentrating funding in the Public Health Service and the National Science Foundation promotes the fear of alienating colleagues at other institutions who may sit in review of one's grant proposals, journal articles, and attempts to organize attractive conferences. This concentration of power and its unfortunate consequences need to be addressed.

Lowered standards of excellence

Fraud is promoted when the graduate student and young scientist see that style is more important than substance, that power and politics count for more than the truth or at least weigh heavily in the advancement of their career. It may often be more important who you know than what you know.

One of the many factors responsible for normative drift, unfortunately, is the democratization of academic life. An "adaptation level" or lowest common denominator effect is at work. When everyone votes on the promotion or merit increase of everyone else, few individuals want high standards because these same standards will be applied against them in the future.

The lowest common denominator may also be at work, within limits, in journal reviews, especially when considering the papers of fellow ideologues. This is not to say that the lowest common denominator effect is invariable. It is to say that peer review in some areas has deteriorated, in part because of the balkanization of psychology and related disciplines. There are large numbers of small new specialized journals and areas of specialization often where editors and reviewers who have risen to positions of power and influence are themselves not truly distinguished. Their standards of excellence tend to match their lesser accomplishments. One does not reject work that is better than one's own. Science and scholarship are necessarily elitist, but the proliferation of small societies and journals has permitted the rise to positions of influence of individuals less than excellent. Standards of excellence are lowered as a consequence. Coupled with ideology, scientists in editorial positions are more likely to do nothing in the face of fraud. I do not claim that these changes characterize all science, since I cannot personally judge all areas of science. It is true of certain areas of psychology and our primary concern here, alcohol studies, especially behavior therapists' alcohol studies .

Publish or perish: A different interpretation

Publish or perish may promote fraud but not for the reasons usually given by the science establishment spokespersons or interpreters. It is not the pressure to publish many articles that induces fraud as much as the cynicism that accompanies publishing so much. It has become apparent that quantity rather that quality is important, because few read other scientists' articles critically. Young scientists - or old - see that only the numbers count because standards of excellence have deteriorated. To have a high standard of excellence requires a value judgment of what is good or bad. Faculty do not wish to make such judgments for a number of reasons. The chilling effect of libel is one. Another is that it takes too much time to read articles carefully and critically. A third reason is networking and ideology. One does not attack a fellow ideologue for having a bad theory, model, orientation, or research design. It is the same as attacking one's self, since you share that theory, model or orientation. Criticisms by individuals outside the fold are construed as an indirect attack upon oneself and can be reasonably discounted as motivated by ideology, dyspepsia or some other irrelevant reason.

There is little collegial feeling or identity with department colleagues in a different area of specialization. One's identity and progress up the academic ranks is dependent to a great extent on the specialized area that extends beyond the department. Furthermore, it may be easier to publish many pedestrian papers than a small number of excellent ones. Papers in one's bibliography are too often merely counted for a promotion or faculty evaluation, not read with care. Differences in quality cannot readily be discerned, therefore there is no need to strive for high quality. If we are not concerned about excellence and standards of excellence, it is one further step - a matter of degree - to excuse fraud. It is only a matter of degree to pass from slipshod work and careless errors that go unnoticed or disregarded in the evaluation process to intentional misrepresentation. The latter is also likely to be accepted, and is therefore acceptable, in the reasoning of the scientist contemplating or completing fraud. If fraud furthers the ends of an ideology, if a greater good is being served, then it is even more likely to be condoned.

Perpetrators of fraud may well reason that they will not be caught because the paper containing fraudulent material will not be read in the necessary detail. There are some exceptions, as suggested by the investigation of Slutsky in the University of California, San Diego Medical School probe of alleged fraud (Engler, Covell, Friedman, Kitcher, & Peters, 1987).

WHAT IS TO BE DONE?

Values in science

Multidetermined and complex phenomena such as fraud, ideology masquerading as empirical issues, and inadequacies in the process of self-correction have no one solution, no more than does the etiology of alcoholism. Several approaches to these problems come to mind. Two are intrinsic to the process of science and education, concerned with influencing character, and three are extrinsic policy recommendations.

(1) There is a parallel between the cohesive family and its characteristics which minimize problems of antisocial behavior and promote prosocial behaviors by its members and the well functioning laboratory. Decreasing the incidence of fraud in science and exposing it when discovered are problems analogous to the general problem of fostering moral development in children. Research in the latter area (Damon, 1988) suggests practices that may reduce the incidence of fraud in science and increase the likelihood of exposing it when discovered. Work together, do things together, establish an identity and esprit de corp. Respect the dignity of the individual, rationally discuss normative conduct and the values of science and ethics and offer support to the individual when needed. Read about and discuss the problem of fraud in science (e.g., Broad & Wade, 1982). A detailed study of "righteous Christians", those people who risked their lives to save Jews during the holocaust as compared to bystanders, showed one or more characteristics and family experiences differentiating the two groups (Oliner & Oliner, 1988). Among the relatively independent differentiating factors were: (a) a strong and cohesive family experience where the family of origin emphasized caring and dependability, and (b) a sense of social commitment. Although the recommendations for inculcating

prosocial behavior summarized by Damon (1988) and others (e.g., Vitz, 1990) may help, there will remain persistent differences among individuals and their norms when they enter a laboratory. These may be too well established to change in some cases. Not all students work in a large laboratory, but all students may be influenced by the moral tone, the nobility of the task confronting psychology. It is possible to return to the depiction of science in general and psychology in particular as it was at the turn of the century, as a profession with a noble mission. Its mission was - and still is - the application of scientific methods to the most complex and important problems on earth: brain-behavior-environment interactions. As noted by various authors in the field of moral development (e.g., Damon, 1988; Vitz, 1990), morality cannot be avoided in the classroom and the laboratory. The problem is to effectively utilize it to foster prosocial behavior in general and in particular moral behavior in accord with the idealized norms of science and society.

(2) Require, or at least strongly encourage, students to take courses in ethics and philosophy taught by the philosophy department, not by psychologists or other scientists, so that students may learn and discuss the various ethical principles that have been proposed and debated over time. Demand a liberal arts education of science students. We need to educate well rounded scientists with knowledge of the values of different civilizations, especially western, not narrow technicians. A PhD should be an honor bestowed upon a student for creative scholarship, not for narrow technical vocational accomplishments. Oscar Wilde's description of a cynic is as apt - or more so - a description of the kind of person we all too often turn loose with a PhD, "One who knows the price of everything and the value of nothing". I suspect that such individuals are at risk for committing fraud, whether in science, business, government, or religion.

(3) There must be a more explicit emphasis upon quality of research rather than quantity. University faculty and administrations must take the initiative in changing criteria for promotion. Each candidate should be asked to indicate their three best publications. These should be read and considered by all members of a review committee and by all faculty who vote. The quality, originality, and significance or importance of the research should be evaluated and the judgment based upon these for explicitly stated reasons. In like fashion qualifications of the principal investigator of a grant proposal should be evaluated in terms of their three best publications not merely the number of publications.

(4) Congressional action is needed to authorize a special prosecutor within the Attorney General's Office that would be responsible for the investigation of fraud in science. They would have judicial powers and the authority to investigate fraud whether or not it has involved government funds. Present federal institutions do not examine fraud per se. They examine the misuse of government funds. The Alcohol Drug and Mental Health Administration (ADAMHA) refused to investigate allegations of misconduct on the part of Caddy et al. because they conducted their research without support from government funds. Their alleged misconduct therefore was not the concern of ADAMHA. Safeguards are essential to protect the individual accused and to provide for due process. Intrusion by the Government should be kept to a minimum. Safeguards must also be in place to protect the whistleblower. These essentially do not exist. Much needs to be done in this area.

(5) A pervasive factor determining the drift in norms is the enormous concentration of funding and concomitant power in federal agencies and their review boards. Scientists do not criticize each other, or blow the whistle, when each may sit in judgment of the other. Conversely, the "old boy network" promotes approval of each other's grant proposals regardless of quality or need. Power must be dispersed. Government funding for research, at least in part, should be distributed in lump sums to the individual universities, research institutes and research hospitals. Research committees appointed by the institutions' academic senate or comparable body should disperse the funds to individual faculty investigators. Every active investigator should receive a basic grant necessary to conduct his or her research which would be renewable as long as research activity is evidenced. If a larger than normal grant is awarded, it is under extraordinary circumstances following careful review by the research committee constituted by diverse members of the university community.

(6) Alcoholism treatment trials must follow the lead of NIMH in reviewing psychiatric clinical studies (Marshall, 1999). Every alcohol efficacy study planning to employ, study, or train, controlled drinking or harm reduction for alcohol misuse problems must be reviewed by a panel that includes a bioethicist and a neuroscientist. The panel must ensure that such studies obtain adequate informed consent from individuals who are not suffering from diminished capacity to provide such consent. It is essential that procedures are initiated to ensure that such studies are conducted according to current ethical guidelines and are in accord with the first principle of care giving: nonmaleficence, do no harm.

(7) At the present time Human Subject Protection Committees or Institutional Review Boards (IRBs) are largely a facade. As long as they do not actually observe the conduct of research at random unannounced times, such committees serve only to control the behavior of compliant ethical investigators. It is a simple matter to verbally comply with all the wishes, rules, and regulations in the written protocol and form of the informed consent. It is another matter to ensure that these are all adopted in the conduct of the research. I could readily agree to have a third-party disinterested observer at each subjects' informed consent and so state in my research protocol submitted to my IRB. It would be impossible for the IRB to know that I had not adhered to the procedure in practice - unless there was a legal action or a complaint brought to the IRB and it was discovered in the discovery phase of a trial or under cross examination that no such procedure was employed.

To be effective in practice, IRBs need a staff of investigators so that one could appear without warning at the time subjects are initiated into a research protocol and given their informed consent to read and sign. An apparent problem with such a procedure is that it would be very expensive. A possible solution is to have the costs of oversight become a regular budget item in grant proposals to the federal government. This is reasonable since the Federal Government is delegating its responsibility in ethics oversight to the university or other research institution. They should not delegate this responsibility without assuming the burden of its costs.

Observers working for IRBs should be drawn from a pool of investigators composed of graduate students in sciences. Students from a department other than the one in which the principal investigator is a member would be selected by the IRB to monitor a particular study. There would be a determination that neither the student nor their advisor is a collaborator or associate of the principal investigator of the project reviewed. Finally, and not to be ignored, the proposed procedure provides a source of financial support for graduate students as well as training in research ethics and a heightened sensitivity to ethical concerns.

Field studies such as the Sobells' follow-up ought to be supervised by IRBs as well as laboratory studies. Names of people interviewed every week are submitted to the IRB with the day and time of the interview. A graduate student working for the IRB randomly selects subjects and calls to confirm the occurrence of an interview corresponding to the one described in the protocol and informed consent form.

Supervision and oversight of IRBs must be placed in the hands of an independent commission. An institute of NIH cannot oversee an IRB review of one of its grantees. An inherent conflict of interest is present. Errors in judgment on the part of an IRB resulting in harm to research subjects is ultimately the responsibility of the NIH institute. If fraud or negligence has occurred, the institute must find itself in part guilty. A safer course is to find no evidence of wrong doing. Supervision of local IRBs must be in the hands of an independent commission rather than the Department of Health and Human Services to avoid any conflict of interest. Katz (1997) has urged such an arrangement for many years.

The first two recommendations, if they would have any influence, are more likely to strengthen the resolve of the potential whistle blower than to dissuade or deter the kind of individual who engages in repeated intentional misrepresentations, the more serious kind of scientific misconduct. Consciousness raising, the discussion of fraud in science and the problems it produces should be a common practice in classrooms and laboratories. Such discussions cannot hurt, and they may produce a change in attitudes that in the long run may serve to deter fraud. If nothing else, such discussions provide the student with a more realistic view of the practice of science than the one obtained in the usual textbook or journal article.

Conclusion

I have learned three lessons as a result of my "ethnographic " experience in the field of alcohol studies:

(1) Truth and the trust that is based on it are essential for a healthy, efficient, and productive society of scientists and society at large. Suppression of dissent, discussion, and controversy is a cancer in the body of behavioral science applied to alcohol studies - as well as society at large.

(2) Freud was right in that there is a psychopathology of every- day life. I have seen it in action.

(3) Behavior of the revisionists is part of a larger syndrome of a troubled society. Their success is possible because a community of individuals, primarily behavior therapists along with pusillanimous publishers, editors, and bureaucrats, aided and abetted them while "otherwise good people" stood by and did nothing.

Science is a social process. It involves people, and therefore necessarily involves values. "Facts", fundamental items of information exchanged, are born, survive, and are transmitted, as a function of the values scientists bring to the profession and those they acquire during their apprenticeship and course of their lives as members of the profession. To promote this process we ought to heed the advice of Brentano (1874/1973):

In science, just as in politics, it is difficult to reach agreement without conflict, but in scientific disputes we should not proceed in such a way as to seek the triumph of this or that investigator, but only the triumph of truth. The driving force behind these battles ought not to be ambition, but the longing for a common subordination to truth, which is one and indivisible. For this reason, just as I have proceeded without restraint to refute and discard the opinions of others whenever they seemed to be erroneous, so I will readily and gratefully welcome any correction of my views which might be suggested to me. (p.xvi).

Finally, there is one thing we can all do, to cite an old Jewish saying: "The way to reform society is to begin by making an honest man of yourself, thereby guaranteeing that there will be one less rascal in the world".

REFERENCES

Abel, E. L. (1984). *Fetal alcohol syndrome and fetal alcohol effects.* New York: Plenum.

Abelson, P. H. (1983). Letter from editor. *Science, 220,* 555-556.

Ader, R. (Ed.) (1981). *Psychoneuroimmunology.* New York: Academic Press.

Adinoff, B., O'Neill, H. K., & Ballenger, J. C. (1995). Alcohol withdrawal and limbic kindling. *The American Journal on Addictions, 4,* 5-17.

Agartz, I., Momenan, R., Rawlings, R. R., Kerich, M. J., & Hommer, D. W. (1999). Hippocampal volume in patients with alcohol dependence. *Archives of General Psychiatry, 56,* 356-363.

Akil, H. D., Mayer, D. J., & Liebeskind, J. C. (1976). Antagonism of stimulation-produced analgesia by naloxone, a narcotic antagonist. *Science, 191,* 961-963.

Alcohol and Health (1997). Ninth Special Report to the U. S. Congress. Washington, DC: U. S. Department of Health and Human Services.

Allport, G. W. (1937). *Personality.* New York: Henry Holt.

American Psychiatric Association. (1994). *Diagnostic and statistical manual of mental disorders* (4th ed.). Washington, DC: Author.

Ames, G. M., & Janes, C. (1992). A cultural approach to conceptualizing alcohol and the workplace. *Alcohol Health & Research World, 16,* 112-119.

Annis, H. M. (1986). Is in-patient rehabilitation of the alcoholic cost-effective? Con position. *Advances in Alcohol and Substance Abuse,5,* 175-190.

Anokhin, P. K. (1965). The role of the orienting exploratory reaction in the formation of the conditioned reflex. In L. G. Voronin, A. N. Leontiev, A. R. Luria, E. N. Sokolov, & O. S. Vinogradova (Eds.), *Orienting reflex and exploratory behavior* (pp. 3-16). Washington, DC: American Institute of Biological Sciences.

Anthenelli, R. M., Smith, T. L., Irwin, M. R., & Schuckit, M. A. (1994). A comparative study of criteria for subgrouping alcoholics: The primary/secondary diagnostic scheme versus variations of the Type 1/Type 2 criteria. *American Journal of Psychiatry, 151,* 1468-1474.

Arendt, T. (1993). The cholinergic deafferentation of the cerebral cortex induced by chronic consumption of alcohol: Reversal by cholinergic drugs and transplantation. In W. A. Hunt & S. J. Nixon (Eds.), *Alcohol-induced brain damage* (pp. 431-460). NIAAA Research Monograph No. 22. NIH Publication No. 93-3549. Rockville, MD: U.S. Department of Health and Human Services.

Armor, D. J., Polich, J. M., & Stambul, H. B. (1976). *Alcoholism and treatment.* Report 1739 NIAAA. Santa Monica, CA: Rand Corporation.

Armor, D. J. Polich, J. M., & Stambul, H. B. (1978). *Alcoholism and treatment.* New York: Wiley.

Babor, T. F., Hofmann, M., DelBoca, F. K., Hesselbrock, V., Meyer, R. E., Dolinsky, Z. S., Rounsaville, B. (1992). Types of alcoholics, I: evidence for an empirically derived typology based on indicators of vulnerability and severity. *Archives of General Psychiatry, 49,* 614-619.

Baer, J. S., Barr, H. M., Bookstein, F. L., Sampson, P. D., & Streissguth, A. P. (1998). Prenatal alcohol exposure and family history of alcoholism in the etiology of adolescent alcohol problems. *Journal of Studies on Alcohol, 59,* 533-543.

Baker, T. (1989). An open letter to Journal readers. *Journal of Studies on Alcohol, 50,* 481-483.

Ballenger, J. C., & Post, R. M. (1978). Kindling as a model for alcohol withdrawal syndromes. *British Journal of Psychiatry, 133,* 1-14.

Banks, W. A., & Kastin, A. J. In S. Zakhari (Ed.), *Alcohol and the endocrine system* (pp. 401-411). NIAAA Research Monograph No. 22. NIH Publication No. 93-3549. Rockville, MD: U. S. Department of Health and Human Services.

Barlow, D. H. (1993). Series Editor's Note. In M. B. Sobell, & L. C. Sobell, *Problem drinkers: Guided self-change treatment.* New York: Guilford.

Barlow, D. H., & Durand, V. M. (1995). *Abnormal psychology: An integrative approach.* Pacific Grove, CA: Brooks/Cole.

Barlow, D. H., Bellack, A.S., Buchwald, A. M., Garfield, S. L., Hartmann, D. P., Herman, C. P., Hersen, M., Miller, P. M., Rachman, S., & Wolpe, J. (1983). Alcoholism studies (Letter to the editor). *Science, 220,* 555.

Barr, C. E., Mednick, S. A., & Munk-Jorgensen, P. (1990). Exposure to influenza epidemics during gestation and adult schizophrenia. *Archives of General Psychiatry, 47,* 869-874.

Bauer, L. O. (1994). Electroencephalographic and autonomic predictors of relapse in alcohol-dependent patients. *Alcoholism: Clinical and Experimental Research, 18,* 755-760.

Baumeister, R. F., Heatherton, T. F., & Tice, D. M. (1994). *Losing control: How and why people fail at self-regulation.* San Diego, CA: Academic Press.

356

Baxter, L. R., Schwartz, J. M., Bergman, K. S., Szuba, M. P., Guze, B. H., Mazziotta, J. C., Alazraki, A., Selin, C. E., Ferng, H-K., Munford, P., & Phelps, M. E. (1992). Caudate glucose metabolic rate changes with both drug and behavior therapy for obsessive-compulsive disorder. *Archives of General Psychiatry, 49,* 681-689.

Beauchamp, T.L. & Waters,L. (Eds.) (1982). *Contemporary issues in bioethics.* 2nd. ed. Belmont, CA: Wadsworth.

Beauchamp, T. L., Faden, R. R., Wallace, R. J., Jr., & Walter, L.(1982). *Ethical issues in social science research.* Baltimore, MD: The Johns Hopkins University Press.

Begleiter, H. (Ed.) (1980). *Biological effects of alcohol.* New York: Plenum.

Begleiter, H., & Kissin, B. (Eds.) (1995). *The genetics of alcoholism.* New York: Oxford University Press.

Begleiter, H., & Kissin, B. (Eds.) (1996). *The pharmacology of alcohol and alcohol dependence.* New York: Oxford University Press.

Begleiter, H., Porjesz, B., Bihari, B., & Kissin, B. (1984). Event-related brain potentials in boys at risk for alcoholism. *Science, 225,* 1493-1496.

Bell, R. G. (1970). *Escape from addiction.* New York: McGraw-Hill.

Belluzzi, J. D., & Stein, L. (1977). Enkephalin may mediate euphoria and drive-reduction reward. *Nature, 266,* 556-558.

Benjamin, J., Li, L., Patterson, C., Greenberg, B. D., Murphy, D. L., & Hamer, D. H. (1996). Population and familial association between the D4 dopamine receptor gene and measures of novelty seeking. *Nature Genetics, 12,* 81-84.

Bennett, L. A., Wolin, S. J., Reiss, D., & Teitelbaum, M. A. (1987). Couples at risk for transmission of alcoholism: Protective influence. *Family Process, 26,* 111-129.

Bernhardt, P. C. (1997). Influences of serotonin and testosterone in aggression and dominance: Convergence with social psychology. *Current Directions in Psychological Science, 6,* 44-48.

Beresford, T. P. (1991). The nosology of alcoholism research. *Alcohol Health and Research World, 15,* 260-265.

Berg, G., Laberg, J. C., Skutle, A., & Öhman, A. (1981). Instructed versus pharmacological effects of alcohol in alcoholics and social drinkers. *Behaviour Research and Therapy, 19,* 55-66.

Bergmann, G. (1954). *The metaphysics of logical positivism.* New York: Longmans, Green.

Berman, K. F., Illowsky, B. P., & Weinberger, D. R. (1988). Physiological dysfunction of dorsolateral prefrontal cortex in schizophrenia. IV. Further evidence for regional and behavioral specificity. *Archives of General Psychiatry, 45,* 616-622.

Bertiere, M. C., Sy, T. M., Baigts, F., Mandenoff, A., & Apfelbaum, M. Stress and sucrose hyperphagia: Role of endogenous opiates. *Pharmacology Biochemsitry & Behavior, 20,* 675-679.

Blakiston's Gould Medical Dictionary. 4th ed. (1970). New York: McGraw-Hill.

Blass, E., Fitzgerald, E., & Kehoe, P. (1987). Interactions between sucrose, pain and isolation distress. *Pharmacology Biochemistry & Behavior, 26,* 483-489.

Blum, K. (with Payne, J. E.) (1991). *Alcohol and the addictive brain.* New York: The Free Press.

Blum, K., Futterman, S., Wallace, J. E., & Schwertner, H. A. (1977). Naloxone-induced inhibition of ethanol dependence in mice. *Nature, 265,* 49-51.

Blum, K., Noble, E. P., Sheridan, P. J., Montgomery, A., Ritchie, T., Jagadeeswaran, P., Nogami, H., Briggs, A. H., & Cohn, J. B. (1990). Allelic association of human dopamine D2 receptor gene in alcoholism. *Journal of the American Medical Associaiton, 263,* 2055-2060.

Blume, S. (1977). The "Rand Report": Some comments and a response. *Journal of Studies on Alcohol, 38,* 163-168.

Boffey, P. M. (1982, June 28). Alcoholism study under new attack. *The New York Times,* p. A12.

Bohman, M., Sogvardsson S., & Cloninger, R. (1981). Maternal inheritance of alcohol abuse: Cross-fostering analysis of adopted women. *Archives of General Psychiatry, 38,* 965-969.

Born, J., Hitzler, V., Pietrowsky, R., Pauschinger, P., Fehm, H. L. (1988). Influences of cortisol on auditory evoked potentials (AEPS) and mood in humans. *Neuropsychobiology, 20,* 145-151.

Bowlby, J. (1982). *Attachment and loss. Vol. 1. Attachment.* 2nd ed. New York: Basic Books.

Bracha, H. S., Torrey, E. F., Gottesman, I. I., Bigelow, L. B., & Cunniff, C. (1992). Second-trimester markers of fetal size in schizophrenia: A study of monozygotic twins. *American Journal of Psychiatry, 149,* 1355-1361.

Brady, J. V. (1972). Emotion revisited. In J. V. Brady & W. J. H. Nauta (Eds.), *Principles, practices, and positions in neuropsychiatric research* (pp. 363-384). Oxford: Pergamon.

Brecher, E. M. (1972). *Licit & illicit drugs.* Boston: Little, Brown.

Goddard, G. V., McIntyre, D. C., & Leech, C. K. (1969). A permanent change in brain function resulting from daily electrical stimulation. *Experimental Neurology, 25,* 295-330.

Gold, M. S. (1994). Neurobiology of addiction and recovery: The brain, the drive for the drug, and the 12-step fellowship. *Journal of Substance Abuse Treatment, 11,* 93-97.

Gold, M. S., & Miller, N. S. (1992). Seeking drugs/alcohol and avoiding withdrawal: The neuroanatomy of drive states and withdrawal. *Psychiatric Annals, 22,* 430-435.

Goldman, D., & Bergen, A. (1998). General and specific inheritance of substance abuse and alcoholism. *Archives of General Psychiatry, 55,* 964-965.

Goldman, M. S. (1983). Cognitive impairment in chronic alcoholics. *American Psychologist, 38,* 1045-1054.

Goldman, M. S., Brown, S. A., & Christiansen, B. A. (1987). Expectancy theory: Thinking about drinking. In H. T. Blane & K. E. Leonard (Eds.), *Psychological theories of drinking and alcoholism* (pp. 181-226). New York: Guilford.

Goldstein, A. (1976). Opioid peptides (endorphins) in pituitary and brain. *Science, 193,* 1081-1086.

Goldstein, M.J., Baker, B.L., & Jamison, K.R. (1986). *Abnormal psychology.* 2nd. ed. Boston, MA: Little, Brown.

Goodwin, D. W., Schulsinger, F., Hermansen, J., Guze, S. B., & Winokur, G. (1973). Alcohol problems in adoptees raised apart from alcoholic biological parents. *Archives of General Psychiatry, 28,* 238-243.

Goodwin, D. W., Schulsinger, F., Knop, J., Mednick, S., & Guze, S. B. (1977a). Alcoholism and depression in adopted-out daughters of alcoholics. *Archives of General Psychiatry, 34,* 751-755.

Goodwin, D. W., Schulsinger, F., Knop, J., Mednick, S., & Guze, S. B. (1977b). Psychopathology in adopted and nonadopted daughters of alcoholics. *Archives of General Psychiatry, 34,* 1005-1009.

Goodwin, D. W., Schulsinger, F., Møller, N., Hermansen, L., Winokur, G., & Guze, S. B. (1974). Drinking problems in adopted and nonadopted sons of alcoholics. *Archives of General Psychiatry, 31,* 164-169.

Gordon, J. P. & Barrett, K. (1993). The codependency movement: Issues of context and differentiation. In J. S. Baer, G. A. Marlatt, & R. J. McMahon (Eds.), *Addictive behaviors across the life span.* Newbury Park, CA: Sage.

Gorski, T. T., & Miller, M. (1986). *Staying sober: A guide for relapse prevention.* Independence, MO: Herald House/Independence.

Gottlieb, G. (1997). *Synthesizing nature-nurture: Prenatal roots of instinctive behavior.* Mahwah, NJ: Erlbaum.

Gottlieb, G. (1998). Normally occurring environmental and behavioral influences on gene activity: From central dogma to probabilistic epigenesis. *Psychological Review, 105,* 792-802.

Gough, H. G. (1960). Theory and measurement of socialization. *Journal of Consulting Psychology, 24,* 23-30.

Gove, W. R. (Ed.) (1980). *The labelling of deviance.* 2nd ed. Beverly Hills, CA: Sage.

Graber, R. A., & Miller, W.R. (1988). Abstinence or controlled drinking goals for problem drinkers: A randomized clinical trial. *Psychology of Addictive Behaviors, 2,* 20-33.

Grahame, N. J., Low, M. J., & Cunningham, C. L. (1998). Intravenous self-administration of ethanol in ß-endorphin-deficient mice. *Alcoholism: Clinical and Experimental Research, 22,* 1093-1098.

Grant, B.F. Toward an alcohol treatment model: A comparison of treated and untreated respondents with DSM-IV alcohol use disorders in the general population. *Alcoholism: Clinical and Experimental Research, 20,* 372-378.

Grant, B.F., Harford, T.C., Dawson, D.A., Chou, P., Dufour, M., & Pickering, R. (1994). Prevalence of DSM-IV alcohol abuse and dependence. *Alcohol Health & Research World, 18,* 243-248.

Greenfield, T. K., & Rogers, J. D. (1999). Who drinks most of the alcohol in the U.S.? The policy implications. *Journal of Studies on Alcohol, 60,* 78-89.

Greenough, W. T. (1977). Experiential modification of the developing brain. In I. L. Janis (Ed.) *Current trends in psychology* (pp. 82-90). Los Altos, CA: William Kaufman.

Griesler, P. C., & Kandel, D. B. (1998). The impact of maternal drinking during and after pregnancy on the drinking of adolescent offspring. *Journal of Studies on Alcohol, 59,* 292-304.

Grisso, T., & Appelbaum, P. S. (1998). *Assessing competence to consent to treatment.* New York: Oxford University Press.

Gruenewald, P. J. (1991). Loss of control drinking among first offender drunk drivers. *Alcoholism: Clinical and Experimental Research, 15,* 634-639.

Gruenewald, P. J., Stewart, K., & Klitzner, M. (1990). Alcohol use and the appearance of alcohol problems among first offender drunk drivers. *British Journal of Addiction, 85,* 107-117.

362

Guilford, J. P. (1936). *Psychometric methods*. New York: McGraw-Hill.

Gustavson, G. R., Garcia, J., Hankins, W. G., & Rusiniak, K. W. (1974). Coyote predation control by aversive conditioning. *Science, 183,* 581-583.

Hall, S. M., Havassy, B. A., & Wasserman, D. A.(1990). Commitment to abstinence and acute stress in relapse to alcohol, opiates, and nicotine. *Journal of Consulting and Clinical Psychology, 58,* 175-181.

Hall, S. M., Havassy, B. E., & Wasserman, D. A. (1991). Effects of commitment to abstinence, positive moods, stress, and coping on relapse to cocaine. *Journal of Consulting and Clinical Psycholology, 59,* 526-532.

Harlow, H. (1958). The nature of love. *American Psychologist, 13,* 673-685.

Harper, C. G., & Kril, J. J. (1990). Neuropathology of alcoholism. *Alcohol & Alcoholism, 25,* 207-216.

Harper, C., Kril, J., & Daly, J. (1987). Are we drinking our neurones away? *British Medical Journal, 294,* 534-536.

Harris, B. (1979). Whatever happened to little Albert? *American Psychologist, 344,* 151-160.

Harris, K. B., & Miller,W. R. (1990). Behavioral self-control training for problem drinkers: Components of efficacy. *Psychology of Addictive Behaviors, 4,* 82-90.

Harrison, A. H., Hoffmann, N. G., & Streed, S. G. (1991). In N. S. Miller (Ed.), *Comprehensive handbook of drug and alcohol addiction* (pp. 1163-1197). New York: Marcel Dekker.

Hasin, D., & Paykin, A. (1998). DSM-IV alcohol abuse: Investigation in a sample of at-risk drinkers in the community. *Journal of Studies on Alcohol, 60,* 181-187.

Hasin, D. S., Grant, B., & Endicott, J. (1990). The natural history of alcohol abuse: Implications for definitions of alcohol use disorders. *American Journal of Psychiatry, 147,* 1537-1541.

Hasin, D., Rossem, R. V., McCloud, S., & Endicott, J. (1997). Alcohol dependence and abuse diagnoses: Validity in community sample heavy drinkers. *Alcoholism: Clinical and Experimental Research, 21,* 213-219.

Heath, A. C. (1995). Genetic influences on drinking behavior in humans. In H. Begleiter & B. Kissin (Eds.), *The genetics of alcoholism* (pp. 82-121). New York: Oxford University Press.

Heather, B. B. (1980). The crisis in the treatment of alcohol abuse. In J. S. Madden, R. Walker, & W. H., Kenyon (Eds.), *Aspects of alcohol and drug dependence* (pp. 252-259). Kent, England: Pitman.

Heather, N. (1989). Psychology and brief interventions. *British Journal of Addiction, 84,* 357-370.

Heather, N., & Robertson, I. (1983). *Controlled drinking* (rev. ed.). London: Methuen.

Heather, N., & Tebbutt, J. (1989). Definitions of non-abstinent and abstinent categories in alcoholism treatment outcome classifications: a review and proposal. *Drug and Alcohol Dependence, 24,* 83-93.

Heather, N., Booth, P., & Luce, A. (1998). Impaired control scale: cross-validation and relationships with treatment outcome. *Addiction, 93,* 761-771.

Heather, N., Tebbutt, J. S., Mattick, R. P., & Azmir, R. (1993). Development of a scale for measuring impaired control over alcohol consumption: a preliminary report. *Journal of Studies on Alcohol, 54,* 700-709.

Hedges, L. V. (1987). How hard is hard science, how soft is soft science? The empirical cumulation of research. *American Psychologist, 42,* 443-455.

Helzer, J. E., & Canino, G. J. (1992). *Alcoholism in North America, Europe, and Asia.* New York: Oxford University Press.

Helzer, J. E., Robins, L. N., Croughan, J. L., & Weiner, A. (1981). Renard diagnostic interview: Its reliability and validity with physicians and lay interviewers. *Archives of General Psychiatry, 38,* 393-398.

Hemmingsson, T., & Lundberg, I. (1998). Work control, work demands, and work social support in relation to alcoholism among young men. *Alcoholism: Clinical and Experimental Research, 22,* 921-927.

Herman, B. H., & Panksepp, J. (1978). Effects of morphine and naloxone on separation distress and approach attachment: Evidence for opiate mediation of social affect. *Pharmacology Biochemistry & Behavior, 9,* 213-220.

Hester, R. K. (1995). Behavioral self-control training. In R. K. Hester & W. R. Miller (Eds.), *Handbook of alcoholism treatment approaches: Effective alternatives.* 2nd ed. (pp. 148-159). Boston: Allyn and Bacon.

Heyser, C. J., Schulteis, G., & Koob, G. F. (1997). Increased ethanol self-administration after a period of imposed ethanol deprivation in rats trained in a limited access paradigm. *Alcoholism: Clinical and Experimental Research, 21,* 784-791.

Higley, J. D., Suomi, S. J., & Linnoila, M. (1996a). A nonhuman primate model of Type II excessive alcohol consumption? Part 1. Low cerebrospinal fluid 5-hydroxyindoleacetic acid concentrations and diminished social competence correlate with excessive alcohol consumption. *Alcoholism: Clinical and Experimental Resesarch, 20,* 629-642.

Higley, J. D., Suomi, S. J., & Linnoila, M. (1996b). A nonhuman primate model of Type II alcoholism? Part 2. Diminished social competence and excessive aggression correlates with low cerebrospinal fluid 5-hydroxyindoleacetic acid concentrations. *Alcoholism: Clinical and Experimental Research, 20,* 643-650.

Higley, J. D., Hasert, M. F., Suomi, S. J., & Linnoila, M. (1991). Nonhuman primate model of alcohol abuse: Effects of early experience, personality, and stress on alcohol consumption. *Proceedings of the National Academy of Science USA, 88,* 7261-7265.

Higley, J. D., King, S. T., Hasert, M. F., Champoux, M., Suomi, S. J., & Linnoila, M. (1996c). Stability of interindividual differences in serotonin function and its relationship to severe aggression and competent social behavior in rhesus macaque females. *Neuropsychopharmacology,14,* 67-76.

Higuchi, S., Matsushita, S., Murayama, M., Takagi, S., & Hayashida, M. (1995). Alcohol and aldehyde dehydrogenase polymorphisms and the risk for alcoholism. *The American Journal of Psychiatry,152,* 1219-1221.

Hill, S. Y. (1995). Early-onset alcoholism in women: Electrophysiological similarities and differences by gender. In W. A. Hunt & S. Zakhari (Eds.), *Stress, gender, and alcohol-seeking behavior* (pp. 61-86). National Institutes of Health Research Monograph No. 29. NIH Publication No. 95-3893. Bethesda, MD: U. S. Department of Health and Human Services.

Hilts, P. J. (1996). *Smoke screen.* Reading, MA: Addison-Wesley.

Hinde, R. A. (1970). *Animal behaviour: A synthesis of ethology and comparative psychology.* 2nd ed. New York: McGraw-Hill.

Hodgson, R., Rankin, H., & Stockwell, T. (1979). Alcohol dependence and the priming effect. *Behaviour Research and Therapy, 17,* 379-387.

Hoffman, H. S. (1996). *Amorous turkeys and addicted ducklings: A search for the causes of social attachment.* Boston, MA: Authors Cooperative.

Hoffman, H. S., & Ratner, A. M. (1973). A reinforcement model of imprinting: Implications for socialization in monkeys and men. *Psychological Review, 80,* 527-544.

Hoffmann, H., Loper, R. G., & Kammeier, M. L. (1974). Identifying future alcoholics with MMPI alcoholism scales. *Quarterly Journal of Studies on Alcohol, 35,* 490-498.

Hoffmann, N. G. & Miller, N. S. (1993). Perspectives of effective treatment for alcohol and drug disorders. *Psychiatric Clinics of North America, 16,* 127-140.

Holden, C.C. (1987). NIMH finds a case of "serious misconduct". *Science,235,* 1566-   1567.

Horvitz, J. C., Stewart, T., & Jacobs, B. L. (1997). Burst activity of ventral tegmental dopamine neurons is elicited by sensory stimuli in the awake cat. *Brain Research, 749,* 251-258.

Hotz, R. L. (1996, September 6). Separate human memory systems found. *Los Angeles Times,* pp. A14, A16.

Hubbell, C. L., Marglin, S. H., Spitalnic, S. J., Abelson, M. L., Wild, K. D., & Reid, L. D. (1991). Opioidergic, serotonergic, and dopaminergic manipulations and rats' intake of a sweetened alcoholic beverage. *Alcohol, 8,* 355-367.

Hudspeth, W. J., & Pribram, K. H. (1992). Psychophysiological indices of cerebral maturation. *International Journal of Psychophysiology, 12,* 19-29.

Humphreys, K., Huebsch, P. D., Finney, J. W., & Moos, R. (1999). A comparative evaluation of substance abuse treatment: V. Substance abuse treatment can enhance the effectiveness of self-help groups. *Alcoholism: Clinical and Experimental Research, 23,* 558-563.

Hunt, M. (1999). *The new know-nothings.* New Brunswick, NJ: Transaction.

Hunt, W. A. (1993). Are binge drinkers more at risk of developing brain damage? *Alcohol, 10,* 559-561.

Hunt, W. A. & Nixon, S. J. (Eds.) (1993). *Alcohol-induced brain damage.* NIAAA Research Monograph No. 22. NIH Publication No. 93-3549. Rockville, MD: U. S. Department of Health and Human Services.

Hunt, W. A., Barnett, L. W., & Branch, J. G. (1971). Relapse rates in addiction programs. *Journal of Clinical Psychology, 27,* 455-456.

Hutchings, D. E. (Ed.) (1989). Prenatal abuse of licit and illicit drugs. *Annals of the New York Academy of Sciences, Vol. 562.* New York: New York Academy of Sciences.

Hyytiä P., & Sinclair, J. D. (1993). Responding for oral ethanol after naloxone treatment by alcohol-preferring AA rats. *Alcoholism: Clinical and Experimental Research, 17,* 631-636.

Iacono, W. G. (1998). Identifying psychophysiological risk for psychopathology: Examples from substance abuse and schizophrenia research. *Psychophysiology, 35*, 621-637.

Ikemoto, S., McBride, W. J., Murphy, J. M., Lumeng, L., & Li, T-K. 1997). 6-OHDA-lesions of the nucleus accumbens disrupt the acquisition but not the maintenance of ethanol consumption in the alcohol-preferring P line of rats. *Alcoholism: Clinical and Experimental Research, 21*, 1042-1046.

Institute of Medicine (1990). *Broadening the base of treatment for alcohol problems.* Washington, DC: National Academy Press.

Israel, Y., Hollander, O., Sanchez-Craig, M., Booker, S., Miller, V., Gingrich, R., & Rankin, J. G. (1996). Screening for problem drinking and counseling by the primary care physician-nurse team. *Alcoholism: Clinical and Experimental Research, 20*, 1443-1450.

Jackson, J. K. (1957). H-technique scales of preoccupation with alcohol and of psychological involvement in alcoholics: Time order of symptoms. *Quarterly Journal of Studies on Alcohol, 18*, 451-467.

Jackson, T. R., & Smith, J. W. (1978). A comparison of two aversion treatment methods for alcoholism. *Journal of Studies on Alcohol, 39*, 187-191.

Jellinek, E. M. (1946). Phases in the drinking history of alcoholics: Analysis of a survey conducted by the official organ of Alcoholics Anonymous. *Quarterly Journal of Studies on Alcohol, 7*, 1-88.

Jellinek, E. M. (1952). Phases of alcohol addiction. *Quarterly Journal of Studies on Alcohol, 13*, 673-684.

Jellinek, E. M. (1960). *The disease concept of alcoholism.* New Brunswik, NJ: Hillhouse.

Jones, M. C. (1924). A laboratory study of fear: The case of Peter. *Pedagogical Seminary, 31*, 308-315.

Jones, M. C. (1974). Albert, Peter, and John B. Watson. *American Psychologist, 29*, 581-583.

Jönsson, E. G., Nöthen, M. M., Gustavsson, J. P., Neidt, H., Brené, S., Tylec, A., Propping, P., Sedvall, G. C. (1997). Lack of evidence for allelic association between personality traits and the dopamine D4 receptor gene polymorphisms. *American Journal of Psychiatry, 154*, 697-699.

Journal Interview (1979). Conversation with D. L. Davies. *British Journal of Addiction, 74*, 239-249.

Joseph, M. H., Young, A. M. J., & Gray, J. A. (1996). Are neurochemistry and reinforcement enough - can the abuse potential of drugs be explained by common actions on a dopamine reward system in the brain. *Human Psychopharmacology,11*, S55-S63.

Kadden, R. M., Cooney, N. L., Getter, H., & Litt, M. D. (1989). Matching alcoholics to coping skills or interactional therapies: Posttreatment results. *Journal of Consulting and Clinical Psychology, 57*, 698-704.

Kalant, H. (1996). Current state of knowledge about the mechanisms of alcohol tolerance. *Addiction Biology, 1*, 133-141.

Kammeier, M. L., Hoffmann, H., & Loper, R. G. (1973). Personality characterisics of alcoholics as college freshmen and at time of treatment. *Quarterly Journal of Studies on Alcohol, 34*, 390-399.

Karni, A. (1997, January/February). Adult cortical plasticity and reorganization. *Science & Medicine, 4*, 24-33.

Katz, J. (1997). Ethics in neurobiological research with human subjects - final reflections. In A. E. Shamoo (Ed.), *Ethics in neurobiological research with human subjects* (pp.329-335). Amsterdam: Gordon and Breach.

Kazdin, A. E. (1983). Psychiatric diagnosis, dimensions of dysfunction, and child behavior therapy. *Behavior Therapy, 14*, 73-99.

Keller, M. (1972). On the loss-of-control phenomenon in alcoholism. *British Journal of Addiction, 67*, 153-166.

Keller, M. (1975). Multidisciplinary perspectives on alcoholism and the need for integration: An historical and prospective note. *Journal of Studies on Alcohol, 36*, 133-147.

Keller, M. (1976) The concept of alcoholism revisited. *Journal of Studies on Alcohol, 37*, 1694-1717.

Keller, M. (1979). The great Jewish drink mystery. In M. Marshall (Ed.), *Beliefs, behaviors, & alcoholic beverages: A cross-cultural survey* (pp. 404-414). Ann Arbor, MI: University of Michigan Press.

Keller, M., & Doria, J. (1991). On defining alcoholism. *Alcohol Health and Research World, 15*, 253-259.

Kemper, T. D. (1990). *Social structure and testosterone.* New Brunswick, NJ: Rutgers University Press.

Kessler, R. C., Sonnega, A., Bromet, E., Hughes, M., Nelson, C. B. (1995). Posttraumatic stress disorder in the National Comorbidity Survey. *Archives of General Psychiatry, 52*, 1048-1060.

Keverne, E. B., Martensz, N. D., & Tuite, B. (1989). Beta-endorphin concentrations in cerebrospinal fluid of monkeys are influenced by grooming relationships. *Psychoneuroendocrinology, 14*, 155-161.

Kiianmaa, P., Hyytiä, P., & Sinclair, D. (1998). Dopamine and alcohol reinforcement in alcohol-preferring AA rats. *Alcoholism: Clinical and Experimental Research, 22*, 155A.

Kiianmaa, K., Nurmi, M., Nykänen, I., & Sinclair, J. D. (1995). Effect of ethanol on extracellular dopamine in the nucleus accumbens of alcohol-preferring AA and alcohol-avoiding ANA rats. *Pharmacology Biochemistry and Behavior, 52*, 29-34.

King, L. S. (1954). What is disease? *Philosophy of Science, 21*, 193-203.

Kishline, A. (1994). *Moderate drinking: The new option for problem drinkers.* Tucson, AZ: See Sharp Press.

Kissin, B., & Begleiter, H. (Eds.) (1983a). *The biology of alcoholism. Vol. 6. The pathogenesis of alcoholism: Psychosocial factors.* New York: Plenum.

Kissin, B., & Begleiter, H. (Eds.) (1983b). *The biology of alcoholism. Vol. 7. The pathogenesis of alcoholism: Biological factors.* New York: Plenum.

Kivlahan, D. R., Marlatt, G. A., Fromme, K., Coppel, D. B., & Williams, K. (1990). Secondary prevention with college drinkers: Evaluation of an alcohol skills training program. *Journal of Consulting and Clinical Psychology, 58*, 805-810.

Kluger, R. (1997). *Ashes to ashes.* New York: Vintage Books.

Knight, L. J., Barbaree, H. E., & Boland, F. J. (1986). Alcohol and the balanced-placebo design: The role of experimenter demands in expectancy. *Journal of Abnormal Psychology, 95*, 335-340.

Koening, H. G. (1997). *Is religion good for your health?* New York: Haworth.

Knorring, A-L. von., Hallman, J., Knorring, L. von., & Oreland, L. (1991). Platelet monoamine oxidase activity in Type 1 and Type 2 alcoholism. *Alcohol & Alcohol, 26*, 409-416.

Knowlton, B. J., Mangels, J. A., & Squire, L. R. (1996). A neostriatal habit learning system in humans. *Science, 273*, 1399-1402.

Köhler, W. (1938). *The place of value in a world of facts.* New York: Liveright.

Kohn, A. (1986). *False prophets: Fraud and error in science and medicine.* Oxford: Basil Blackwell.

Korenman, S. G., & Barchas, J. D. (Eds.) (1993). *Biological basis of substance abuse.* New York: Oxford University Press.

Korytnyk, N. X., & Perkins, D. V. (1983). Effects of alcohol versus expectancy for alcohol on the incidence of graffiti following an experimental task. *Journal of Abnormal Psychology, 92*, 382-385.

Küfner, H., & Feuerlein, W. (1989). *In-patient treatment for alcoholism.* Berlin: Springer-Verlag.

Kuhn, T. S. (1962). *The structure of scientific revolutions.* Chicago: University of Chicago Press.

Kurtines, W. M., Azmitia, M., & Gewirtz, J. L. (1992). *The role of values in psychology and human development.* New York: Wiley.

Laberg, J. C. (1986). Alcohol and expectancy: Subjective, psychophysiological and behavioral responses to alcohol stimuli in severely, moderately and non-dependent drinkers. *British Journal of Addiction, 81*, 797-808.

Lakatos, I. (1970). Falsification and the methodology of scientific research programmes. In I. Lakatos & A. Musgrave (Eds.), *Criticism and the growth of knowledge* (pp. 91-195). London: Cambridge University Press.

Langenbucher, J. W., & Martin, C. S. (1996). Alcohol abuse: Adding content to category. *Alcoholism: Clinical and Experimental Research, 20*, 270A-275A.

Lappalainen, J., Long, J. C., Eggert, M., Ozaki, N., Robin, R. W., Brown, G. L., Naukkarinen, H., Virkkunen, M., Linnoila, M., & Goldman, D. (1998). Linkage of antisocial alcoholism to the serotonin 5-HT1B receptor gene in 2 populations. *Archives of General Psychology, 55*, 989-994.

Larimer, M. E., Marlatt, G. A., Baer, J. S., Quigley, L. A., Blume, A. W., & Hawkins, E. H. (1998). Harm reduction for alcohol problems. In G. A. Marlatt (Ed.), *Harm reduction: Pragmatic strategies for managing high-risk behaviors* (pp.69-121). New York: Guilford.

Lashley, K. S. (1923). The behavioristic interpretation of consciousness. *Psychological Review, 30*, 237-272, 329-353.

Lashley, K. S. (1951). The problem of serial order in behavior. In L. A. Jeffress (Ed.), *Cerebral mechanisms in behavior* (pp. 112-136). New York: Wiley.

Laudan, L. (1977). *Progress and its problems.* Berkeley, CA: University of California Press.

Laundergan, J. C. (1982). *Easy does it.* na. Hazelden.

Lemere, F. (1956). The nature and significance of brain damage from alcoholism. *American Journal of Psychiatry, 113*, 361-362.

Lemere, F., & O'Hollaren, P. (1950). Thiopental U. S. P. (Pentothal®) treatment of alcoholism. *Archives of Neurology and Psychiatry, 63*, 579-585.

Lemere, F., & Voegtlin, W. L. (1950). An evaluation of the aversion treatment of alcoholism. *Quarterly Journal of Studies on Alcohol, 11*, 199-204.

Leonard, K. E., & Blane, H. T. (1987) Conclusion. In H. T. Blane & K. E. Leonard (Eds.). *Psychological theories of drinking and alcoholism* (pp.388-395). New York: Guilford.

Levine, R. J. (1988). *Ethics and regulation of clinical research.* 2nd. ed. New Haven, CT: Yale University Press.

Lewis, J. W., Cannon, J. T., & Liebeskind, J. C. (1980). Opioid and nonopioid mechanisms of stress analgesia. *Science, 208,* 623-625.

Lhermitte, F. (1986). Human autonomy and the frontal lobes. Part II: Patient behavior in complex and social situations: the "environmental dependency syndrome." *Annals of Neurology, 19,* 335-343.

Lilienfeld, S. O. (1995a). Reply to Maltzman's "Why alcoholism is a disease". *Journal of Psychoactive Drugs, 27,* 287-291.

Lilienfeld, S. O. (1995b). *Seeing both sides.* Pacific Grove, CA: Brooks/Cole.

Lindsley, D. (1951). Emotion. In S. S. Stevens (Ed.), *Handbook of experimental psychology* (pp. 473-516). New York: Wiley.

Lindstrom, L. (1992). *Managing alcoholism: Matching clients to treatments.* Oxford: Oxford University Press.

Linnoila, M., Mefford, I., Nutt, D., & Adinoff, B. (1987). Alcohol withdrawal and noradrenergic function. *Annals of Internal Medicine, 107,* 875-889.

Litt, M. D., Babor, T. F., DelBoca, F. K., Kadden, R. M., & Cooney, N. L. (1992). Types of alcoholics, II: application of an empirically derived typology to treatment matching. *Archives of General Psychiatry, 49,* 609-614.

Logue, A. W. (1986). *The psychology of eating and drinking.* New York: W. H. Freeman.

Longabaugh, R., Wirtz, P. W., Zweben, A., & Stout, R. L. (1998). Network support for drinking, alcoholics anonymous and long-term matching effects. *Addiction, 93,* 1313-1333.

Loper, R. G., Kammeier, M. L., & Hoffmann, H. (1973). MMPI characteristics of college freshman males who later became alcoholics. *Journal of Abnormal Psychology, 82,* 159-162.

Lovaas, O. I. (1993). The development of a treatment-research project for developmentally disabled and autistic children. *Journal of Applied Behavior Analysis, 26,* 617-630.

Lovibond, S. H., & Caddy, G. (1970). Discriminated aversive control in the moderation of alcoholics' drinking behavior. *Behavior Therapy, 1,* 437-444.

Ludwig, A. M., & Stark, L. H. (1974). Alcohol craving: subjective and situational aspects. *Quarterly Journal of Studies on Alcohol, 35,* 899-905.

Ludwig, A. M., Wikler, A., & Stark, L. H. (1974). The first drink: Psychobiological aspects of craving. *Archives of General Psychiatry, 30,* 539-547.

Luria, A. R. (1980). *Higher cortical functions in man.* 2nd ed. New York: Basic Books.

Lyons, D., Whitlow, C. T., Smith, H. R., & Porrino, L. J. (1998). Brain imaging: Functional consequences of ethanol in the central nervous system. In M. Galanter (Ed.), *Recent developments in alcoholism. Vol. 14. The consequences of alcoholism* (pp. 253-284). New York: Plenum.

Lyvers, M. (1998). Drug addiction as a physical disease: The role of physical dependence and other chronic drug-induced neurophysiological changes in compulsive drug self-administration. *Experimental and Clinical Psychopharmacology, 6,* 107-125.

Lyvers, M. (in press). "Loss of control" in alcoholism and drug addiction: A neuroscientific interpretation.

Lyvers, M. F., & Maltzman, I. (1991a). Selective effects of alcohol on Wisconsin card sorting test performance. *British Journal of Addiction, 86,* 399-407.

Lyvers, M. F., & Maltzman, I. (1991b). The balanced placebo design: Effects of alcohol and beverage instructions cannot be independently assessed. *The International Journal of the Addictions, 26,* 963-972.

Lyvers, M., Boyd, G., & Maltzman, I. (1988). Effects of cigarette smoking on bilateral electrodermal measures of the orienting reflex. *Psychophysiology, 25,* 408-417.

Maier, S. F., & Watkins, L. R. (1998). Cytokines for psychologists: Implications of bidirectional immune-to-brain communication for understanding behavior, mood, and cognition. *Psychological Review, 105,* 83-107.

Maier, S. F., Watkins, L. R., & Fleshner, M. (1994). Psychoneuroimmunology: The interface between behavior, brain, and immunity. *American Psychologist, 49,* 1004-1017.

Makanjuola, R. O. A., Dow, R. C., & Ashcroft, G. W. (1980). Behavioural responses to stereotactically controlled injections of monamine neurotransmitters into the accumbens and caudate-putamen nuclei. *Psychopharmacology, 71,* 227-235.

Malhotra, A. K., Virrkkunen, M., Rooney, W., Eggert, M., Linnoila, M., & Goldman, D. (1996). The association between the dopamine D4 receptor (DRD4) 16 amino acid repeat polymorphism and novelty seeking. *Molecular Psychiatry, 1,* 388-391.

Maltzman, I. (unpublished a). A reply to the Sobells: You did not do what you said you did; you did not find what you said you found.

Maltzman, I. (unpublished b). The Sobells and alchemy.

Maltzman, I. (unpublished c). Criticisms of the Dickens Committee Enquiry into the Sobells' alleged fraud and Doob's effort at their defense.

Maltzman, I. (unpublished d). A reply to Nathan, the Sobells, Baker and Cook: The truth of the matter.

Maltzman, I. (unpublished e). The place of facts in a world of values: With comments on the disease concept of alcoholism and its revisionist critics.

Maltzman, I. (1976). *Affidavit of Irving Maltzman in support of motion to dismiss complaint.* United States District Court. Central District of California.

Maltzman., I. (1979a). Orienting reflexes and classical conditioning in humans. In H. D. Kimmel, E. H. van Olst, & J. F. Orlebeke (Eds.), *The orienting reflex in humans* (pp. 323-351). New York: Erlbaum.

Maltzman, I. (1979b). Orienting reflexes and significance: A reply to O'Gorman. *Psychophyioslogy, 16,* 274-283.

Maltzman, I. (1984). More on: "Controlled drinking versus Abstinence: Where do we go from here?" *Bulletin of the Society of Psychologists in Addictive Behaviors, 3,* 71-73.

Maltzman, I. (1987a). Controlled drinking and the treatment of alcoholism (Letter to the Editor). *Journal of the American Medical Association, 257,* 927, 3229.

Maltzman, I. (1987b). A neo-Pavlovian interpretation of the OR and classical conditioning in humans: With comments on alcoholism and the poverty of cognitive psychology. In G. Davey (Ed.), *Cognitive processes and Pavlovian conditioning in humans* (pp. 211-249). Chichester: John Wiley.

Maltzman, I. (1988). The rise and decline of controlled drinking. *XXI International Congress of Psychology.* Sydney, Australia, February 1988.

Maltzman, I. (1989). A reply to Cook, "Craftsman versus professional: Analysis of the controlled drinking controversy". *Journal of Studies on Alcohol, 50,* 466-472.

Maltzman, I. (1990). The OR and significance. With a comment by E. N. Sokolov. *The Pavlovian Journal of Biological Science, 25,* 111-122.

Maltzman, I. (1991). Is alcoholism a disease? A critical review of a controversy. *Integrative Physiology and Behavioral Science, 26,* 200-210.

Maltzman, I. (1992, October). The winter of scholarly science journals. *Professional Counselor, 7(2),* 38-39, 41-43.

Maltzman, I. (1994). Why alcoholism is a disease. *Journal of Psychoactive Drugs, 26,* 13-31.

Maltzman, I. (1998). Reply to Lilienfeld: Why alcoholism is a disease. *Journal of Psychoactive Drugs, 30,* 99-104.

Maltzman, I., & Marinkovic, K. (1996). Alcohol, alcoholism, and the autonomic nervous system: A critical account. In H. Begleiter, & B. Kissin (Eds.), *The pharmacology of alcohol and alcohol dependence* (pp. 248-306). New York: Oxford University Press.

Maltzman, I., & Raskin, D. C. (1965). Effects of individual differences in the orienting reflex on conditioning and complex processes. *Journal of Experimental Research and Personality, 1,* 1-16.

Maltzman, I. & Schweiger, A. (1991). Individual and family characteristics of middle-class adolescents hospitalized for alcohol and other drug use. *British Journal of Addiction, 86,* 1435-1447.

Maltzman, I., & Wolff, C. (1970). Preference for immediate versus delayed noxious stimulation and the concomitant GSR. *Journal of Experimental Psychology, 83,* 76-79.

Maltzman, I., Weissbluth, S., & Wolff, C. (1978). Habituation of orienting reflexes in repeated GSR semantic conditioning. *Journal of Experimental Psychology: General, 107,* 309-333.

Maltzman, I., Gould, J., Pendery, M., & Wolff, C. (1977). Semantic conditioning and generalization of the galvanic skin response-orienting reflex with overt and covert activity. *Journal of Experimental Psychology: General, 106,* 172-184.

Maltzman, I., Harris, L., Ingram, E., & Wolff, C. (1971). A primacy effect in the orienting reflex to stimulus change. *Journal of Experimental Psychology, 87,* 202-206.

Maltzman, I., Smith, M. J., Kantor, W., & Mandell, M. P. (1971). Effect of stress on habituation of the orienting reflex. *Journal of Experimental Psychology, 87,* 207-214.

Maltzman, I., Gould, J., Barnett, O. J., Raskin, D. C., & Wolff, C. (1977). Classical conditioning components of the orienting reflex to words using innocuous and noxious unconditioned stimuli under different conditioned stimulus-unconditioned stimulus intervals. *Journal of Experimental Psychology: General, 106,* 171-212.

Mann, M. (1950). *Primer on alcoholism.* New York: Rinehart.

368

Marinkovic, K. (1993). Effects of alcohol on event-related potentials and skin conductance in two discrimination tasks. Unpublished Ph.D Dissertation, University of California, Los Angeles.

Margolis, J. (1976). The concept of disease. *Journal of Medical Philosophy, 1,* 238-255.

Marlatt, G. A. (1979). Alcohol use and problem drinking: A cognitive-behavioral analysis. In P. C. Kendall, & S. D. Hollon (Eds.), *Cognitive-behavioral interventions: Theory, research, and procedures* (pp. 319-355). New York: Academic Press.

Marlatt, G. A. (1983). The controlled-drinking controversy: A commentary. *American Psychologist, 38,* 1097-1110.

Marlatt, G. A. (1984a). Reply to Maltzman (letter to editor). *Contemporary Psychology, 29,* 175.

Marlatt, G. A. (1984b). President's message. *Bulletin of the Society of Psychologists in Addictive Behaviors, 3,* 67.

Marlatt, G. A. (1985a). Controlled drinking: The controversy rages on. (Comment) *American Psychologist, 40,* 374-376.

Marlatt, G. A. (1985b). Relapse prevention: Theoretical rationale and overview of the model. In G. A. Marlatt & J. R. Gordon (Eds.), *Relapse prevention* (pp. 3-70). New York: Guilford.

Marlatt, G. A. (1992). Substance abuse: Implications of a biopsychosocial model for prevention, treatment, and relapse prevention. In J. Grabowski & G. R. VandenBos (Eds.), *Psychopharmacology: Basic mechanisms and applied interventions* (pp. 131-162). Washington, DC: American Psychological Association.

Marlatt, G. A., & Forseth, R. (1991). Theatrical defenses: A conversation. *Dionysos, 2,* 19-29.

Marlatt, G. A., & Gordon, J. R. (Eds.) (1985). *Relapse prevention: Maintenance strategies in the treatment of addictive behaviors.* New York: Guilford.

Marlatt, G. A., Baer, J. S., & Larimer, M. (1995). Preventing alcohol abuse in college students: A harm-reduction approach. In G. M. Boyd, J. Howard, and R. A. Zucker (Eds.), *Alcohol problems among adolescents* (pp. 147-172). Hillsdale, NJ: Erlbaum.

Marlatt, G. A., Demming, B., & Reid, J. B. (1973). Loss of control drinking in alcoholics: An experimental analogue. *Journal of Abnormal Psychology, 81,* 233-241.

Marlatt, G. A., Larimer, M. E., Baer, J. S., & Quigley, L. A. (1993). Harm reduction for alcohol problems: Moving beyond the controlled drinking controversy. *Behavior Therapy, 24,* 461-504.

Marlatt, G. A., Baer, J. S., Kivlahan, D. R., Dimeff, L. A., Larimer, M. E., Quigley, L. A., Somers, J. M., & William, E. (1998). Screening and brief intervention for high-risk college student drinkers: Results from a 2-year follow-up assessment. *Journal of Consulting and Clinical Psychology, 66,* 604-615.

Marlatt, G. A., Miller, W. R., Duckert, F., Gotestam, G., Heather, N., Peele, S., Sanchez-Craig, M., Sobell, L. C., & Sobell, M. B. (1985). Abstinence and controlled drinking: Alternative treatment goals for alcoholism and problem drinking? *Bulletin of the Society of Psychologists in Addictive Behaviors, 4,* 123-150.

Marshall, E. (1999). NIMH to screen studies for science and human risks. *Science, 283,* 464-465.

Martin, C. S., & Sayette, M. A. (1993). Experimental design in alcohol administration research: Limitations and alternatives in the manipulation of dosage-set. *Journal of Studies on Alcohol, 54,* 750-761.

Martin, C. S., Earlywine, M., Finn, P., & Young, R. (1990). Some boundary conditions for effective use of alcohol placebos. *Journal of Studies on Alcohol, 51,* 500-505.

Masterman, M. (1970). The nature of a paradigm. In I. Lakatos & A. Musgrave (Eds.), *Criticism and the growth of knowledge* (pp. 59-89). London: Cambridge University Press.

Mayr, E. (1969). *Principles of systematic zoology.* New York: McGraw-Hill.

Mayr, E. (1982). *The growth of biological thought.* Cambridge, MA: Harvard University Press.

McBride, W. J., Murphy, J. M., Lumeng, L., & Li, T-K. (1990). Serotonin, dopamine and GABA involvement in alcohol drinking of selectively bred rats. *Alcohol, 7,* 199-205.

McCabe, R. J. R. (1986). Alcohol-dependent individuals sixteen years on. *Alcohol & Alcoholism, 21,* 85-91.

McConnell, J. V. (1989). *Understanding human behavior.* 6th ed.. New York: Holt, Rinehart and Winston.

McCready, W. C., Greeley, A. M., & Thiesen, G. (1983). Ethnicity and nationality in alcoholism. In B. Kissin & H. Begleiter (Eds.), *The biology of alcoholism. Vol. 6. The pathogenesis of alcoholism: Psychosocial factors* (pp.309-340). New York: Plenum.

McDonald, K. A. (1989, September). Rutgers journal forced to publish paper despite threats of libel lawsuit. *The Chronicle of Higher Education, 36,* pp. A5, A13.

McEwen, B. S., Angulo, J., Cameron, H., Chao, H. M., Daniels, D., Gannon, M. N., Gould, E., Mendelson, S., Sakai, R., Spencer, R., & Woolley, C. (1992). Paradoxical effects of adrenal steroids on the brain: Protection versus degeneration. *Biological Psychiatry, 31,* 177-199.

McGue, M. (1993). From proteins to cognitions: The behavioral genetics of alcoholism. In R. Plomin & G. E. McClearn (Eds.), *Nature Nurture & Psychology* (pp.245-268). Washington, DC: American Psychological Association.

McKinzie, D.L., Nowak, K.L., Yorger, L., McBride, W.J., Murphy,J.M., Lumeng, L., & Li, T.-K. The alcohol deprivation efffect in the alcohol-preferring P rat under free-drinking and operant access conditions. *Alcoholism: Clinical and Experimental Research, 212,* 1170-1176.

McLachlan, J. F. C. (1974). Therapy strategies, personality orientation and recovery from alcoholism. *Canadian Psychiatric Association Journal, 19,* 25-30.

McLellan, A. T., Luborsky, L., Woody, G. E., & O'Brien, C. P. (1980). An improved diagnostic evaluation instrument for substance abuse patients: The Addiction Severity Index. *The Journal of Nervous and Mental Disease, 168,* 26-33.

McLellan, A. T., Grisson, G. R., Brill, P., Durell, J., Metzger, D. S., & O'Brien, C. P. (1993). Private substance abuse treatments: Are some programs more effective than others? *Journal of Substance Abuse Treatment, 10,* 243-254.

Mendelson, J. H., & Mello, N. K. (1966). Experimental analysis of drinking behavior of chronic alcoholics (pp.828-845). *Annals of the New York Academy of Science, 133.* New York: New York Academy of Sciences.

Mendelson, J. H., & Mello, N. K. (1985). *Alcohol use and abuse in America.* Boston: Little, Brown.

Mennella, J. A. (1998). Short-term effects of maternal alcohol consumption on lactational performance. *Alcoholism: Clinical and Experimental Research, 22,* 1389-1392.

Merton, R. (1968). *Social theory and social structure* (enlarged ed.) New York: The Free Press.

Miller, P. M., Hersen, M., Eisler, R. M., & Hemphill, D. P. (1973). Electrical aversion therapy with alcoholics: An analogue study. *Behaviour Research & Therapy, 11,* 491-497.

Miller, W. R. (1983). Controlled drinking: A history and critical review. *Journal of Studies on Alcohol, 44,* 68-83.

Miller, W. R. (1987). Behavioral alcohol treatment research advances: Barriers to utilization. *Advances in Behaviour Research and Therapy, 9,* 145-171.

Miller, W. R. (1988a). Abstinence or controlled drinking goals for problem drinkers: A randomized clinical trial. *Psychology of Addictive Behaviors, 2,* 20-33.

Miller, W. R. (1988b, June 21). Hearing before Senate Governmental Affairs Committee. *Alcoholism Report, 3.*

Miller, W. R. (1990). Alcohol treatment alternatives: What works? In H. B. Milkman & L. I. Sederer (Eds.), *Treatment choices for alcoholism and substance abuse* (pp. 253-264). Lexington, MA: Lexington.

Miller, W. R., & Caddy, G. R. (1977). Abstinence and controlled drinking in the treatment of problem drinkers. *Journal of Studies on Alcohol, 38,* 986-1003.

Miller, W. R., & Hester, R. K. (1980). Treating the problem drinker: Modern approaches. In W. R. Miller (Ed.), *The addictive behaviors* (pp.11-141). Oxford: Pergamon.

Miller, W. R., & Hester, R. K. (1986). The effectiveness of alcoholism treatment methods. What research reveals. In W. R. Miller & N. Heather (Eds.), *Treating addictive behaviors: Processes of change* (pp. 121-174). New York: Plenum.

Miller, W. R., & Joyce, M. A. (1979). Prediction of abstinence, controlled drinking, and heavy drinking outcomes following behavioral self-control training. *Journal of Consulting and Clinical Psychology, 47,* 773-775.

Miller, W. R. & Munoz, R. F. (1982). *How to control your drinking.* rev.ed. Albuquerque, NM: University of New Mexico Press.

Miller, W.R., & Rollnick, S. (Eds.)(1991), *Motivational interviewing.* New York: Guilford.

Miller, W. R., & Taylor, C. L. (1980). Relative effectiveness of bibliotherapy, individual and group self-control training in the treatment of problem drinkers. *Addictive Behaviors, 5,* 13-24.

Miller, W. R., Leckman, A. K., & Tinkcom, M. (1987). Controlled drinking and the treatment of alcoholism (Letter to the editor). *Journal of the American Medical Association, 257,* 3228-3229.

Miller, W. R., Taylor, C. A., & West, J. C. (1980). Focused versus broad-spectrum behavior therapy for problem drinkers. *Journal of Consulting and Clinical Psychology, 48,* 590-601.

Miller, W. R., Leckman, A. L., Delaney, H. D., & Tinkcom, M. (1992). Long-term follow-up of behavioral self-control training. *Journal of Studies on Alcohol, 53,* 249-261.

Miller, W. R., Leckman, A. L., Tinkcom, M., & Rubenstein, J. (1986). Long-term follow-up of controlled drinking therapies. Paper presented at the American Psychological Association Convention. Washington, D. C.

Miller, W. R., Brown, J. M., Simpson, T. L., Handmaker, N. S., Bien, T. H., Luckie, L. F., Montgomery, H. A., Hester, R. K., & Tonigan, J. S. (1995). What works? A methodological analysis of the alcohol treatment outcome literature. In R. K. Hester & W. R. Miller (Eds.), *Handbook of alcoholism treatment approaches: Effective alternatives* 2nd ed. (pp.12-44). Boston: Allyn and Bacon.

Milner, B. (1963). Effects of different brain lesions on card sorting: The role of the frontal lobes. *Archives of Neurology, 9,* 100-110.

Mirenowicz, J., & Schultz, W. (1994). Importance of unpredictability for reward responses in primate dopamine neurons. *Journal of Neurophysiology, 72,* 1024-1027.

Modell, J. G., Mountz, J. M., Glaser, F. B., & Lee, J. Y. (1993). Effect of haloperidol on measures of craving and impaired control in alcoholic subjects. *Alcoholism: Clinical and Experimental Research, 17,* 234-240.

Monahan, S. C., & Finney, J. W. (1996). Explaining abstinence rates following treatment for alcohol abuse: a quantitative synthesis of patient, research design and treatment effects. *Addiction, 91,* 787-805.

Monteiro, M. G., Klein, J., & Schuckit, M. A. (1991). High levels of sensitivity to alcohol in young adult Jewish men: A pilot study. *Journal of Studies on Alcohol, 52,* 464-469.

Moos, R. H. (1997a). *Evaluating treatment environments.* 2nd ed. New Brunswick, NJ: Transaction.

Moos, R. H. (1997b). How to become a true scientist: A guide to minimizing pesky treatment effects (Letter to editor). *Addiction, 92,* 481-482.

Moos, R. H., & Humphrey, B. (1974). *Group environment scale.* Palo Alto, CA: Consulting Psychologists.

Moos, R. H., & Moos, B. S. (1981). *Family environment scale manual.* Palo Alto, CA: Consulting Psychologists.

Moos, R. H., Finney, J. W., Ouimette, P. C., & Suchinsky, R. T. (1999). A comparative evaluation of substance abuse treatment: I. Treatment orientation, amount of care, and 1-year outcomes. *Alcoholism: Clinical and Experimental Research, 23,* 529-536.

Morse, R. M., & Flavin, D. K. (1992). The definition of alcoholism. *Journal of the American Medical Association, 268,* 1012-1014.

Mulford, H. A., & Miller, D. E. (1960a). Drinking in Iowa: III. A scale of definitions of alcohol related to drinking behavior. *Quarterly Journal of Studies on Alcohol, 21,* 267-278.

Mulford, H. A., & Miller, D. E. (1960b). Drinking in Iowa. IV. Preoccupation with alcohol and definitions of alcohol, heavy drinking and trouble due to drinking. *Quarterly Journal of Studies on Alcohol, 21,* 279-291.

Muuronen, A., Bergman, H., Hindmarsh, T., & Telakivi, T. (1989). Influence of improved drinking habits on brain atrophy and cognitive performance in alcoholic patients: A 5-year follow-up study. *Alcoholism: Clinical and Experimental Research, 13,* 137-141.

Myers, R. D. (1990). Anatomical "circuitry" in the brain mediating alcohol drinking revealed by THP-reactive sites in the limbic system. *Alcohol, 7,* 449-459.

Myers, R. D., & Melchior, C. L. (1977). Alcohol drinking: Abnormal intake caused by tetrahydropapaveroline in brain. *Science, 196,* 554-556.

Nathan, P. E. (1985). Alcoholism: A cognitive social learning approach. *Journal of Substance Abuse Treatment, 2,* 169-173.

Nathan, P. E. (1989). A prefatory comment. *Journal of Studies on Alcohol, 50,* 465.

Nathan, P. E., & Lipscomb, T. R. (1979). Behavior therapy and behavior modification in the treatment of alcoholism. In J. H. Mendelson, & N. K. Mello (Eds.), *The diagnosis and treatment of alcoholism* (pp. 306-357). New York: McGraw-Hill.

Nathan, P. E., & Niaura, R. S. (1985). Behavioral assessment and treatment of alcoholism. In J. H. Mendelson & N. K. Mello (Eds.), *The diagnosis and treatment of alcoholism.* (pp. 391-455). 2nd ed. New York: McGraw-Hill.

Nathan, P. E., & Skinstad, A-H. (1987). Outcomes of treatment for alcohol problems: Current methods, problems, and results. *Journal of Consulting and Clinical Psychology, 55,* 332-340.

Neal, A. (1988, February 1). Is alcoholism a disease? *American Bar Association Journal,* 58-62.

Neisser, U. (1982). *Memory observed. Remembering in natural contexts.* San Francisco, CA: W. H. Freeman.

371

Nelson, C. B., Little, R. J. A., Heath, A. C., & Kessler, R. C. (1996). Patterns of DSM-III-R alcohol dependence symptom progression in a general population survey. *Psychological Medicine, 26,* 449-460.

Neumark, Y., Friedlander, Y., Thomasson, H. R., & Li, T-K. (1998). Association of the *ADH2*2* allele with reduced ethanol consumption in Jewish men in Israel: A pilot study. *Journal of Studies on Alcohol, 59,* 133-139.

Newlin, D. B., & Pretorius, M. B. (1991). Prior exposures to the laboratory enhance the effect of alcohol. *Journal of Studies on Alcohol, 52,* 470-473.

Nicolás, J. M., Catafau, A. M., Estruch, R., Lomeña, F. J., Salamero, M., Herranz, R., Monforte, R., Cardenal, C., & Urban-Marquez, A. (1993). Regional cerebral blood flow-SPECT in chronic alcoholism: Relation to neuropsychological testing. *Journal of Nuclear Medicine, 34,* 1452-1459.

Nordstrom, G., & Berglund, M. (1967). A prospective study of successful long-term adjustment in alcohol dependence: Social drinking versus abstinence. *Journal of Studies on Alcohol, 48,* 95-103.

O'Connor, M. J., Sigman, M., & Brill, N. (1987). Disorganization of attachment in relation to maternal alcohol consumption. *Journal of Consulting and Clinical Psychology, 55,* 831-836.

Office of Applied Studies (1998). *Prevalence of substance use among racial and ethnic subgroups in the United States 1991-1993.* SAMHSA Analytic Series: A-6. Rockville, MD: U. S. Department of Health and Human Services.

Olausson, P., Ericson, M., Petersson, A., Kosowski, A., Söderpalm, B., & Engel, J. A. (1998). Nefazodone attenuates the behavioral and neurochemical effects of ethanol. *Alcohol, 15,* 77-86.

Olds, J., & Travis, R. P. (1960). Effects of chlorpromazine, meprobamate, pentobarbital and morphine on self-stimulation. *Journal of Pharmacology and Experimental Therapeutics, 128,* 397-404.

O'Malley, S. S., Jaffe, A. J., Rode, S., & Rounsaville, B. J. (1996). Experience of a "slip" among alcoholics treated with naltrexone or placebo. *American Journal of Psychiatry, 153,* 281-283.

O'Malley, S. S., Jaffe, A. J., Chang, G., Schottenfeld, R. S., Meyer, R. E., & Rounsaville, B. (1992). Naltrexone and coping skills therapy for alcohol dependence. *Archives of General Psychiatry, 49,* 881-887.

Orford, J., & Edwards, G. (1977). *Alcoholism: A comparison of treatment and advice, with a study of the influence of marriage, Maudsley Monograph No. 26.* Oxford: Oxford University Press.

Orford, J., & Hawker, A. (1974). Note on the ordering of onset of symptoms in alcohol dependence. *Psychological Medicine, 4,* 281-288.

Orford, J., & Keddie, A. (1986). Abstinence or controlled drinking in clinical practice: A test of the dependence and persuasion hypotheses. *British Journal of Addiction, 81,* 495-504.

Orford, J., Oppenheimer, E., & Edwards, G. (1976). Abstinence or control: the outcome for excessive drinkers two years after consultation. *Behaviour Research and Therapy, 14,* 409-418.

Orne, M. T. (1962). On the social psychology of the psychological experiment: With particular reference to demand characteristics and their implications. *American Psychologist, 17,* 776-783.

Orwell, G. (1949/1950). *1984.* New York: Harcourt, Brace.

Oscar-Berman, M., McNamara, P., & Freedman, M. (1991). Delayed response tasks: Parallels between experimental ablation studies and findings in patients with frontal lesions. In H. S. Levin, H. M. Eisenberg, & A. L. Benton (Eds.), *Frontal lobe function and dysfunction* (pp. 230-255). New York: Oxford University Press.

Osgood, C. E., Suci, G. J., & Tannenbaum, P. H. (1957). *The measurement of meaning.* Urbana, IL: University of Illinois Press.

Panksepp, J., Herman, B., Conner, R., Bishop, P., & Scott, J. P. (1978). The biology of social attachments: Opiates alleviate separation distress. *Biological Psychiatry, 13,* 607-618.

Park, P. (1973). Developmental ordering of experiences in alcoholism. *Quarterly Journal of Studies on Alcohol, 34,* 473-488.

Parker, D. A., & Harford, T. C. (1992). The epidemiology of alcohol consumption and dependence across occupations in the United States. *Alcohol Health & Research World, 16,* 97-105.

Parkinson, C. N. (1957). *Parkinson's law.* Boston: Houghton Mifflin.

Parsons, O. S. (1994). Neuropsychological measures and event-related potentials in alcoholics: Interrelationships, long-term reliabilities, and prediction of resumption of drinking. *Journal of Clinical Psychology, 50,* 37-46.

Patel, V. A., & Pohorecky, L.A. (1989). Acute and chronic ethanol treatment on beta-endorphin and catecholamine levels. *Alcohol, 6,* 59-63.

Paton, A. (1996). Thoughts on 'alcohol problems into the next century'. *Alcohol & Alcoholism, 31,* 231-234.

Pattison, E. M., Sobell, M. B., & Sobell, L. C. (1977). *Emerging concepts of alcohol dependence.* New York: Springer.

Paula-Barbosa, M. M., Brandão, F., Madeira, M. D., & Cadete-Leite, A. (1993). Structural changes in the hippocampal formation after long-term alcohol consumption and withdrawal in the rat. *Addiction, 88,* 237-247.

Pavlov, I. P. (1955). *Selected works.* (Edited under the supervision of Kh. S. Koshtoyants, translated by S. Belsky) Moscow: Foreign Languages Publishing House.

Pearlman, S., Zweben, A., & Li, S. (1989). The comparability of solicited versus clinic subjects in alcohol treatment research. *British Journal of Addiction, 84,* 523-532.

Peele, S. (1983, April). Through a glass darkly. *Psychology Today,* 38-42.

Peele, S. (1984, March/April). The new prohibitionists. *The Sciences,* 14-19.

Peele, S. (1985). *The meaning of addiction.* Lexington, MA: Lexington.

Peele, S. (1988). Can alcoholism and other drug addiction problems be treated away or is the current treatment binge doing more harm than good? *Journal of Psychoactive Drugs, 20,* 375-383.

Peele, S. (1989). *Diseasing of American.* Lexington, MA: Lexington.

Peele, S., & Brodsky, A. (with M. Arnold) (1991). *The truth about addiction and recovery: The life process program for outgrowing destructive habits.* New York: Simon & Schuster.

Peele, S. (1992). Alcoholism, politics, and bureaucracy: The consensus against controlled-drinking therapy in America. *Addictive Behaviors, 17,* 49-62.

Pendery, M. L. (1976). *Affidavit of Mary Pendery in support of motion to dismiss complaint.* United States District Court. Central District of California.

Pendery, M., & Maltzman, I. (1977). Instructions and the orienting reflex in "semantic conditioning" of the galvanic skin response in an innocuous situation. *Journal of Experimenal Psychology: General, 106,* 120-140.

Pendery, M. L., Maltzman, I. M., & West, L. J. (1982). Controlled drinking by alcoholics? New findings and a reevaluation of a major affirmative study. *Science, 217,* 169-175.

Perry, A. (1973). The effect of heredity on attitudes toward alcohol, cigarettes, and coffee. *Journal of Applied Psychology, 58,* 275-277.

Pettinati, H. M., Sugerman, A., & Maurer, H. S. (1982). Four year MMPI changes in abstinent and drinking alcoholics. *Alcoholism: Clinical and Experimental Research, 6,* 487-494.

Pettinati, H. M., Sugerman, A. A., DiDonato, N., & Maurer, H. S. (1982). The natural history of alcoholism over four years after treatment. *Journal of Studies on Alcohol, 43,* 201-215.

Phillips, R. O. (1995, July/August). Miller and Hester: Taking research to new heights, providing new insights. *The Counselor,* pp.14-15.

Phillips, S. C., & Craig, B. G. (1984). Alcohol withdrawal causes a loss of cerebellar Purkinje cells in mice. *Journal of Studies on Alcohol, 45,* 475-480.

Piazza, N. J., & Wise, S. L. (1988). An order-theoretic analysis of Jellinek's disease model of alcoholism. *International Journal of the Addictions, 23,* 387-397.

Piazza, N. J., Vrbka, J. L., & Yeager, R. D. (1989). Telescoping of alcoholism in women alcoholics. *International Journal of Addictions, 24,* 19-28.

Piazza, N. J., Peterson, J. S., Yates, J. W., & Sundgren, A. S. (1986). Progression of symptoms in women alcoholics: Comparison of Jellinek's model with two groups. *Psychological Reports, 56,* 367-370.

Pliner, P., & Cappell, H. (1974). Modification of affective consequences of alcohol: A comparison of social and solitary drinking. *Journal of Abnormal Psychology, 83,* 418-425.

Pokorny, A. D., & Kanas, T. E. (1980). Stages in the development of alcoholism. In W. E. Fann, I. Karacan, A. D. Pokorny, & R. L. Williams (Eds.), *Phenomenology and treatment of alcoholism* (pp.445-68). New York: Spectrum.

Pokorny, A., Kanas, T., & Overall, J. E. (1981). Order of appearance of alcohol symptoms. *Alcoholism: Clinical and Experimental Research, 5,* 216-220.

Poldrugo, F., & Snead III, O. C. (1984). Electroencephalographic and behavioral correlates in rats during repeated ethanol withdrawal syndromes. *Psychopharmacology, 83,* 140-146.

Polich, J. M., Armor, D. J., & Braiker, H. B. (1980). *The course of alcoholism: Four years after treatment.* Santa Monica, CA: Rand Corporation.

Polich, J. M., Armor, D. J., & Braiker, H. B. (1981). *The course of alcoholism: Four years after treatment.* New York: Wiley.

Porto, J. A. D., & Masur, J. (1984). The effects of alcohol, THC and diazepam in two different social settings. A study with human volunteers. *Research Communications in Psychology, Psychiatry and Behavior, 9,* 201-212.

Project MATCH Research Group (1993). Project MATCH: Rationale and methods for a multisite clinical trial matching patients to alcoholism treatment. *Alcoholism: Clinical and Experimental Research, 17,* 1130-1145.

Project MATCH Research Group (1997). Matching alcoholism treatments to client heterogeneity: Project MATCH posttreatment drinking outcomes. *Journal of Studies on Alcohol, 58,* 7-29.

Project MATCH Research Group (1998). Matching alcoholism treatments to client heterogeneity: Project MATCH three-year drinking outcomes. *Alcoholism: Clinical and Experimental Research, 22,* 1300-1311.

Prytula, R. E., Oster, G. D., & Davis, S. F. (1977). The "rat rabbit" problem: What did John B. Watson really do? *Teaching of Psychology, 4,* 444-445.

Raine, A. (1993). *The psychopathology of crime.* San Diego, CA: Academic Press.

Raine, A., & Lencz, T. (1993). Brain imaging research on electrodermal activity in humans. In J-C Roy, W. Boucsein, D. C. Fowles, & J. H. Gruzelier (Eds.), *Progress in electrodermal research* (pp. 115-135). New York: Plenum.

Raleigh, M. J., McGuire, M. T., Brammer, G. L., Pollack, D. B., & Yuwiler, A. (1991). Serotonergic mechanisms promote dominance acquisition in adult male vervet monkeys. *Brain Research, 559,* 181-190.

Rancurello, A. C. (1968). *A study of Franz Brentano.* New York: Academic Press.

Rankin, H., Hodgson, R., & Stockwell, T. (1979). The concept of craving and its measurement. *Behaviour Research and Therapy, 17,* 389-396.

Razran, G. (1961). The observable unconscious and the inferable conscious in current Soviet psychophysiology: Interoceptive conditioning, semantic conditioning, and the orienting reflex. *Psychological Review, 68,* 81-147.

Reichenbach, H. (1938). *Experience and prediction.* Chicago: University of Chicago Press.

Reznek, L. (1987). *The nature of disease.* London: Routledge & Kegan Paul.

Resnick, H. S., Yehuda, R., Pitman, R. K., & Foy, D. W. (1995). Effect of previous trauma on acute plasma cortisol level following rape. *American Journal of Psychiatry, 152,* 1675-1677.

Richards, R. J. (1992). *The meaning of evolution: The morphological construction and ideological reconstruction of Darwin's theory.* Chicago: The University of Chicago Press.

Richards, R. J.(1993). Ideology and the history of science. *Biology and Philosophy, 8,* 103-108.

Rilke, O., May, T., Oehler, J., & Wolffgramm, J. (1995). Influences of housing conditions and ethanol intake on binding characteristics of D2, 5-HT1A, and benzodiazepine receptors of rats. *Pharmacology Biochemistry and Behavior, 52,* 23-28.

Riley, D. R., Sobell, L. C., Leo, G. I., Sobell, M. B., & Klajner, F. (1987). Behavioral treatment of alcohol problems: A review and a comparison of behavioral and nonbehavioral studies. In M. W. Cox (Ed.), *Treatment and prevention of alcohol problems: A resource manual* (pp. 73-115). New York: Academic Press.

Roberts, A. J., Chu, H-P., Crabbe, J. C., & Keith, L. D. Differential modulation by the stress axis of ethanol withdrawal seizure expression in WSP and WSR mice. *Alcoholism: Clinical and Experimental Research, 15,* 412-417.

Robertson, I., Heather, N., Dzialdowski, A., Crawford, J., & Winton, M. (1986). A comparison of minimal versus intensive controlled drinking treatment interventions for problem drinkers. *British Journal of Clinical Psychology, 25,* 185-194.

Robinson, T. E., & Berridge, K. C. (1993). The neural basis of drug craving: An incentive-sensitization theory of addiction. *Brain Research Reviews, 18,* 247-291.

Roediger, III., J. L., Capaldi, E.D., Paris, S. G., & Polivy, J. (1991).*Psychology.* 3rd.ed. New York: HarperCollins.

Roehrs, T., Zwyghuizen-Doorenbos, A., Knox, M., Moskowitz, H., & Roth, T. (1992). Sedating effects of ethanol and time of drinking. *Alcoholism: Clinical and Experimental Research, 16,* 553-557.

Roizen, R. (1987). The great controlled-drinking controversy. In M. Galanter (Ed.), *Recent developments in alcoholism: Vol. 5* (pp. 245-279). New York: Plenum.

Rokeach, M., & Ball-Rokeach, S. J. (1989). Stability and change in American value priorities, 1968-1981. *American Psychologist, 44,* 775-784.

Ron, M. A. (1984). Brain damage in chronic alcoholism. In N. Krasner, J. S. Madden, & R. J. Walker (Eds.), *Alcohol related problems: Room for manoeuvre* (pp. 243-249). Chichester: Wiley.

Rosch, E. H. (1973). Natural categories. *Cognitive Psychology, 4,* 328-350.

Rosch, E. & Mervis, C. B. (1975). Family resemblances: Studies in the internal structure of categories. *Cognitive Psychology, 7,* 573-605.

374

Rosen, J. B., & Schulkin, J. (1998). From normal fear to pathological anxiety. *Psychological Review, 105,* 325-350.

Rosenthal, R. (1994). Science and ethics in conducting, analyzing, and reporting psychological research. *Psychological Science, 5,* 127-134.

Rosenthal, R. (1995). Ethical issues in psychological science: Risk, consent, and scientific quality. *Psychological Science, 6,* 322-323.

Ross, D. F., & Pihl, R. O. (1989). Modification of the balanced placebo design for use at high blood alcohol levels. *Addictive Behaviors, 14,* 91-97.

Rotgers, F. (1996a, September/October). Empowering clients with respect to drinking goals. *The Counselor,* 33-36.

Rotgers, F. (1996b). Book Review. *Handbook of alcoholism treatment approaches: Effective alternatives.* 2nd ed. by Reid K. Hester and William R. Miller (Eds.). Boston: Allyn and Bacon, 1995, 307 + xx pages. *Journal of Studies on Alcohol, 57,* 101-102.

Rusinov, V. S. (1973). *The dominant focus..* New York: Consultants Bureau.

Rychtarik, R. G., Foy, D. W., Scott, T., Lokey, L., & Prue, D. M. (1987). Five- to six-year follow-up of broad-spectrum behavioral treatment for alcoholism: Effects of training controlled drinking skills. *Journal of Consulting and Clinical Psychology, 55,* 106-108.

Ryle, G. (1949). *The concept of mind.* New York: Barnes & Noble.

Salamone, J. D. (1994). The involvement of nucleus accumbens dopamine in appetitive and aversive motivation. *Behavioural Brain Research, 61,* 117-133.

Samelson, F. (1980). J. B. Watson's little Albert, Cyril Burt's twins, and the need for a critical science. *American Psychologist, 35,* 619-625.

Sanchez-Craig, M. (1980). Random assignment to abstinence or controlled drinking in a cognitive-behavioral program: Short-term effects on drinking behavior. *Addictive Behaviors, 5,* 35-39.

Sanchez-Craig, M. (1986). How much is too much? Estimates of hazardous drinking based on clients' self-reports. *British Journal of Addiction, 81,* 251-256.

Sanchez-Craig, M., Wilkinson, A., & Davila, R. (1995). Empirically based guidelines for moderate drinking: 1-Year results from three studies with problem drinkers. *American Journal of Public Health, 85,* 823-828.

Sanchez-Craig, M., Annis, H. M., Bornet, A. R., & MacDonald, K. R. (1984). Random assignment to abstinence and controlled drinking: Evaluation of a cognitive-behavioral program for problem drinkers. *Journal of Consulting and Clinical Psychology, 52,* 390-403.

Sannibale, C., & Hall, W. (1998). An evaluation of Cloninger's typology of alcohol abuse. *Addiction, 93,* 1241-1249.

Sapolsky, R. M. (1993). Glucocorticoid neurotoxicity: Is this effect relevant to alcoholic neurotoxicity? In S. Zakhari (Ed.), *Alcohol and the endocrine system* (pp. 271-280). NIAAA Research Monograph No. 22. NIH Publication No. 93-3549. Rockville, MD: U. S. Department of Health and Human Services.

Sapolsky, R. M., Krey, L. C., & McEwen, B. S. (1985). Prolonged glucocorticoid exposure reduces hippocampal neuron number: Implications for aging. *The Journal of Neuroscience, 5,* 1221-1227.

Sayette, M. A., Breslin, F. C., Wilson, G. T., & Rosenblum, G. D. (1994). An evaluation of the balanced placebo design in alcohol administration research. *Addictive Behaviors, 19,* 333-342.

Schaler, J. A. (1990). Alcoholism, disease, and myth. *Skeptical Inquirer, 14,* 198-201.

Schall, M., Kemeny, A., & Maltzman, I. (1992). Factors associated with alcohol use in university students. *Journal of Studies on Alcohol, 53,* 122-136.

Schandler, S. L., Brannock, J. C., Cohen, M. J., & Mendez, J. (1993). Spatial learning deficits in adolescent children of alcoholics. *Experimental and Clinical Psychopharmacology,1,* 207-214.

Schmahmann, J. D. (Ed.) (1997). *The cerebellum and cognition.* San Diego, CA: Academic Press.

Schore, A. N. (1994). *Affect regulation and the origin of the self: The neurobiology of emotional development.* Hillsdale, NJ: Erlbaum.

Schuckit, M. A. (1994). Low level of response to alcohol as a predictor of future alcoholism. *American Journal of Psychiatry, 151,* 184-189.

Schuckit, M. A. (1998). Biological, psychological and environmental predictors of the alcoholism risk: A longitudinal study. *Journal of Studies on Alcohol, 59,* 485-494.

Schuckit, M. A., & Smith, T. L. (1996). An 8-year follow-up of 450 sons of alcoholic and control subjects. *Archives of General Psychiatry, 53,* 202-210.

Schuckit, M. A., Gold, E. O., & Risch, S. C. (1987). Plasma cortisol levels following ethanol in sons of alcoholics and controls. *Archives of General Psychiatry, 44,* 942-943.

Schuckit, M. A., Risch, S. C., & Gold, E. O. (1988). Alcohol consumption, ACTH level, and family history of alcoholism. *American Journal of Psychiatry, 145,* 1391-1395.

Schuckit, M., Smith, T. L., Anthenelli, R., & Irwin, M. (1993). Clinical course of alcoholism in 636 male inpatients. *American Journal of Psychiatry, 150,* 786-792.

Schuckit, M. A., Tipp, J. E., Smith, T. L., & Bucholz, K. K. (1997). Periods of abstinence following the onset of alcohol dependence in 1,853 men and women. *Journal of Studies on Alcohol, 58,* 581-589.

Schuckit, M. A., Tsuang, J. W., Anthenelli, R. M., Tipp, J. E., & Nurnberger, J. I., Jr. (1996). Alcohol challenges in young men from alcoholic pedigrees and control families: A report from the COGA project. *Journal of Studies on Alcohol, 57,* 368-377.

Schuckit, M. A., Smith, T. L., Daeppen, J-B., Eng, M., Li, T-K., Hesselbrock, V. M., Nurnberger, J. I., Jr., & Bucholz, K. K. (1998). Clinical relevance of the distinction between alcohol dependence with and without a physiological component. *American Journal of Psychiatry, 155,* 733-740.

Schultz, W., Dayan, P., & Montague, P. R. (1997). A neural substrate of prediction and reward. *Science, 275,* 1593-1599.

Schwartz, J. M., Stoessel, P. W., Baxter, L. R., Martin, K. M., & Phelps, M. E. (1996). Systematic changes in cerebral glucose metabolic rate after successful behavior modification treatment of obsessive-compulsive disorder. *Archives of General Psychiatry, 53,* 109-113.

Searles, J. S. (1993). Science and fascism: Confronting unpopular ideas. *Addictive Behaviors, 18,* 5-8.

Segal, B. (1987). Forward. In M. B. Sobell, & L. C. Sobell (Eds.), *Moderation as a goal or outcome of treatment for alcohol problems: A dialogue* (pp. xi-xiii). New York: Haworth.

Seligman, M. E. P. (1995). The effectiveness of psychotherapy. *American Psychologist, 50,* 965-974.

Seligman, M. E. P. (1996). Science as an ally of practice. *American Psychologist, 51,* 1072-1088.

Selvaggio, K. (1983, November). WHO bottles up alcohol study. *Multinational Monitor,* 9-16.

Selzer, M. L., Vinokur, A., & van Rooijen, L., (1975). A self-administered short Michigan Alcoholism Screening Test (SMAST), *Journal of Studies on Alcohol, 36,* 117-126.

Senter, R. J., & Richman, C. L. (1969). Induced consumption of high-concentration ethanol solution in rats. *Quarterly Journal of Studies on Alcohol, 30,* 330-335.

Shapere, D. (1964). The structure of scientific revolutions. *Philosophical Review, 73,* 383-394.

Shear, P. K., Jerrigan, T. L., & Butters, N. (1994). Volumetric magnetic resonance imaging quantification of longitudinal brain changes in abstinent alcoholics. *Alcoholism: Clinical and Experimental Research, 18,* 172-176.

Sher, K. J. (1985) Subjective effects of alcohol: The influence of setting and individual differences in alcohol expectancies. *Journal of Studies on Alcohol, 46,* 137-146.

Shiffman, S., Hickox, M., Paty, J. A., Gnys, M., Kassel, J. D., & Richards, T. J. (1997). The abstinence violation effect following smoking lapses and temptations. *Cognitive Therapy and Research, 21,* 497-522.

Siegfried, B., Netto, C. A., & Izquierdo, I. (1987). Exposure to novelty induces naltrexone-reversible analgesia in rats. *Behavioral Neuroscience, 101,* 436-438.

Sigvardsson, S., Bohman, M., & Cloninger, C. R. (1996). Replication of the Stockholm adoption study of alcoholism. *Archives of General Psychiatry, 53,* 681-687.

Simpson, G. G. (1961). *Principles of animal taxonomy.* New York: Columbia University Press.

Sinclair, J. D., & Senter, R. J. (1968). Development of an alcohol-deprivation effect in rats. *Quarterly Journal of Studies on Alcohol, 29,* 863-867.

Skinner, B. F. (1938). *The behavior of organisms.* New York: Appleton-Century-Crofts.

Skinner, B. F. (1976). *About behaviorism.* New York: Vintage Books.

Skinner, B. F. (1987, July/August). A humanist alternative to A.A.'s twelve steps: A human-centered approach to conquering alcoholism. *Humanist, 47,* 5.

Skinner, H. A., & Horn, J. L. (1984). *Alcohol dependence scale (ADS): Users Guide.* Toronto: Addiction Research Foundation.

Smith, D. I. (1983). Evaluation of an inpatient alcohol rehabilitation programme. *Drug and Alcohol Dependence, 11,* 333-352.

Smith, D. I. (1985a). The criminal justice system and alcohol rehabilitation: A pilot evaluation study. *Australian and New Zealand Criminology, 18,* 206-214.

Smith, D. I. (1985b). Evaluation of a residential AA programme for women. *Alcohol & Alcoholism, 20,* 315-327.

Smith, D. I. (1986). Evaluation of a residential AA program. *The International Journal of the Addictions, 21,* 33-49.

Smith, E. L. P., Coplan, J. D., Trost, R. C., Scharf, B. A., & Rosenblum, L.A. (1997). Neurobiological alterations in adult nonhuman primates exposed to unpredictable early rearing. In R. Yehuda & A.

C. McFarlane (Eds.), Psychobiology of posttraumatic stress disorder (pp. 545-548). *Annals of the NY Academy of Sciences, 821.* New York: New York Academy of Sciences.

Smith, J. W. (1980). Abstinence-oriented alcoholism treatment approaches. In J. M. Ferguson & C. B. Taylor (Eds.), *The comprehensive handbook of behavioral medicine. Vol 3* (pp. 223-236). New York: Spectrum.

Smith, J. W. (1994). Relevant biological factors in the etiology and treatment of alcohol misuse and abuse. In G. S. Howard & P. E. Nathan (Eds.), *Alcohol use and misuse by young adults* (pp.25-40). Notre Dame, IN: University of Notre Dame Press.

Smith, J. W., & Frawley, P. J. (1993). Treatment outcome of 600 chemically dependent patients treated in a multimodal inpatient program including aversion therapy and pentothal interviews. *Journal of Substance Abuse Treatment, 10,* 359-369.

Smith, J. W., Frawley, P. J., & Polissar, L. (1991). Six- and twelve-month abstinence rates in inpatient alcoholics treated with aversion therapy compared with matched inpatients from a treatment registry. *Alcoholism: Clinical and Experimental Research, 15,* 862-870.

Smith, J. W., Frawley, P. J., & Polissar, N. L. (1997). Six- and twelve-month abstinence rates in inpatient alcoholics treated with either faradic aversion or chemical aversion compared with matched inpatients from a treatment registry. *Journal of Addictive Diseases, 16,* 5-24.

Sobell, L. C. (1987). Introduction. *Advances in Behaviour Research and Therapy, 9,* 53-58.

Sobell, L. C., Cunningham, J. A., & Sobell, M. B. (1996). Recovery from alcohol problems with and without treatment: Prevalence in two populations surveys. *American Journal of Public Health, 86,* 966-972.

Sobell, L. C., Maisto, S. A., Sobell, M. B., & Cooper, A. M. (1979). Reliability of alcohol abuser's self-reports of drinking behavior. *Behaviour Research and Therapy, 17,* 157-160.

Sobell, L. C., Sobell, M. B., Maisto, S. A., & Cooper, A. M. (1985). Time-line follow-back assessment method. In D. J. Lettieri, J. E. Nelson, & M. A. Sayers (Eds.), *NIAAA Treatment Handbook Series, 2. Alcoholism treatment assessment research instruments* (pp. 530-534). Rockville, MD.: National Institute on Alcohol Abuse and Alcoholism.

Sobell, M. B. (1978). Alternatives to abstinence: Evidence, issues and some proposals. In P. E. Nathan, G. A. Marlatt, & T. Loberg (Eds.), *Alcoholism: New directions in behavioral research and treatment* (pp. 177-209). New York: Plenum.

Sobell, M. B. (1987). Behavioral research: The particularly unwanted child of conventional wisdom in the alcohol field. *Advances in Behaviour Research and Therapy, 9,* 59-72.

Sobell, M. B., & Sobell, L. C. (1972). Individualized behavior therapy for alcoholics: Rationale, procedures, preliminary results and appendix. *California Mental Health Research Monograph, No. 13.* Sacramento, CA: Department of Mental Hygiene.

Sobell, M. B., & Sobell, L. C. (1973a). Alcoholics treated by individualized behavior therapy: One year treatment outcome. *Behaviour Research and Therapy, 11,* 599-618.

Sobell, M. B., & Sobell, L. C. (1973b). Individualized behavior therapy for alcoholics. *Behavior Therapy, 4,* 49-72.

Sobell, M. B., & Sobell, L. C. (1975). The need for realism, relevance and operational assumptions in the study of substance dependence. In H. D. Cappell & A. E. LeBlanc (Eds.), *Biological and behavioural approaches to drug dependence* (pp.133-167). Toronto: Addiction Research Foundation.

Sobell, M. B., & Sobell, L. C. (1976). Second year treatment outcome of alcoholics treated by individualized behavior therapy: Results. *Behaviour Research and Therapy, 14,* 195-215.

Sobell, M. B., & Sobell, L. C. (1978). *Behavioral treatment of alcohol problems: Individualized therapy and controlled drinking.* New York: Plenum.

Sobell, M. B., & Sobell, L. C. (1984a). The aftermath of heresy: A response to Pendery et al.'s (1982) critique of "individualized behavior therapy for alcoholics." *Behaviour Research and Therapy, 22,* 413-440.

Sobell, M. B., & Sobell, L. C. (1984b). Under the microscope yet again: A commentary on Walker and Roach's critique of the Dickens Committee's enquiry into our research. *British Journal of Addiction, 79,* 157-168.

Sobell, M. B., & Sobell, L. C. (1987a). Conceptual issues regarding goals in the treatment of alcohol problems. In M. B. Sobell & L. C. Sobell (Eds.), *Moderation as a goal or outcome of treatment for alcohol problems: A dialogue* (pp.1-37). New York: Haworth.

Sobell, M. B., & Sobell, L. C. (1987b). Stalking white elephants. *British Journal of Addiction, 82,* 245-247.

Sobell, M. B., & Sobell, L. C. (1989). Moratorium on Maltzman: An appeal to reason. *Journal of Studies on Alcohol, 50,* 473-480.

Sobell, M. B., & Sobell, L. C. (1993). *Problem drinkers: Guided self-change treatment.* New York: Guilford.

Sobell, M. B., & Sobell, L. C. (1995a). Controlled drinking after 25 years: How important was the great debate? (Editorial). *Addiction, 90,* 1149-1153.

Sobell, M. B., & Sobell, L. C. (1995b). Moderation, public health and paternalism. *Addiction, 90,* 1175-1177.

Sokolov, E. N. (1960). Neuronal models and the orienting reflex. In M. A. B. Brazier (Ed.), *The central nervous system and behavior* (pp.187-276). New York: Josiah Macy, Jr. Foundation.

Sokolov, E. N. (1963). *Perception and the conditioned reflex.* New York: Macmillan.

Sonnenstuhl, W. J. (1996). *Working sober.* Ithaca, NY: Cornell University Press.

Spinrad, S. (1993). The use of antabuse as an adjunct to alcoholism treatment: A focus on patient compliance. Unpublished Doctoral Dissertation. University of California, Los Angeles.

Starkstein, S. E., & Robinson, R. G. (1997). Mechanism of disinhibition after brain lesion. *The Journal of Nervous and Mental Disease, 185,* 108-114.

Stewart, R. B., & Grupp, L. A. (1985). Some determinants of the motivational properties of ethanol in the rat: Concurrent administration of food or social stimuli. *Psychopharmacology, 87,* 43-50.

Stewart, R. B., Gatto, G. J., Lumeng, L., Li, T-K., & Murphy, J. M. (1993). Comparison of alcohol-preferring (P) and nonpreferring (NP) rats on tests of anxiety and for the anxiolytic effects of ethanol. *Alcohol, 10,* 1-10.

Stewart, S. H. (1996). Alcohol abuse in individuals exposed to trauma: A critical review. *Psychological Bulletin, 120,* 83-112.

Stimmel, B., Cohen, M., Sturiano, V., Hanbury, R., Kortis, D., & Jackson, G. (1983). Is treatment of alcoholism effective in persons on methadone maintenance? *American Journal of Psychiatry,140,* 862-866.

Stinchfield, R., & Owen, P. (1998). Hazelden's model of treatment and its outcome. *Addictive Behaviors, 23,* 669-683.

Stockwell, T., Murphy, D., & Hodgson, R. (1983). The severity of alcohol dependence questionnaire: its use, reliability and validity. *British Journal of Addiction, 78,* 145-155.

Stockwell, T. R., Hodgson, R. J., Rankin, H. J., & Taylor, C. (1982). Alcohol dependence, beliefs and the priming effect. *Behavioural Research and Therapy, 20,* 513-522.

Stockwell, T., Hodgson, R., Edwards, G., Taylor, C., & Rankin, H. (1979). The development of a questionnaire to measure severity of alcohol dependence. *British Journal of Addiction, 74,* 79-87.

Straus, R., & Bacon, D. (1953). *Drinking in college.* New Haven, CT: Yale University Press.

Streissguth, A. P., Sampson, P. D., Olson, H. C., Bookstein, F. L., Barr, H. M., Scott, M., Feldman, J., & Mirsky, A. F. (1994). Maternal drinking during pregnancy: Attention and short-term memory in 14-year-old offspring - a longitudinal prospective study. *Alcoholism: Clinical and Experimental Research, 18,* 202-218.

Stuss, D. T., & Benson, D. F. (1984). Neuropsychological studies of the frontal lobes. *Psychological Bulletin, 95,* 3-28.

Stuss, D. T. & Benson, D. F. (1986). *The frontal lobes.* New York: Raven.

Stuss, D. T., Gow, C. A., & Hetherington, C. R. (1992). "No longer Gage": Frontal lobe dysfunction and emotional changes. *Journal of Consulting and Clinical Psychology, 60,* 349-359.

Suddath, R. L., Christison, G. W., Torrey, E. F., Casanova, M. F., & Weinberger, D. R. (1990). Anatomical abnormalities in the brains of monozygotic twins discordant for schizophrenia. *The New England Journal of Medicine, 322,* 789-794.

Sullivan, J. L., Baenziger, J. C., Wagner, D. L., Rauscher, F. P., Nurnberger, J. I., Jr., & Holmes, J. S. (1990). Platelet MAO in subtypes of alcoholism. *Biological Psychiatry, 27,* 911-922.

Sullivan, P. F., Fifield, W., Kennedy, M. A., Mulder, R. T., Sellman, J. D., & Joyce, P. R. (1998). No association between novelty seeking and the type 4 dopamine receptor gene (DRD4) in two New Zealand samples. *American Journal of Psychiatry, 155,* 98-101.

Susser, M. (1989). The challenge of causality: Human nutrition, brain development and mental performance. *Bulletin of the New York Academy of Medicine, 65,* 1032-1049.

Susser, M., Neugebauer, R., Hoek, H. W., Brown, A. S., Lin, S., Labovitz, D., & Gorman, J. M. (1996). Schizophrenia after prenatal famine. *Archives of General Psychiatry, 53,* 25-31.

Szasz, T. S. (1972). Bad habits are not diseases: A refutation of the claim that alcoholism is a disease. *The Lancet, 2,* 83-84.

Tangney, J. P. (1987). Fraud will out - or will it? *New Scientist, 115,* 62-63.

378

Taylor, J. R. (1987). Controlled drinking studies: Methodological issues. In M. B. Sobell & L. C. Sobell (Eds.), *Moderation as a goal or outcome of treatment for alcohol problems: A dialogue* (pp. 83-107). New York: Haworth.

Taylor, J. R., Helzer, J. E., & Robins, L. N. (1986). Moderate drinking in ex-alcoholics: Recent studies. *Journal of Studies on Alcohol, 47,* 116-121.

Tershner, S. A., & Helmstetter, F. J. (1996). Injections of corticotropin-releasing factor into the periaqueductal gray enhance Pavlovian fear conditioning. *Psychobiology, 24,* 49-56.

Tey, J. (1951). *The daughter of time.* New York: Macmillan.

Thiagarajan, A. B., Mefford, I. N., & Eskay, R. L. (1989). Single-dose ethanol administration activates the hypothalamic-pituitary-adrenal axis: Exploration of the mechanism of action. *Neuroendocrinology, 50,* 427-432.

Thomasson, H. R., & Li, T-K. (1993). How alcohol and aldehyde dehydrogenase genes modify alcohol drinking, alcohol flushing, and the risk for alcoholism. *Alcohol Health & Research World, 17,* 167-172.

Thombs, D. L. (1994). *Introduction to addictive behaviors.* New York: Guilford.

Thompson, R. F. (1994). Behaviorism and neuroscience. *Psychological Review, 101,* 259-265.

Thomsen, R. (1975). *Bill W.* New York: Harper & Row.

Tiihonen, J., Kuikka, J., Hakola, P., Paanila, J., Airaksinen, J., Eronen, M., & Hallikainen, T. (1994). Acute ethanol-induced changes in cerebral blood flow. *American Journal of Psychiatry, 151,* 1505-1508.

Tolman, E.C. (1925a/1951). Behaviorism and purpose. In *Collected papers in psychology* (pp. 32-37). Berkeley, CA: University of California Press.

Tolman, E. C. (1925b/1951). Purpose and cognition: The determiners of animal learning. In *Collected papers in psychology* (pp.38-47). Berkeley, CA: University of California Press.

Tolman, E. C. (1932). *Purposive behavior in animals and men.* New York: Appleton-Century-Crofts.

Tolman, E. C. (1935/1951). Psychology versus immediate experience. In *Collected papers in psychology* (pp. 94-114). Berkeley, CA: University of California Press.

Toulmin, S. E. (1970). Does the distinction between normal and revolutionary science hold water? In I. Lakatos & A. Musgrave (Eds.), *Criticism and the growth of knowledge* (pp. 39-47). London: Cambridge University Press.

Trachtenberg, R. L. (1984). *Report of the Steering Group to the Administrator Alcohol, Drug Abuse, and Mental Health Administration Regarding its Attempts to Investigate Allegations of Scientific Misconduct Concerning Drs. Mark and Linda Sobell.* Rockville, MD: Alcohol, Drug Abuse, and Mental Health Administration.

Tsai, G., Gastfriend, D. R., & Coyle, J. T. (1995). The glutamatergic basis of human alcoholism. *American Journal of Psychiatry, 152,* 332-340.

Turner, C. F., Ku, L., Rogers, S. M., Lindberg, L. D., Pleck, J. H., & Sonenstein, F. L. (1998). Adolescent sexual behavior, drug use, and violence: Increased reporting with computer survey technology. *Science, 280,* 867-873.

Ullman, A. D. (1953). The first drinking experience of addictive and of "normal" drinkers. *Quarterly Journal of Studies on Alcohol, 14,* 181-191.

Valenstein, E. S. (1986). *Great and desperate cures.* New York: Basic Books.

Vaillant, G. M. (1995). *The natural history of alcoholism revisited.* Cambridge, MA: Harvard University Press.

Veatch, L. M., & Gonzalez, L. P. (1996). Repeated ethanol withdrawal produces site-dependent increases in EEG spiking. *Alcoholism: Clinical and Experimental Research, 20,* 262-267.

Venables, P. Maternal exposure to influenza in pregnancy and electrodermal activity: A further study from Mauritius. *Psychophysiology, 35,* 438-442.

Virkkunen, M., Rawlings, R., Tokola, R., Poland, R. E., Guidotti, A., Nemeroff, C., Bissette, G., Kalogeras, K., Karonen, S-L., & Linnoila, M. (1994). CSF biochemistries, glucose metabolism, and diurnal activity rhythms in alcoholic, violent offenders, fire setters, and healthy volunteers. *Archives of General Psychiatry, 51,* 20-27.

Vitz, P. C. (1990). The use of stories in moral development. *American Psychologist, 45,* 709-720.

Vogler, R. E., Lunde, S. E., Johnson, G. R., & Martin, P. L. (1970). Electrical aversion conditioning with chronic alcoholics. *Journal of Consulting and Clinical Psychology, 34,* 302-307.

Volkow, N. D., Hitzemann, R., Wang, G-J., Fowler, J. S., Burr, G., Pascani, K., Dewey, S. L., & Wolf, A. P. (1992). Decreased brain metabolism in neurologically intact healthy alcoholics. *American Journal of Psychiatry, 149,* 1016-1022.

Volpicelli, J. R. (1987). Uncontrollable events and alcohol drinking. *British Journal of Addiction, 82*, 381-392.

Volpicelli, J. R., & Ulm, R. R. (1990). The influence of control over appetitive and aversive events on alcohol preference in rats. *Alcohol, 7*, 133-136.

Volpicelli, J. R., Alterman, A. I., Hayashida, M. & O'Brien, C. P. (1992). Naltrexone in the treatment of alcohol dependence. *Archives of General Psychiatry, 49*, 876-880.

Walker, D. W., Barnes, D. E., Zornetzer, S. F., Hunter, B. E., & Kubanis, P. (1980). Neuronal loss in hippocampus induced by prolonged ethanol consumption in rats. *Science, 209*, 711-712.

Walker, K. D., & Roach, C. A. (1984). A critique of the report of the Dickens' enquiry into the controlled drinking research of the Sobells. *British Journal of Addiction, 79*, 147-156.

Walker, N. D. (1987). Long term outcome for alcoholic patients treated in a hospital based unit. *New Zealand Medical Journal, 1000*, 554-556.

Wallace, J. (1989a) *Writings: The alcoholism papers*. Newport, RI: Edgehill Publications.

Wallace, J. (1989b). Can Stanton Peele's opinions be taken seriously? A reply to Peele. *Journal of Psychoactive Drugs, 21*, 259-271.

Wallace, J. (1990). Controlled drinking, treatment effectiveness, and the disease model of addiction: A commentary on the ideological wishes of Stanton Peele. *Journal of Psychoactive Drugs, 22*, 261-284.

Wallace, J., McNeill, D., Gilfillan, D., MacLeon, K., & Fanella, F. I. (1988). Six-month treatment outcomes in socially stable alcoholics: Abstinence rates. *Journal of Substance Abuse Treatment, 5*, 247-252.

Wallace, P., Cutler, S., & Haines, A. (1988). Randomised controlled trial of general practitioner intervention in patients with excessive alcohol consumption. *British Medical Journal, 297*, 663-668.

Walsh, D. C., Hingson, R. W., Merrigan, D. M., Levenson, S. M., Cupples, A., Herren, T., Coffman, G. A., Becker, C. A., Barker, T. A., Hamilton, S. K., McGuire, T. G., & Kelly, C.A. (1991). A randomized trial of treatment options for alcohol-abusing workers. *The New England Journal of Medicine, 325*, 775-806.

Wand, G. S., Mangold, D., El Deiry, S., McCaul, M. E., & Hoover, D. (1998). Family history of alcoholism and hypothalamic opioidergic activity. *Archives of General Psychiatry, 55*, 1114-1119.

Watson, J. B. (1913). Psychology as the behaviorist views it. *Psychological Review, 20*, 158-177.

Watson, J. B. (1916). Behavior and the concept of mental disease. *Journal of Philosophy Psychology and Scientific Method, 13*, 589-597.

Watson, J. B. (1930). *Behaviorism*. Chicago: University of Chicago Press.

Watson, J. B., & Raynor, R. (1920). Conditioned emotional reactions. *Journal of Experimental Psychology, 3*, 1-13.

Watson, R. R., & Watzl, B. (1992). *Nutrition and alcohol*. Boca Raton, LA: CRC.

Webster's New World Dictionary (1984) 2nd. Abbreviated Edition. New York: Simon & Schuster.

Wechsler, H., Dowdall, G. W., Davenport, A., & Castillo, S. (1995). Correlates of college student binge drinking. *American Journal of Public Health, 85*, 921-926.

Wechsler, H., Davenport, A., Dowdall, G., Moeykens, B., & Castillo, S. (1994). Health and behavioral consequences of binge drinking in college: A national survey of students at 140 campuses. *Journal of the American Medical Association, 272*, 1672-1677.

Weinberg, J., Taylor, A. N., & Gianoulakis, C. (1996). Fetal ethanol exposure: Hypothalamic-pituitary-adrenal and ß-endorphin responses to repeated stress. *Alcoholism: Clinical and Experimental Research, 20*, 122-131.

Weinberger, D. R., Berman, K. P., & Zec, R. F. (1986). Physiologic dysfunction of dorsolateral prefrontal cortex in schizophrenia. *Archives of General Psychiatry, 43*, 114-124.

Weisman, C. P. (1994). Factors affecting severity of alcohol withdrawal. Unpublished doctoral dissertation. University of California, Los Angeles.

Welte, J. W., Lyons, J. P., & Sokolow, L. (1983). Relapse rates for former clients of alcoholism rehabilitation units who are drinking without symptoms. *Drug and Alcohol Dependence, 12*, 25-29.

Werner, E. E. (1986). Resilient offspring of alcoholics: A longitudinal study from birth to age 18. *Journal of Studies on Alcohol, 47*, 34-40.

Whitbeck, C. (1977). Causation in medicine: The disease entity model. *Philosophy of Science, 44*, 619-637.

Whitehead, P. C., & Simpkins, J. (1983). Occupational factors in alcoholism. In B. Kissin & H. Begleiter (Eds.), *The biology of alcoholism, Vol. 6. The pathogenesis of alcoholism: Psychosocial factors* (pp. 406-553). New York: Plenum.

Wigmore, S. W., & Hinson, R. E. (1991). The influence of setting on consumption in the balanced placebo design. *British Journal of Addiction, 86,* 205-215.

Wilkinson, D.A., & Sanchez-Craig, M. (1981). Relevance of brain dysfunction to treatment objectives: Should alcohol-related cognitive deficits influence the way we think about treatment? *Addictive Behaviors, 6,* 253-260.

Williams, A. F. (1967). Validation of college problem-drinking scale. *Journal of Projective Techniques and Personality Assessment, 31,* 33-40.

Williams, C. L., & Perry, C. L. (1998). Lessons from project Northland. *Alcohol Health & Research World, 22,* 107-116.

Williams, C. L., Perry, C. L., Farbakhsh, K., & Veblen-Moftenson, S. (1999). Project Northland: Comprehensive alcohol use prevention for young adolescents, their parents, schools, peers and communities. *Journal of Studies on Alcohol, Supplement No. 13,* 112-124

Williams, J. B. W., Gibbon, M., First, M. B., Spitzer, R. L., Davies, M., Borus, J., Howes, M. J., Kane, J., Pope, H. G., Jr., Rounsaville, B., & Wittchen, H-U. (1992). The structured clinical interview for DSM-III-R (SCID). II. Multisite test-retest reliability. *Archives of General Psychiatry, 49,* 630-636.

Wilson, G. T. (1978). Alcoholism and aversion therapy: Issues, ethics and evidence. In G. A. Marlatt & P. E. Nathan (Eds.), *Behavioral approaches to alcoholism* (pp. 90-113). New Brunswick, NJ: Rutgers Center of Alcohol Studies.

Wilson, J. Q., & Herrnstein, R.J. *Crime and human nature.* New York: Simon & Schuster.

Wingard, J. A., & Maltzman, I. (1980). Interest as a predeterminer of the GSR index of the orienting reflex. *Acta Psychologica, 46,* 153-160.

Winokur, G., Rimmer, J., & Reich, T. (1971). Alcoholism IV: Is there more than one type of alcoholism? *British Journal of Psychiatry, 118,* 515-531.

Wise, R.A., & Bozarth, M. A. (1987). A psychomotor stimulant theory of addiction. *Psychological Review, 94,* 469-492.

Wittgenstein, L. (1953). *Philosophical investigations.* Oxford: Basil Blackwell.

Wolff, P. H. (1972). Ethnic differences in alcohol sensitivity. *Science, 175,* 449-450.

Wolffgramm, J. (1991). An ethopharmacological approach to the development of drug addiction. *Neuroscience & Biobehavoral Reviews, 15,* 515-519.

Wolffgramm, J., & Heyne, A. (1991). Social behavior, dominance and social deprivation of rats determine drug choice. *Pharmacology Biochemistry & Behavior, 38,* 389-399.

Wolffgramm, J., & Heyne, A. (1995). From controlled drug intake to loss of control: the irreversible development of drug addiction in the rat. *Behavioural Brain Research, 70,* 77-94.

Wolin, S., Bennett, L. A., Noonan, D. L. & Teitelbaum, M. A. (1980). Disrupted family rituals: A factor in the intergenerational transmission of alcoholism. *Journal of Studies on Alcohol, 41,* 199-214.

Wolpe, J. *Psychotherapy by reciprocal inhibition.* Stanford, CA:Stanford University Press.

Wortman, C. B., Loftus, E. F., & Marshall, M. E. (1988). *Psychology* 3rd. ed.. New York: Knopf.

Wundt, W. (1897). *Outlines of psychology.* Leipzig: Wilhelm Engelmann.

Wurtman, R. J., & Wurtman, J. J. (Eds.) (1987). *Human Obesity. Annals of the New York Academy of Sciences, 499.* New York: The New York Academy of Sciences.

Yates, W. R., Cadoret, R. J., Troughton, E. P., Stewart, M., & Giunta. T. S. (1998). Effect of fetal alcohol exposure on adult symptoms of nicotine, alcohol, and drug dependence. *Alcoholism: Clinical and Experimental Research, 22,* 914-920.

Yeager, R. D., Piazza, N. J., & Yates, J. W. (1992). Testing the progressive nature of alcoholism. *International Journal of Addictions, 27,* 947-959.

Yehuda, R. (1997). Sensitization of the hypothalamic-pituitary-adrenal axis in posttraumatic stress disorder. In R. Yehuda & A. McFarlane (Eds.), Psychobiology of posttraumatic stress disorder (pp.57-75). *Annals of the New York Academy of Sciences, 821.* New York: New York Academy of Sciences.

Yehuda, R., Kahana, B., Binder-Brynes, K., Southwick, S. M., Mason, J. W., & Giller, E. L. (1995). Low urinary cortisol excretion in holocaust survivors with posttraumatic stress disorder. *American Journal of Psychiatry, 152,* 982-986.

Yoshimoto, K., McBride, W. J., Lumeng, L., Li, T-K. (1992). Ethanol enhances the release of dopamine and serotonin in the nucleus accumbens of HAD and LAD lines of rats. *Alcohol: Clinical and Expermental Research, 16,* 781-785.

Zuckerman, M. (1979). *Sensation seeking: Beyond the optimal level of arousal.* Hillsdale, NJ: Erlbaum.

Zuckerman, M. (Ed.) (1983). *Biological bases of sensation seeking, impulsivity, and anxiety.* Hillsdale, NJ: Erlbaum.

Author Index

Subject Index